DISEASE, WAR, AND THE IMPERIAL STATE

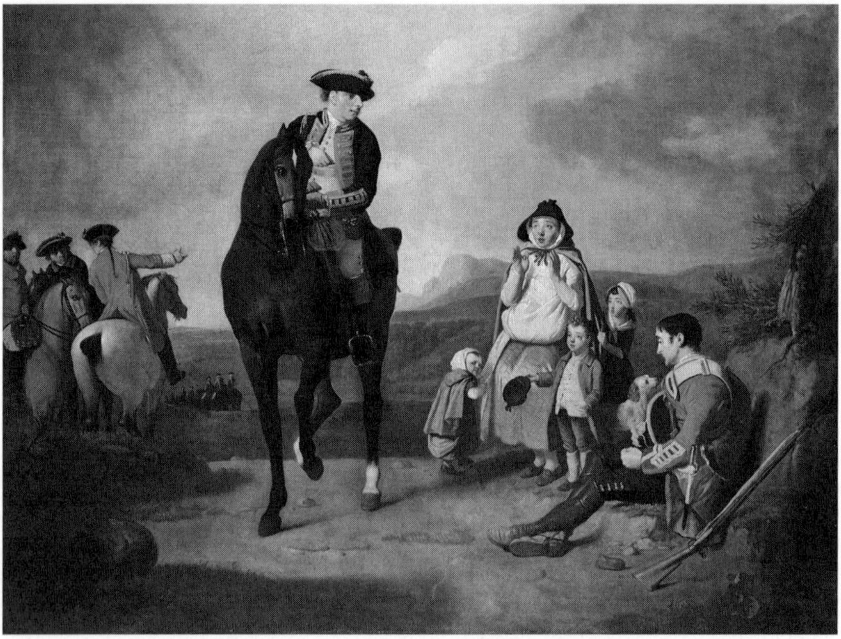

Frontispiece. Edward Penny (1714–91), *The Marquis of Granby Giving Alms to a Sick Soldier and His Family* (1764). Ashmolean Museum, University of Oxford.

DISEASE, WAR, AND THE IMPERIAL STATE

The Welfare of the British Armed Forces during the Seven Years' War

ERICA CHARTERS

THE UNIVERSITY OF CHICAGO PRESS
CHICAGO AND LONDON

ERICA CHARTERS is associate professor in the history of medicine and a fellow of Wolfson College at the University of Oxford.

The University of Chicago Press, Chicago 60637
The University of Chicago Press, Ltd., London

Printed in the United States of America

23 22 21 20 19 18 17 16 15 14   1 2 3 4 5

ISBN-13: 978-0-226-18000-7 (cloth)
ISBN-13: 978-0-226-18014-4 (e-book)
DOI: 10.7208/chicago/9780226180144.001.0001

Charters, Erica M. (Erica Michiko), 1978– author.

Disease, war, and the imperial state : the welfare of the British armed forces during the Seven Years' War / Erica Charters.
pages cm
Includes bibliographical references and index.
ISBN 978-0-226-18000-7 (cloth : alkaline paper) — ISBN 978-0-226-18014-4 (e-book) 1. Great Britain—Armed Forces—Medical care—History—18th century. 2. Armed Forces—Diseases—Great Britain—History—18th century. 3. Medicine, Military—Great Britain—History—18th century. 4. Seven Years' War, 1756–1763—Medical care. I. Title.
DA67.C47 2014
940.2'534—dc23

2014006591

♾ This paper meets the requirements of ANSI/NISO Z39.48-1992 (Permanence of Paper).

CONTENTS

List of Illustrations *vii*
List of Abbreviations *ix*
Acknowledgments *xi*

Introduction *1*
1. Wilderness Warfare, American Provincials, and Disease in North America *18*
2. The Black Vomit and the Provincial Press: The Campaigns in the West Indies *53*
3. Flux, Fever, and Politics: The European Theater of War *86*
4. The Royal Navy's Western Squadron: Trials, Innovation, and Medical Efficacy *120*
5. Adaptation and Hot Climates: Fighting in India *142*
6. Imperial War at Home: The Welfare of French Prisoners of War *172*

Epilogue *191*
Notes *201*
Bibliography *241*
Index *281*

ILLUSTRATIONS

Figures

Frontispiece	Edward Penny (1714–91), *The Marquis of Granby Giving Alms to a Sick Soldier and His Family* (1764)	ii
3.1	Return, "Weekly State of the Army under the Command of Lieut. Earl of Albemarle on the Island of Cuba Aug 16th 1762"	105
5.1	*Officer of the East India Company, Probably the Surgeon William Fullerton, on a Terrace, Smoking a Huqqa Directing a Servant,* by Dip Chand, ca. 1760–63	147

Map

Map	The global scope of the Seven Years' War	2

Table

2.1	Returns of rank-and-file British forces at Havana under Albemarle, 1762	75

ABBREVIATIONS

Add. MS	Additional Manuscripts, British Library
ADM	Admiralty Board Papers
ANF	Archives Nationales de la France, Paris
APAC	Asia, Pacific and Africa Collections, British Library
BL	British Library, London
CO	Colonial Office Papers
CP, MFR	Cumberland Papers, Microform Research Collection, British Library
HL	Huntington Library, San Marino, CA
HRO	Hampshire Record Office, Winchester, UK
IOR	India Office Records, British Library
KHLC	Kent History and Library Centre, Maidstone, UK
LO	Loudoun Papers, Huntington Library, San Marino, CA
NAC	National Archives of Canada, Ottawa
NAM	National Army Museum, London
NLS	National Library of Scotland, Edinburgh
NMM	National Maritime Museum, London
PA	Parliamentary Archives, London
Pringle MS	John Pringle's Medical Annotations, Royal College of Physicians of Edinburgh, Edinburgh
RCHM	Royal Commission on Historical Manuscripts, Great Britain
SHD	Service Historique de la Défense, Vincennes, France
SP	State Papers
SRO	Suffolk Record Office, Ipswich, UK
TNA	The National Archives, London
WO	War Office Papers

ACKNOWLEDGMENTS

I began research on this topic at the University of Oxford, during which time I enjoyed financial support from Canada's Social Science and Humanities Research Council, the Wellcome Trust, and the Canadian Centennial Scholarship Fund, as well as through an Overseas Research Scholarship. Later, I was fortunate to receive support from a number of institutions, which allowed me to transform my research into this book. A Price Fellowship from the William L. Clements Library at the University of Michigan and a W. M. Keck Foundation Fellowship from the Huntington Library provided me with access to relevant archival materials and stimulating research environments. An award from the University of Oxford's Fell Fund granted me precious research leave to write and complete final revisions.

A number of institutions and individuals have provided crucial assistance. I am grateful to archivists at the British Library; the Caird Library at the National Maritime Museum; the National Archives, London; the Royal College of Physicians, Edinburgh; and many other archives scattered throughout the United Kingdom and overseas. I am also grateful to the librarians at the Bodleian Library, especially those at the History Faculty, the Wellcome Unit for the History of Medicine, and the Upper Reading Room. The University of North Texas provided assistance during the final stages of writing, particularly the History Department and the Library Services. Versions of parts of this study were presented to various seminars and conferences, and I am grateful for the feedback I received from the Eighteenth-Century Seminar in London, the history of medicine seminars at the universities of Birmingham, Cambridge, and Newcastle, and workshops and conferences organized by BSECS, the Imperial War Museum, McGill University, the National Army Museum, the National

Maritime Museum, OIEAHC, SMU, SSHM, the University of Leeds, and the University of Liverpool.

I have been fortunate to enjoy feedback and support from colleagues at the University of Newcastle, the University of Liverpool, the University of Bath Spa, and the University of Oxford. In particular, I am grateful to Holger Hoock, who enthusiastically read over earlier versions; William J. Ashworth, who encouraged me to think more precisely about the state and scientific practice; and Elaine Chalus, for her warmth and wisdom. At Oxford, the Eighteenth-Century Seminar has long been a source of both intellectual stimulation and companionship, and Perry Gauci and Kathryn Gleadle have become delightful mentors as well as colleagues. Joanna Innes in particular has helped me in conceptualizing eighteenth-century Britain and the state, while encouraging me to become a more thoughtful historian in many ways. Laurence Brockliss has long provided helpful guidance and insight into historical research, and Pietro Corsi has taught me much about thinking and doing the history of science. I am also grateful to Eric Ash, Heather Beatty, Sophie Burton, Stephen Conway, Brian Cowan, Patricia Crimmin, James Davey, Huw David, Angela Davis, Joyce Taylor Dawson, John Donoghue, Denis Galligan, Victoria Gardner, Alan J. Guy, Stephen Hague, Richard Harding, Bob Harris, Ben Heller, Julian Hoppit, Geoffrey Hudson, Catherine Kelly, Roger Knight, Peter MacLeod, Tabitha Marshall, John McAleer, Matthew McCormack, Henry Meier, Iain Milne, Renaud Morieux, Matthew Neufeld, Sorcha Norris, Jacomien Prins, Nicholas Rodger, Matt Schumann, Eric Seeman, Kevin Siena, Peter Silver, Paul Slack, Hannah Smith, Todd Smith, Glenn Steppler, Hew Strachan, Eric Gruber von Arni, Rosemary Wall, Jennifer Wallach, Katherine Watson, and Peter H. Wilson as generous scholars and friends who have shared unpublished work, read drafts, offered helpful comments, or were willing to discuss ideas, findings, and arguments.

At Oxford, I have had the good fortune to be a fellow at Wolfson College, which has provided financial and moral support, alongside true collegiality and intellectual stimulation. As well as enjoying the support of the History Faculty, I have found myself lucky in returning to Oxford's Wellcome Unit for the History of Medicine as faculty. The Unit's research fellows, particularly Richard Biddle, Jeong-Ran Kim, Tim McEvoy, Saurabh Mishra, and Elise Smith, have shared research material and ideas, while also providing good fun. The Monday history of medicine seminar has helped to refine my ideas and arguments, as have numerous students who have made doing history more lively, rewarding, and tangible. I am grateful to my colleague Sloan Mahone for her guidance and unstinting level-headedness, to Belinda Michaelides for her constant good cheer and assistance, and to Margaret Pelling for her generosity, historical expertise, and friendship. My work owes an obvious debt to Mark Harrison, whose own research and teaching on military and colonial medicine whetted my interest, guided my research, and helped to refine my historical arguments. It has been my good fortune to have him first as a supervisor and now as a colleague.

My family has been a constant source of support and encouragement, and I am thankful that they planted and then nourished my academic interests. In Guy Chet I have been lucky to find someone willing to endlessly discuss eighteenth-century warfare and the nature of modern state formation. His critiques, comments, and companionship have made me a more thoughtful and happy historian.

I have been fortunate to work with knowledgeable and practical editors at the University of Chicago Press, notably Russell Damian, Robert Devens, and Timothy Mennel, and I am grateful to them for their support and advice. I am also grateful for the sharp eye of Marian Rogers, my copy editor. I also thank the reviewers who helped to tighten and clarify my research and argument, and Alex Mendoza for his map design.

I would like to thank the Ashmolean Museum for granting me permission to publish *The Marquis of Granby Giving Alms to a Sick Soldier and His Family*, and Colin Harrison for discussing the painting with me. I would also like to thank the National Archives for granting me permission to publish an image of a military return and the Victoria and Albert Museum for granting me permission to publish a portrayal of William Fullerton. Portions of chapters 1, 3, and 4 have previously been published, but these chapters have been substantially reworked and adapted for this volume, presenting significantly different arguments as part of a whole. I am grateful to the editors of the *Historical Journal* for granting me permission to publish portions of an article that first appeared in volume 52 (2009); to the editors of *War in History* for permission to publish part of an article that first appeared in volume 16 (2009), DOI 10.1177/0968344508097615; and to the editors of the *Canadian Bulletin of Medical History/Bulletin canadien d'histoire de la médecine* for permission to publish part of an article that first appeared in volume 27 (2010). I am also grateful to Peter Clifford and Boydell Press for granting me permission to publish a revised version of a chapter that I contributed to the volume *Health & Medicine at Sea, 1700–1900*, edited by Sally Archer and David Boyd Haycock (2009), and to the committee members of the Sir Julian Corbett Prize in Modern Naval History for their support.

INTRODUCTION

The frontispiece of this book is Edward Penny's painting *The Marquis of Granby Giving Alms to a Sick Soldier and His Family*, completed in 1764. Here, in an intimate moment, we see the popular officer responding to the plight of an individual soldier and his family, gently looking down to give the soldier money from his private purse. Granby the hero is not fighting a battle, but rather is a benevolent and humane commander. As art historian David Solkin points out, this image unites the public and private spheres: Granby's "modest act of charity brings the military man and the man of feeling together as one," and was widely appreciated.[1] First displayed in London in 1765, Penny's painting was disseminated throughout Britain in the form of engravings, and was the most popular painting of the Seven Years' War—with more copies sold than Benjamin West's later *The Death of Wolfe*.[2]

While *The Death of Wolfe* is today the most recognizable image of the Seven Years' War, it is useful to compare these two popular portrayals of British success. West's glorious painting, marking British conquest of the French in North America and showing the coordination of Native Americans, Highlanders, marines, Anglo-American provincial soldiers, and British regulars, illustrates all that was necessary for the impressive British victory. With naval power underpinning British military might, British forces and native troops were able to crush the most powerful European nations of that time—imperial France and Spain—in India, the Caribbean, the Philippines, North America, and Europe. Britain had reason to be proud of its achievements. Its victory was spectacular, ensuring the establishment of the British Empire: securing Canada and the American colonies, gaining strategic islands in the West Indies and bases along the west coast of Africa, and also expanding its involvement in India. With the Peace of

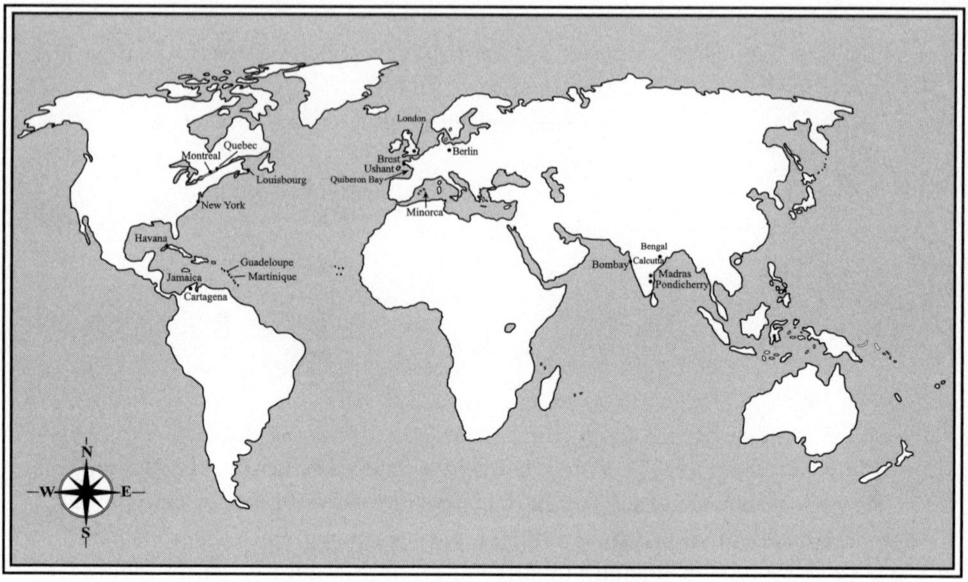

Map. The global scope of the Seven Years' War.

Paris in 1763, Britain emerged as the greatest military and imperial power of the modern age, together with a debt of £133 million.

West's *The Death of Wolfe* was not displayed until 1771, almost ten years after the end of the war. Its focus on a North American victory says more about later preoccupations with American troubles than about the Seven Years' War. In contrast, Penny's painting does not highlight imperial glory, but a caring relationship. Along with Francis Hayman's immensely popular representations of the war, shown in Vauxhall Gardens, Penny's *The Marquis of Granby* represented a new style of history painting, showing recent events and contemporary dress. On display were the humane virtues of Britain's great military leaders, directed at a wide public audience.[3] *The Marquis of Granby* illustrates the way in which the British public understood its imperial success: Britain had won the Seven Years' War, and hence a modern empire, not just through military force, but also because of genuine care for the welfare of troops under its command. As in Hayman's depictions of benevolent imperial governance in India and America, British prowess is portrayed here as rooted in enlightened humanity. Empire was earned, not simply conquered.

These images of the war were not only colorful patinas, meant to assuage British imperial anxieties. It was no accident that Penny's popular painting showed an officer's response to a sick soldier: as in all premodern wars, disease was far more deadly than combat in the Seven Years' War, particularly in its foreign, colonial environments. Given that population was considered one of the state's most precious resources in early modern Europe, the welfare of troops was an object of official and public scrutiny, with national as well as military relevance. In a war that spanned diverse environments and involved more troops than ever before, disease played a major role in campaigning, British state policy, and imperial relations.

This study examines the nature of British responses to disease during the Seven Years' War with a particular focus on the role of the state and its relationship to the welfare of the armed forces. Britain's fiscal-military power was necessary for victory, but it was also the conservation of manpower and the prudent use of resources that ensured global success.[4] Besides fiscal and logistical capability, British success required consistent and well-publicized attention to the welfare of troops to maintain manpower strength, support recruitment, and retain public support and public financing for the war. As the British political pamphleteer Israel Mauduit claimed in 1760, "Money may, in a qualified sense, be allowed to be the sinews of war; but it must find men to make up the flesh and substance of our armies."[5] A focus on the "flesh and substance" provides insight into the British eighteenth-century state in action, particularly as it consolidated and extended its imperial reach.

Historians have long recognized the relationship between war and the state.[6] The "military revolution" and ensuing debates have extensively outlined how the demands of war shaped the development of the early modern European state.[7] Eighteenth-century Britain has long been considered an exceptional case, given its ability to wage war across four continents and yet remain, compared with most other European states, relatively decentralized. John Brewer's concept of the fiscal-military state, drawing on the work of various economic historians, demonstrates how Britain's public administration and its system of taxation and public debt allowed it to wage large-scale war efficiently and effectively.[8] For historians, the fiscal-military state has become fundamental to understanding the development of the modern state, not least in acknowledging the formative role of European warfare.[9] At the same time, many British historians of the state have resisted equating modernization and power with centralization, noting that the successful waging of war did not necessarily depend on the buildup of central power.[10] Given the key role of Parliament and the vibrancy of Britain's public sphere, the nature of British state authority in the eighteenth century has been characterized as strikingly dependent on support from local authorities and the public.

Brewer acknowledged that the power of a fiscal-military state required public legitimacy. Recent works, especially Tim Blanning's magisterial *The Culture of Power and the Power of Culture*, have examined in detail the role of public opinion and political culture in the establishment of modern European states. As Blanning points out, the power and success of the state "is not just a question of military might and the means to finance it, however important they might be. Power depends as much on perception as reality."[11] Accordingly, Britain and Prussia won the Seven Years' War because of their ability to adapt to the new public sphere and to sustain the legitimacy of their power. The consolidation and expansion of power were seen as products of paternalistic care, rather than corrupt ambition; thus, they were accepted as credible and just. The successful fiscal-military state was a caring fiscal-military state, one that paid attention to and invested in the welfare of its armed forces. Granby, similarly, was a successful military commander precisely because it was well known that he took good care of his men.

Disease provides a key analytical tool in this respect. According to eighteenth-century medical theory, disease was not simply a product of contagious pathogens. Rather, contemporaries held that disease arose because of disorder in an individual's constitution, as well as from unhealthy environments lacking proper sanitation and adequate provisions. Thus, troops remained healthy when commanders paid close attention to the physical and moral state of their men, and provided them regular supplies of fresh provisions and salubrious accommodation. An outbreak of disease among the troops, therefore, pointed to a failure of leadership. Not surprisingly, reports of disease among troops were used in partisan politics, as they still are today.

The welfare of armed forces was essential to the state for a variety of reasons. At the practical level, disease among troops led to manpower shortages and hence to defeat, especially during sieges and colonial campaigns, both highly characteristic of eighteenth-century warfare. While death as a result of battle is an unsurprising end for a soldier or sailor, contemporaries viewed death due to disease as both inglorious and objectionable. Reports of disease among troops, therefore, led to recruitment problems, caused friction among colonial and allied civilian populations, engendered doubt in the minds of allied governments and commanders, and were a powerful weapon in the hands of opposition politicians on the home front. On a broader scale, disease among the armed forces could be seen as a symptom of disorder: physical, social, political, and moral.

Because disease was widely recognized as resulting from administrative failure and political weakness, this study is concerned with the role of political debates and public opinion concerning war policy and, hence, focuses on representations and reports of military operations in both the colonies and Britain. As Francis Hayman's portrayals of the Seven Years' War make clear, eighteenth-century Britons were adept manipulators of narratives and events in the midst of a society that was willing to challenge any form of political authority deemed illegitimate, particularly during the turbulent period of the mid-eighteenth century. Public opinion, "a presence and pressure at once nebulous and effective," played a significant role in eighteenth-century Britain, exerting particular pressure on state officials during times of war.[12] Such pressure was felt by officers and administrators with regard to troop health. The popularity of Penny's depiction of Granby was symptomatic of the British public's interest in and concern for the welfare of its armed forces.

Disease during war thus provides another historical avenue to consideration of the relationship between war and society, and is particularly useful in uncovering societal attitudes toward the armed forces. Soldiers and sailors were deemed worth the cost of fresh provisions, as well as the expense of nursing through illness and injury, and officials could quickly become unpopular should they display disdain for the welfare of British troops. This reinforces studies showing that Britain's armed forces in the eighteenth century were not shunned or suited only to the desperate and socially marginal, but rather that soldiers and sailors were well regarded and well trained, as well as an integral part of society.[13] The medical care provided to British troops and the extent of public attention devoted to their welfare indicate that they were considered a valuable resource by both state and society.

In this history of the Seven Years' War, the strength and success of the British state are judged not by its administrative capabilities such as taxation, but by its ability to portray itself as a credible and just imperial authority. It secured public approval and support through its attention to the welfare of its armed forces, accomplished by applying medical knowledge and adapting to local conditions around the globe. This study, then, is not an analysis of the effectiveness of eighteenth-century medicine, nor is it an account of how medicine won the war. Instead, medicine is used to assess the extent to which authorities were willing to invest time, energy, and resources in the welfare of the armed forces, regardless of whether modern biomedicine vindicates the methods of eighteenth-century medicine. Whereas historians can be distracted by outdated and harmful medical treatments such as bleeding and purging, this study examines eighteenth-century medicine as a concern for welfare. Rather than identifying drugs or techniques that were precursors to modern biomedicine, it focuses on prevention, hygiene, diet, exercise, and rest. These were all central components of early modern medicine, and often (such as in the case of fresh foodstuffs) the most troublesome and expensive as well. As contemporaries did not approach disease statistically, and as comprehensive quantitative records of disease rates do not exist, disease is here predominantly examined through social and cultural history, which also clarifies disease's political and military importance.

This study demonstrates that the incidence of disease played a significant role in the formation of wartime strategy and policy in the eighteenth century, and that the Seven Year's War, in turn, stimulated new ways of thinking about disease and medicine, particularly in colonial environments. Applying the methods of social and cultural histories of medicine, this analysis of disease is informed by modern scientific medicine, providing a biological basis with which to examine how cultural understandings of disease coincided with biological phenomena. Although sensitive to the dangers of retro-diagnosis, this study approaches disease as a tangible, physical reality, using disease rates and causation in order to understand the problems facing eighteenth-century contemporaries and to explain the complexity and dynamism of medicine during the mid-eighteenth century. Medical writings, published and unpublished, provide the basis for understanding contemporary medical thought and practice. Unlike many histories of military medicine, this study also relies extensively on the records and correspondence of military and political officials, tracing how medical observations and theories were transformed into medical practices, as well as military strategy and policy. Alongside this, published accounts in newspapers and pamphlets demonstrate the extent to which eighteenth-century Britons were concerned with the welfare of the armed forces.

More specifically, this analysis of the Seven Years' War traces how imperial warfare shaped the development of British medical expertise. Defined as "technical or scientific competence in the service of a public administration," expertise refers not only to the knowledge that sets one apart from laypeople, but also to knowledge derived from experience or skill, in contrast to theoretical or abstract knowledge.[14] Eric Ash has demonstrated the linkages between early modern state formation and the development of expertise, describing how developing states required experts who could control and manipulate nature, to "collect and digest useful information, give dependable advice . . . and otherwise mediate between the centre and the localities."[15] Such knowledge and mediation were necessary for the consolidation and expansion of state power and authority. At the same time, political authorities legitimized the position of experts, thereby validating experts' claims to knowledge and authority. Delineating the development of expertise allows a focus on how contemporaries evaluated knowledge: rather than fixating on modern-day applicability, this focus on expertise demonstrates whether eighteenth-century officials used, applied, and endorsed medical theories and practices.

In studies on eighteenth-century Britain, the role of the state in shaping medicine and science is often overlooked in favor of a focus on the role of the public, whether in the marketplace, as consumers, or as members of learned societies. This stems in part from the influence of Roy Porter, who invigorated the study of the history of medicine both generally and particularly for eighteenth-century Britain. By combining his interests in the eighteenth-century commercial revolution and the British Enlightenment with the history of medicine, Porter produced seminal studies on voluntary hospitals, consumer-driven medicine, and sociable scientific investigation: subjects that preclude noticeable state activity.[16] In broad surveys of eighteenth-century science, British government support is described as "tending to be modest," if not weak.[17] This narrative of insubstantial state involvement in science is shown more broadly in histories of eighteenth-century British innovation, including the Industrial Revolution, in which the state often merits little mention, if any.[18]

By contrast, this examination of disease and medicine during imperial war highlights the central role that the British state played in the shaping of eighteenth-century medicine and scientific innovation. This study builds on research on the history of military and naval medicine, as well as histories of science and medicine in Britain's burgeoning empire.[19] Tropical medicine, a discipline that would prove integral to modern imperial expansion and consolidation, had its roots in the experiences of the Seven Years' War. The structure of the British armed forces and the opportunity that the army and navy provided for observation and experimentation shaped the nature, practices, and research methods of eighteenth-century scientific medicine. The experience of war allowed medical practitioners in the army and navy to claim authority and status, becoming experts in their field. At the same time, medicine became a form of expertise in the service of the British Empire, applied during campaigning and influencing the nature of imperial policy. By the same token, contemporaries viewed outbreaks of disease among troops not as evidence of the failure of medical science, but of state infrastructure.

As the activity and structure of the armed forces reflect the capabilities, practices, and aims of the state, military surgeons and physicians hired to serve and preserve British manpower on land and sea were regarded as agents of the state.[20] The source of their expertise was their service to the state, and their primary allegiance was to the British state, even if they combined private and public interests while employed (as did many officeholders).[21] Although central bureaucratic offices, such as the Royal Navy's Sick and Hurt Board, are easily identified as state structures, individuals working on their behalf were also part of the state's network of agencies, exercising military and political power.[22] In their position as medical experts responsible for keeping soldiers and sailors fit for overseas service, military medical practitioners played a key role in the expansion of the British Empire, implementing measures for the welfare of troops, advising officers and officials, and even directly shaping policy. Indeed, the provision of welfare to the lower orders is a central focus of social histories of state development.[23] As a consequence, military medicine, especially in wartime, provides a salient opportunity to analyze the mechanics and ideology of state formation.

Like military medical practitioners, army and naval officers were clearly serving the Crown and, when sent overseas, acted as imperial authorities, by either implementing imperial policy or negotiating on behalf of the British state with representatives of local, allied, or enemy governments. Although not bureaucrats, military officers spent most of their time dealing with the logistical and administrative demands of warfare, especially in the colonies.[24] During the Seven Years' War, when thousands of British regulars were sent to all key overseas theaters in unprecedented numbers (over 20,000 to North America, 7,500 to the Caribbean, nearly 4,000 to India, along with around 80,000 deployed at sea), officers were likely the most common, if not the only, contact point between British settlers abroad and their imperial government. Whereas few British (regular) forces reached India or were stationed in the American colonies in the first part of the eighteenth century, the Seven Years' War marked a turning point in terms of the presence and activity of the British Army and Royal Navy overseas.[25]

Although the wars of the 1740s featured fighting overseas as well as in Europe, in the Seven Years' War Britain's colonies remained principal theaters of conflict throughout the war. Overseas settlements and naval bases played a central role in British and French strategy during the war. The Seven Years' War thus provides an excellent opportunity to examine the functioning of Britain's imperial state, building on studies that consider the mid-eighteenth century as crucial in evaluating the nature of British imperial rule. As P. J. Marshall notes, by the time formal fighting ended in 1763, "what had begun as a defensive war had become a war of conquest."[26] This study is not concerned with revising the history of the war with regard to decisive battles, debates over maritime and Continental strategies, or the role of nonstate or indigenous forces. It instead uses the prism of disease and medicine to examine Britain's activity as an imperial state. The campaigns covered in the six chapters that follow reflect Britain's confrontations with its imperial rivals in theaters central to British interests.

While the Seven Years' War is often accurately described as the first world war, there are remarkably few studies of it that examine British progression on all key continents: Europe, America (including the Caribbean), and India.[27] American historians have long been interested in the war as the precursor to American identity and independence.[28] British and European historians have reminded Americanists of the role of the European balance of power in this war, while the relationship between the two provides rich resources for Atlantic historians.[29] The war is also taken as the first major step in the consolidation of British power in India.[30] And as the basis of all colonial campaigns and the nature of modern British maritime power, the Royal Navy during the war enjoys much attention.[31] While these regional analyses offer important insights on the war and on colonial and international dynamics, they examine the progression of the war in isolation. As Britain's success in this war—the foundation of its global empire—was due to its impressive coordination of transcontinental policy, this atomized approach is all the more remarkable.

A global approach to the war provides a comprehensive understanding of this war's significance. Rather than considering the Seven Years' War as a precursor to the American War of Independence or to British rule in India, the examination here accentuates the overarching similarities of British warfare in India, North America, the Caribbean, and Europe at midcentury. It is fitting that historians have been interested in the Seven Years' War as the foundation of American independence and identity or of the British Empire in India or of the decline of French power in Europe. Yet these developments were intertwined, and detailed examinations demonstrate that they were indeed processes, not inevitable outcomes.[32] The inclusion of Europe is integral to this approach. Although the Seven Years' War is acknowledged as central to the study of colonial warfare, examining the waging of war in all theaters demonstrates the underlying coherence of colonial and Continental warfare.[33] Indeed, the category of "colonial warfare" is often self-defining: it demands that non-European warfare be studied separately, most often as a subsection of American exceptionalism. As Jeremy Black has pointed out, this distinction obscures the similarities between warfare on the Continent and warfare abroad, thereby encouraging preoccupation with, on the one hand, Frederician linear warfare, and on the other, wilderness, ranger-style American warfare.[34] The colonial experience was not necessarily more challenging than was the waging of war in more conventional environments, and a comprehensive overview of how this global war was waged demonstrates common foundations, while acknowledging regional divergences.

At first glance, it is not surprising that no British global history of the war exists. After all, contemporaries of the war did not necessarily see it as one coherent conflict. When news of the official declaration of war between Britain and France reached the British East India Company in Bengal, its first response was to broker neutrality with the French. Not only was it already embroiled in an expensive conflict with local authorities, but it saw no reason to start fighting against the French just because the metropole had decreed as much.[35] Likewise, fighting in the American colonies erupted long before ministers declared war. Just as the war could not be given its name until well after it had concluded, it was not necessarily a unified war while under way.[36] The success of wartime politicians, such as William Pitt, was not due to a holistic policy across seas and continents; rather, they exploited opportunities as they arose in different theaters, and weaved a comprehensible version of foreign policy afterward.[37]

While British foreign policy may not appear planned, it was coherent in its approach, particularly in its flexibility. The British state here examined was one that adapted to local environments and conditions, responded well to problems, and instituted new solutions for the sake of both operational success and political legitimacy. As studies of the British fiscal-military state have demonstrated, its strength lay not in its size or resources, but rather in the effectiveness with which it mobilized and deployed resources. This, in turn, depended on authority wielded in the localities: it was precisely the decentralized nature of the regime that maintained its legitimacy and efficiency.[38] As this study makes clear, this was also the case beyond Britain. Officials negotiated with local authorities in India and North America in similar fashion to their negotiations in the English provinces and in Scotland. These were not simply partnerships:

representatives of the British state responded to the demands of local authorities, as well as instituting their own measures and initiatives.[39] The British state, both imperial and domestic, is shown here to be an adaptive body, rather than a deterministic one.

Indeed, the experience of the Seven Years' War changed the nature of British imperial governance, demonstrating how this global conflict was fundamental to the long-term development of the British imperial state. Wars are processes, influenced by and influencing local conditions; they do not emerge fully formed, as static entities. Because of the wartime effectiveness of the Western Squadron, and more generally, the success and popularity of a blue-water strategy, Britain would always aim to rule the waves—a strategy that was vindicated by the experience of the Seven Years' War. Similarly, the physical experience of campaigning in the West and East Indies led medical and military officials to draw conclusions about the relationship between Europeans and discipline, simultaneously physical, military, and cultural. The Seven Years' War was an integral, and thus responsive, part of eighteenth-century British society, politics, and culture. By the end of the war, Britain had consolidated its hold on a global empire; it had also crystallized the procedures that would characterize the nature of British imperial governance for years to come.

PREVENTING DISEASE, DISCIPLINING BODIES, AND DEVELOPING EXPERTISE

Although military historians have generally not paid much attention to the role of disease in war, those engaged in battle were well aware that disease killed far more men than did the enemy, and that disease outbreaks influenced the outcome of campaigns. Siege warfare, characteristic of Continental and colonial warfare during this period, produced high rates of sickness, as troops on both sides were crowded into small holdings with limited provisions and fragmented sanitary and medical arrangements.[40] Eighteenth-century medical theory claimed that disease was caused by miasma: a concept that originally related to ideas of pollution and referred to putrefaction of the air by decaying matter and the sick, and generally associated with bad smells. Epidemic disease thus arose when bodies and their effluvia were crowded into unventilated environments. Miasmatic theories seemed vindicated by these instances of sickness during sieges.[41]

Officers were cognizant of hazards and uses of disease during campaigns. Prince William Augustus, Duke of Cumberland, while commander of the German-allied army in western Europe, remarked in 1757 to Lord John Ligonier after a two-month siege: "I expect in very few days the good news of the surrender of *Prague*. Famine & sickness has executed what Bombs & red hot Balls could not."[42] In the West Indies, the aptly named "black vomit" (yellow fever) was more feared than battle, and its consequences were taken into account when forming military strategy. Given that yellow fever fatally struck only newcomers, the disease seemed to offer French and Spanish garrisons a natural defense against besiegers.[43]

Colonial warfare thus accentuated difficulties associated with disease. Not only did British forces have to contend with a foreign climate and its specific diseases, but traditional supplies and adequate supply routes were often deficient or nonexistent, which facilitated the outbreak of disease. Moreover, the transportation of reinforcements also proved difficult. Although lacking a modern grasp of medical complexities, contemporaries recognized that epidemic disease encountered on campaign arose from a lack of order and, hence, poor care for troop welfare. More specifically, the most common diseases of the army and navy—scurvy, "fevers" (usually typhus), and the "flux" (dysentery or diarrheal diseases)—arose when provisions were lacking, accommodation inadequate, and when an initial outbreak was not quickly isolated and given sufficient attention. Given this, it is understandable that contemporaries associated disease outbreaks, especially among troops, with the breakdown of military order. Orders from military officials repeatedly stressed the importance of discipline and cleanliness in camp to avoid what was often termed "disorder"—meaning both disease as disorder within an individual, and the lack of discipline in camp directly related to an outbreak of disease. Preventing disease required discipline, an orderly camp, and a well-ordered logistical system, and hence was part of the responsibilities of military officers.

In understanding and treating foreign diseases, military medical practitioners made use of indigenous knowledge and practices, but also shaped these practices and interpreted this knowledge according to their own cultural background. Recruitment of native and colonial men into the army was informed by theories of native resistance to local diseases. Once they were part of the armed forces, these men were provided with British medical services. They were also expected to conform to British military discipline, something that Anglo-American provincials notably failed to do. British troops also carried with them their own contagious diseases, as armies and navies always do, which spread among colonial soldiers and settlements, causing resentment toward imperial forces. Disease was thus a locus for civilian and military interaction, especially in colonial theaters. Military administrators thus managed the war effort not only by preventing disease, but also by ensuring civilian support, both in colonial locales and at home, through demonstrated care for troops.

Examining efforts aimed at disease prevention and troop welfare lays bare the mechanisms, and complexity, of imperial relations and identities. Historians have studied medicine as an instrument of social control, applied to both the lower classes of society and colonial populations; similarly, influenced by Foucault and Said, imperial and postcolonial historians have examined how networks of power construct medical knowledge and expertise.[44] The body has been a much-explored site of imperial power and scientific culture, especially through histories of public health and hygiene, as well as through histories of bodily discipline as it relates to military practice.[45] Yet the physical experience of colonial warfare makes clear that disciplining bodies was not only about power relations and Foucauldian order, but was also necessary—according to contemporary medical science—for health and survival. In histories of the body, as Nancy Stepan rightly observes, the body's "materiality often seems to disappear into textuality and words."[46] Officials in the field and soldiers on campaign could not ignore the thousands of contagious, sickly, and stinking bodies in the midst of a siege; they were an inescapable threat to military victory, physical survival, and morale. By the same token, theories on what caused such sickness, as well as why some became sick while others did not, provide fascinating cultural and political insights, linking visible physical characteristics—disease and death—to inner properties.

For contemporaries of the Seven Years' War, the relationship between physical and moral constitutions was direct. In the tropical climates of the West Indies and India, disease was a result of intemperance: too much alcohol, rich foods (including exotic fruits), sexual indulgence, and excessive physical exertion all encouraged disease among European troops. Self-control—the proverbial English stiff upper lip—could prevent the danger of disease in foreign climates. The colonial environment itself could also become healthier if ordered, as medical practitioners recommended that troops be stationed in drained and cultivated settlements, thereby avoiding the wild and damp malaria-ridden locations. In Germany, disease outbreaks were identified with the breakdown of camp order and military discipline, when provisions ran short and soldiers resorted to plunder. More particularly, disease arose and spread when hospitals were disordered, especially because of overcrowding. On board ships and in naval squadrons, disease was prevented by regulating provisions and cleanliness, while naval hospitals developed cures and prevented disease through regulated medical trials and observations.[47]

Sanitation and hygiene are obvious examples of rules of order that prevent and control disease. Military sanitation has thus been identified as the earliest form of colonial medicine, which attempted to control what was seen as a disordered colonial environment and population, just as institutional rules of sanitation and hygiene imposed order on soldiers, sailors, and hospital patients. Discipline and order were also seen as key to British military superiority in combat: as warfare in North America and in India had demonstrated, British victory rested on maintaining discipline during and after battles. It was therefore hardly surprising to contemporaries that the less-disciplined Anglo-American provincials made better laborers than soldiers, and that their relaxed constitutions also resulted in higher rates of sickness than among British-born troops. In other words, theories of constitutional differences were based on observations of physical and cultural differences. By the later eighteenth century, ideas of these differences were hardening into theories of biological racial fixedness, and hierarchies of civility and hygiene.[48] These conclusions were drawn from observations garnered during the eighteenth century, when thousands of bodies came together to interact on and off the battlefield, across the Americas, India, Europe, and Africa. As this global history of the Seven Years' War shows, the war's experiences gave rise to theories of the modern body and European biological, ethical, and military superiority.

The exigencies of imperial war, alongside the demands of Parliament and a vocal public, helped to mold what can be called an expertise of manpower. Because a state's population was considered the basis of national wealth, the health of the lower orders was a key political concern, as eighteenth-century political arithmetic and medical charities evince. In times of war, conserving manpower, particularly given the cost of trained sailors and soldiers, was an issue vital to military and national strength. Military administrators were not alone in demanding regular reports on the state of manpower; both Parliament and political officeholders also requested such information. During the Seven Years' War, British officials regularly collected unusually quantitative data on the state of manpower in all theaters of the war, including detailed rates of sickness. This data not only guided British strategy and policy, but also molded military and colonial medicine, informing medical theories on how to best preserve manpower during war and in foreign climates. Medicine and state administration shaped one another, both striving toward methods by which manpower could be used more efficiently. A detailed examination of disease and medicine during imperial war demonstrates the fundamental role played by the state in eighteenth-century medicine, particularly through the state's most tangible articulations of authority: the making and sustaining of war and empire.

The structure of this study reflects the physical scope of the war. Each chapter focuses on a theater of operations, demonstrating the significance of responding to local conditions, knowledge, and practices. By the same token, each chapter also details one aspect of disease or troop welfare and how the British state responded to such challenges. Throughout, the nature of British imperial warfare and the structure of the British armed forces are linked to medical theories and practice, tracing how these interacted. Medical knowledge is analyzed not only in terms of content, but also in terms of structure and method, showing the nature of research and innovation, as well as the way that theories were translated into practice and policy.

Chapter 1 examines the North American campaigns and the impact of scurvy and smallpox. Partly a consequence of the logistical problems inherent in wilderness warfare, these diseases differentiated between British regulars and American provincial soldiers, encouraging suggestions that British-born soldiers were physically different from their Anglo-American counterparts. In chapter 2 these differences are examined during the West Indian campaigns, showing how adaptation to the disease environment there played a role in the conquest of Guadeloupe, Martinique, and Spanish-held Havana. Regardless of victory, reports of mortality and sickness circulated freely in American colonial newspapers, demonstrating the role of disease in generating colonial hostility to participation in imperial campaigns. At the same time, the experience of war in the American and West Indian colonies contributed to empirical methodology and theories on the distinctiveness of tropical climates, showing the influence of the Seven Years' War on emerging medical practice and thought.

Chapter 3 focuses on the traditional diseases of army camps (typhus and dysentery) and their role in campaigns in Germany and in military hospitals. Given that committing resources to the Continental campaign was a target for the British parliamentary opposition, reports of disease among troops were used for partisan political purposes. More broadly, the threat that disease posed to national manpower and vigor was made explicitly clear in mercantilist theories of political arithmetic. Chapter 4 examines the Royal Navy and its response to scurvy in the main operation in which it acted without the army, an operation integral to British victory in the war: the Western Squadron. Contemporary medicine and naval administration informed one another's practices; as a result, naval medicine developed procedures that had far-reaching implications for science in general, such as clinical trials.

Chapter 5 outlines the campaigns and diseases of Royal troops and British East India Company forces stationed in India. Although contemporary medical theory claimed that British-born soldiers should have been able to acclimatize to India and thus become inured to its diseases, experience accrued during the war suggested otherwise. The Seven Years' War was thus a turning point not only in terms of Britain becoming a political and territorial power in India, but also regarding theories on physical adaptation and climate. Chapter 6 focuses on prisoners of war and how British authorities and civilians responded to the 20,000 enemy soldiers and sailors held captive during hostilities. Care for French prisoners, by both the British state and local communities, illustrates the fundamental relationship between the welfare of troops, military victory, and the legitimacy of British state authority.

This book is novel in its global approach to the British experience of the Seven Years' War, and in its detailed examination of disease, medicine, and eighteenth-century imperial war. It is not an exhaustive history of the British side of the war, but rather a study of the nature of the British imperial state in action. This state was responsive to physical realities: it adapted to foreign environments and countenanced local and colonial concerns. It also responded to the demands of the public by, for example, publicizing the care given to its own forces or to enemy prisoners of war and censoring reports on poor health among troops. The British state was not only a fiscal war-machine, but was also concerned with the development of scientific knowledge. It strove to manage manpower effectively through the application of medical expertise, and at the same time played a central role in the development of scientific medicine.

More broadly, the course of disease reveals the precariousness of victory, as well as the potential fissures within what would become the formal British Empire. Examining how politicians responded to reports of disease on campaigns and how disease itself was reported in both the metropolitan and the colonial press clarifies that disease was not merely a physical entity. It was not only a military and logistical stumbling block for commanders, but also dangerous in the political and diplomatic arenas—an occurrence that opened the door to damaging charges of incompetence and malfeasance at the highest levels. The ill health of American provincials frustrated British officials, while also discouraging provincial contributions to future military campaigns. This suggests that disease played a significant role in emerging tensions and hostilities between Britain and its colonies. Similarly, the difference in disease rates between British soldiers and native troops in India encouraged not only the enlistment of large numbers of native troops into British forces, but also their differentiation based on physical characteristics, both of which contrasted with previous theories of acclimatization. This had long-term consequences for the nature of British rule in India, most obviously in the military uprisings of the nineteenth century and in the emergence of racial doctrines and policies.

At home, in the reporting on the campaigns in Europe and at sea, disease became a political issue linked to debates over British foreign policy, and a means for evaluating the administrative capabilities of officials. Disease and the reporting on disease brought the war into the lives of civilian populations in a morally and politically meaningful way. The physical, palpable presence of disease was a threat to military operations, to the lives of soldiers and sailors, and also to the health of civilians in port towns and villages in Britain and its colonies. It intensified public scrutiny of military strategy and officer conduct, and pressured imperial authorities to understand and tackle the causes of outbreaks. In the process, the responses to wartime outbreaks of disease enhanced state authority, elevated the status and refined the expertise of medical practitioners, and transformed the nature and practice of medical science.

CHAPTER ONE

Wilderness Warfare, American Provincials, and Disease in North America

In North American campaigns during the Seven Years' War, British forces found themselves struggling to maintain, and then extend, their hold on settlements and trading forts in a challenging environment. Not only did the climate seem unduly harsh, with its long, bitterly cold winters, but fighting in the immense expanses of wilderness alongside provincials (Anglo-American colonists) and against Native Americans presented British authorities with varied problems. In the first few years of the war, Britain suffered disastrous military and naval defeats. Yet by 1758, British troops and provincial regiments, supported by the Royal Navy, began winning the victories that would ensure British control of North America by the end of 1760.

Over the course of the war, British imperial military strategy showed itself to be responsive to North American environmental and colonial challenges—a crucial aspect of its success during the war.[1] Depending on colonial officials and constituents for the recruitment of provincial troops and a reliable supply of provisions, British officials negotiated with colonial authorities and tried to dampen sites of potential colonial friction. Yet the experience of warfare did strain imperial relations: colonial officials complained about British demands and resisted recruitment, while British officials in turn complained about colonists' military inexperience and lack of vigor. Disease reinforced these imperial differences, often acting as a physical manifestation of the logistical obstacles of warfare in North America and the social differences between provincial and British regular troops.[2]

This chapter focuses on scurvy and smallpox in North America, two diseases that constrained and shaped British colonial military strategy during the war, examining the military, medical, and political responses to disease by British officials. Scurvy is a salient example of the logistical challenges of North American warfare, as it was common during the long winters, when no fresh provisions could be found or easily transported across large and uncharted distances. The British garrison at Quebec suffered devastating rates of scurvy in the winter of 1759–60, resulting in British defeat at the battle of Sainte-Foy in April 1760. While 58 British soldiers lost their lives at the battle on the Plains of Abraham, over 500 British soldiers died from disease between the battle on the Plains and the battle of Sainte-Foy. Thus, the history of disease, contextualized by eighteenth-century theories of scurvy, allows a reconsideration of what is the most famous battle of the Seven Years' War: the conquest of Canada in 1759.

Smallpox highlights the social context of disease. Most likely brought from Europe by French and British troops at the opening of the war, smallpox affected provincial troops more so than British regulars, and was likewise particularly feared among colonial populations. As its spread was associated with the movement of troops, smallpox encouraged colonial resentment and resistance to British military endeavors, while also physically distinguishing between provincial and British-born troops. Moreover, contemporary medical theory posited that lifestyle and constitution predisposed some individuals to disease more than others. Thus, laziness and intemperance, for instance, were seen to encourage scurvy and smallpox. Disease thus appeared to bear out widely held beliefs about physical and temperamental differences between provincial and British soldiers.

Responses to scurvy and smallpox are here evaluated not solely through the prism of modern biomedicine, but also according to contemporary medical theory. Military and colonial records are examined for evidence of the application of eighteenth-century understandings of disease and medicine. As a result, what emerges is a vibrant network of medical observations and experimentation. Military medicine in the colonies afforded even lowly regimental surgeons the opportunity to develop medical expertise and contribute to the broader understanding of disease by leading figures such as James Lind (1716–94) and John Pringle (1707–82). This reinforces recent studies that have defended eighteenth-century British military medicine against accusations of poor or insufficient care, and that establish eighteenth-century military medicine, particularly in the colonies, as innovative and influential.[3] This study reveals that medicine was an important component of military campaigns in the eighteenth century as well as a tangible demonstration of the adaptability and responsiveness of British officials to the physical and social difficulties of

North American campaigns. Even though scurvy and smallpox were not always prevented, British officers were genuinely concerned with the welfare of soldiers under their command. Various preventative methods and cures for disease, informed by current medical theories and observations, were instituted by military and medical officials while on campaign in North America. These responses demonstrate not only the vast scope of resources dedicated to combating disease in colonial military operations and the expertise with which these resources were invested, but also contemporary preoccupation with disease.

This is not an overview of British operations in North America during the war; various studies offer a comprehensive view of the military operations, politics, and diplomacy of the Seven Years' War in North America, or, as it is known in America, the French and Indian War. These studies richly detail the war's transformative effect on colonial governments and societies, as well as on Native American political alliances, tactics, and society.[4] By contrast, this study presents the British perspective on the war, one that was not interested in the minutiae of regional and tribal distinctions—indiscriminately grouping American colonists and colonial forces under the heading of "provincials," and referring to various Native American groups as "Indians'—but a perspective nonetheless concerned with the long-term welfare of allied populations.

This chapter introduces the significance of disease in warfare, and demonstrates the cultural and social frameworks that shaped responses to it, while providing an overview of the structure of medical care in the British Army in the mid-eighteenth century. In doing so, it elucidates the nature of eighteenth-century warfare, which was not neatly confined to battles and combatants. As contemporaries recognized, early modern warfare took place within a broad social context and had a significant impact on civilian populations, and—particularly in colonial contexts—is best described as unlimited in its scope. Focusing on the history of soldiers' bodies and the interpretation of disease demonstrates the symbiotic relationship between the very physicality of warfare and its conduct.

The chapter opens with a discussion of the role scurvy played in British warfare in North America during the Seven Years' War, beginning with an overview of modern and eighteenth-century understandings of the disease. It then considers the prevalence of scurvy during North American land campaigns and the measures that British military officials adopted in response. A detailed examination of the siege of Quebec City in 1760, in which the British garrison suffered from such high rates of scurvy that it risked losing control of New France's center of operations, offers a pertinent example of the significance of disease in warfare. The medical responses to scurvy in both the colonies and the metropole provide insight into the nature of eighteenth-century medicine in the British Army, demonstrating that colonial military medicine was an influential component of eighteenth-century medical theory. In the final section, a discussion of smallpox explains how disparate social backgrounds resulted in different rates of disease between provincials and British soldiers, exacerbating social and imperial political tensions in the British American colonies.

EIGHTEENTH-CENTURY NOTIONS OF SCURVY

We know now that scurvy is caused by a lack of vitamin C, or ascorbic acid. It was not until the early 1910s, however, that researchers suggested a specific dietary deficiency as the cause for scurvy. With the successful isolation of vitamin C in 1932, scientists established that scurvy was indeed caused by a deficiency of that vitamin.[5] This relatively late discovery can be partly explained by scurvy's abnormality. Not only is a disease with such a simple cause uncommon, but most animals can synthesize their own vitamin C, so that it is impossible for them to suffer from scurvy. Thus, laboratory research, especially on rats, was often unhelpful. Human societies have also been remarkably efficient at avoiding scurvy by adapting to a variety of food environments. People who live in climates with little greenery, such as the Inuit in northern Canada, obtain their vitamin C from raw meat, and newborn children obtain it through breast milk. Certain nomadic tribes in North Africa remain scurvy-free on their traditional diet, which contains little or no vitamin C, yet develop symptoms of scurvy if they change to a nontraditional diet also lacking vitamin C.[6]

It takes very little ascorbic acid to prevent scurvy: European Union guidelines suggest thirty milligrams as a daily amount; ten milligrams, or four teaspoons of orange juice, is sufficient to avoid any health problems. A person also needs to forgo vitamin C for many days before symptoms develop. Because vitamin C is needed for cell development, tissue growth and repair, and the immune system, symptoms of its deficiency are wide-ranging. After thirty days without any vitamin C, slight skin problems appear. Resistance to infections is reduced, and one feels tired and worn-out. Small hemorrhages in out-of-the-way places, such as under the tongue, also develop. In anywhere from eleven to thirty weeks, the gums begin to soften, wounds have problems healing or reopen, and diseases such as tuberculosis can reappear. Death is usually caused by the complications from other diseases, or by heart hemorrhages brought on by the breakdown of connective internal tissue.[7]

Eighteenth-century medical texts recounted similar symptoms of scurvy: soft, spongy gums, healed wounds reopening, and general fatigue and lassitude, until sufferers became too weak to get out of bed. Death occurred when an individual tried to vigorously exert him- or herself (by getting out of bed, for example), causing internal hemorrhage. Scurvy was a disease not surprisingly associated with unusual circumstances, such as famines, sieges, long voyages, and especially sailing. In Britain, George Anson's celebrated voyage around the world in the 1740s, though successful in terms of plunder, was also infamous at the time for the hundreds of sailors who died from scurvy.

In 1753, James Lind published his famous *Treatise of the Scurvy*, and dedicated it to Anson. He explained in the preface:

> The subject of the following sheets is of great importance to this nation; the most powerful in her fleets, and the most flourishing in her commerce, of any in the world. Armies have been supposed to lose more of their men by sickness, than by the sword. But this observation has been much more verified in our fleets and squadrons; where the scurvy alone, during the last war, proved a more destructive enemy, and cut off more valuable lives, than the united efforts of the *French* and *Spanish* arms.[8]

Lind had served as a naval surgeon during the wars of the 1740s, and then became head physician of the Haslar Royal Naval Hospital. Using his naval and hospital experience, throughout his lifetime Lind published a number of works on the health of sailors and soldiers, becoming a famous medical figure not only in Britain but throughout Europe. His early work on scurvy ensured that Lind was also considered the leading authority on scurvy, and even today he is judged a hero in the battle against this disease.[9] Lind's treatise is best remembered for its account of the so-called clinical trial conducted on board the HMS *Salisbury*, and today he is hailed for discovering that oranges and lemons cured scurvy. Yet a careful reading of Lind's treatise challenges this straightforward version of events. Rather than suggesting a single and simple cure for scurvy, Lind's theory of the disease was far more complex.

In his explanation of the mechanism of the disease, Lind describes a state of health as arising from constant evacuations and consumption, which prevent the body from developing its otherwise natural descent into putrefaction and corruption:

> An animal body is composed of solid and fluid parts; and these consist of such various and heterogeneous principles, as render it, of all substances, the most liable to corruption and putrefaction. . . . Hence the necessity of throwing out of the body, by different outlets, these acrimonious and putrescent juices, rendered thus unfit for the animal uses and functions, together with the abraded particles of the solids. And a daily supply of food, or fresh nourishment, is required to recruit this constant waste, both of the solid and fluid parts. Thus the bodies of all animals are in a constant state of change and renovation, by which they are preserved from death and putrefaction.[10]

The main evacuation so necessary to rid the body of its putrescent juices was perspiration. The Italian physiologist Sanctorius found, when weighing everything he ate and drank over a controlled period of time, as well as everything evacuated from his body, that five-eighths of everything he consumed was expelled from the body in the form of perspiration, and more specifically insensible perspiration (perspiration of which we are unaware). If one's perspiration was blocked, then disease, in the form of putrefaction, was sure to follow.

Cold, according to Lind's empirically grounded theory, "obstructs or diminishes insensible perspiration."[11] Moist air was also to blame for putrid diseases, as it impeded perspiration and made digestion more difficult by interfering with breathing and encouraging the natural process of putrefaction. More dangerous still was the combination of moist air with a diet that was difficult to digest and break down into a substance that could be mixed "with the blood, and all the rest of our humours."[12] The diet most difficult to break down, Lind noted, was one based on salt meats and unleavened breads, such as the biscuits used as bread rations by the army and navy.

All hope was not lost for those forced to subsist on army rations of salted meat and biscuits, and live in cold and damp conditions. Such evils could be corrected by substances and practices that preserved the body from putrefaction and corrected putrid tendencies. In cold climates, Lind recommended exercise to encourage insensible perspiration. Vegetables and acids, such as vinegar, and especially acidic fruits, such as lemons and oranges, helped break down what Lind called "a gross and viscid [viscous] diet."[13] Even more helpful were those substances that preserved the body from putrefaction by their "fermentative tendency." This tendency Lind identified not only as common to vegetables, but as found also in wine, beer, cider, and spruce beer, as demonstrated in his various trials and experiments.[14]

By the symptoms of swollen limbs, spongy gums, and the fetid smell of urine, ulcers, and breath, Lind thus diagnosed scurvy to be a disease of putrefaction, caused by the blockage of perspiration and a diet that both impeded proper digestion and encouraged putrefaction. Such a theory was by no means radical or controversial, as respected men of science, such as Robert Boyle, had already investigated putrefaction. Furthermore, other authoritative physicians agreed with Lind in their writings and experiments. John Pringle, another celebrated military physician and president of the Royal Society from 1772 to 1778, was eager to find substances that would retard the putrefaction of animal humors, especially for medical purposes. Like Lind, Pringle believed that putrefaction was at the root of many diseases, and not just scurvy. Scurvy itself could degenerate into a flux, or into hospital fever if improperly managed.

In his experiments, Pringle attempted to recreate the natural human processes of digestion and putrefaction. He mixed animal substances (usually meat) with saliva in a sealed container, and placed the container by a furnace at the same temperature as human blood. After a few days, he observed the result, looking for evidence of putrefaction. Such experiments were repeated, adding various "antiseptics" (as eighteenth-century contemporaries called them), to observe their effect on the rate of putrefaction. As in Lind's experiments, Pringle found that acids, wine, and what he called "the hotter antiscorbutic plants," such as mustard and horseradish, were useful in retarding this process.[15]

SCURVY IN THE NORTH AMERICAN THEATER

In North America, British troops were all too vulnerable to this natural process of putrefaction, especially during the long winters, when they had only salted meats and army biscuits on which to survive. Early letters from commanding officers during the winter months struck an optimistic tone, but by January and February, the troops were repeatedly described as showing signs of scurvy. By April and May, when the ground had thawed and the campaigning season commenced, many soldiers had died from scurvy, and many more were languishing in temporary hospitals, waiting for recovery in the spring.[16]

The connection between spring's fresh produce and the men's recovery was not lost on Pringle, Lind, and army officers. Soldiers were expected to forage for fresh fruits and vegetables to supplement their standard rations. Yet in North America fresh produce could not be found during the long winter; also small foraging parties were easy prey for Native American raiding parties. John Johnson, the clerk of the Fifty-Eighth Regiment, reported his horror at hearing that three of his comrades had been found scalped when they had "straggled to a small distance, into a wood on the flank of their camp to gather some vegetable herbs to eat with their salt meat; and which are good for several disorders, and with which the woods abound in the summer season."[17] Moreover, British officials had constant difficulties in obtaining fresh provisions from local suppliers at what they considered reasonable prices. Colonial officials such as Massachusetts governor Thomas Pownall thus spent much time and money trying to "perswade the People of the County of Hampshire" to provide the army with "fresh provisions & all other refreshments that the Country affords."[18]

To remedy this situation, the army began the practice of planting gardens within its forts. At Halifax, such a garden was first tended in 1757, beside the general hospital, in preparation for the siege of Louisbourg.[19] Camped at Fort Niagara during 1759 and 1760, William Eyre wrote to Jeffrey Amherst, commander in chief of the forces in North America, requesting seeds for the fort's vegetable garden, to be planted in the spring. James Murray, head of the garrison at Quebec in 1760, also asked Amherst for garden seeds, pleading with him in mid-May: "We are very low, the scurvy makes terrible havock. For gods sake send us up molasses, and seeds which may produce vegetables."[20] When the garrison at Fort William Augustus reported early signs of scurvy in March 1762, Governor Gage of Montreal reported to Amherst that he had "directed Major Christie to collect some Garden Seeds which I shall also send up thither immediately."[21] In the course of the war, gardens became a standard British military practice throughout the American colonies, even among smaller outposts. By 1760, the practice was standard enough that the prosecutor at Major General Lord Charles Hay's court-martial asked witnesses whether they had "heard [Hay] represent the design of raising greens for the health of the sick and Scorbutick soldiers as a great Grievance to the men employ'd in clearing Ground" as evidence of his contempt for the conduct and authority of commanders.[22]

Yet fresh vegetables were not the only remedies and preventatives used for scurvy. The soldiers were also given various foodstuffs that had been classified as "antiscorbutic" by Lind and Pringle. Vinegar was regularly issued to the men to prevent scurvy, and wine was given to sick men as a cure. The most common, and most popular, preventative and cure for scurvy was spruce beer. Contrary to what its name suggests, it was not traditionally made from spruce trees. Kenneth Carpenter suggests that the name stems from the German *sprossen-bier*, made from *sprossen* (sprouts)—the buds of fir trees. It was reported as a drink used by sailors in the Baltic Sea as early as the sixteenth century. In North America, a customary story credits the expedition of Jacques Cartier in 1535 and Amerindians with the use of spruce beer. According to Cartier's account, he and his men suffered severely from scurvy during their winter explorations near what became Quebec City. Meeting with a band of Native Americans after many of his men had died, Cartier learned how to boil the leaves and bark of a certain tree in water, and then drink the infused water and place it on the affected parts of his body. Following the instructions of the Native Americans, all of Cartier's remaining party recovered.[23] Unfortunately, Cartier is not very clear on what type of tree the natives recommended, leaving historians to debate about various types of spruce, pine, and cedar trees native to Canada.[24]

According to Canadian legend, Native Americans showed Cartier how to brew spruce beer, therefore initiating and legitimating that country's love of beer. Today, spruce beer is still sold in parts of Canada, and can be bought at supermarkets in Quebec. Yet Native Americans almost certainly did not brew beer. Their tree-infused water, however, soon became the tradition of spruce beer for Europeans in North America. Both Lind and Pringle recommended spruce beer as an antiscorbutic; Lind stated that "a simple decoction of the tops, cones, leaves or even bark and wood of these trees, is antiscorbutic: but it becomes much more so when fermented, as in making spruce beer."[25] Spruce beer remained popular for many years: it was used to prevent scurvy during the California gold rush and was brought on the ships searching for the Franklin expedition in the Arctic in the 1850s.[26] By the early nineteenth century, spruce beer had become a respectable drink among British polite society: in *Emma*, Jane Austen has Mr. Knightley teach the charming Frank Churchill how to brew spruce beer.[27]

In North America during the Seven Years' War, spruce beer was considered essential for the health of the troops, not only because it helped prevent scurvy, but also because it replaced rum and its ill effects.[28] Officers constantly requested molasses, which was necessary for the brewing of beer, and one boasted: "Our Brewery succeeds Extremely Well, the Beer grows better every week; . . . the Soldiers are all fond of it. Indeed, I fancy it has help'd to put Many of them upon their Legs, who little Expected it some time ago."[29] Soldiers were regularly sent out on expeditions to fetch spruce; Samuel Jenks, a captain from Massachusetts, reported on 19 July 1760, "This day about 500 troops went across the lake to git spruce; nothing meterial hapned."[30] John Knox, a British captain of the Forty-Third Regiment, reported in his diary in 1757:

> The troops of this province are supplied with spruce beer, which was first introduced, during the late war, in the garrison of Louisbourg when we were in possession of it; and then the melasses were issued from the store gratis, this liquor being thought necessary for the preservation of the healths of our men, as they were confined to salt provisions, and it is an excellent antiscorbutic:—It is made of the tops and branches of the Spruss-tree, boiled for three hours, then strained into casks, with a certain quatity of melasses; and, as soon as cold, it is fit for use.
>
> When we were incamped at Halifax, the allowance was two quarts *per* day to each man, or three gallons and a half *per* week, for which he paid seven pence New-York currency. . . . Here [in central North America] the soldiers are obliged to draw five pints *per* day, or four gallons and three pints per week, for which they are charged nine-pence half-penny currency of this province . . . the paymaster of the 43rd regiment assured me, that the spruce account for that corps, in the space of about seven weeks, amounted to eighty pounds currency.[31]

The commander in chief, Jeffrey Amherst, was also a supporter of spruce beer. He recorded in his diary in 1759, "Fresh provisions now and then and a constant supply of spruce beer keeps the army in good health and they work well which helps much towards the health of the provincials, who if left to themselves would eat fryed pork and lay in their tents all day long." Amherst recorded the recipe for spruce beer at the back of his journal:

> Take 7 pounds of good spruce and boil it well until the bark peels off, then take the spruce out and put 3 gallons of molasses to the liquor and boil it again, scum it well as it boils, then take it out of the kettle and put it into a cooler, boil the remainder of the water sufficient for a barrel of 30 gallons, if the kettle is not large enough to boil it together, when milkwarm in the cooler put a pint of ye[a]st into it and mix it well, then put it in the barrel, and let it work for two or three days, keep filling it up as it works out: when done working, bung it up with

> a tent peg in the barrel, to give it vent every now and then, it may be used in two or three days after. If wanted to be bottled it should stand a fortnight in the cask. It will keep a great while.[32]

The method used by the British officers is not just of idle interest: the water-infused drinks made from the leaves of spruce, pine, or cedar trees all contain large amounts of vitamin C, which would certainly cure and protect soldiers from scurvy. Once turned into beer through fermentation or left to sit for any length of time, however, the amount of vitamin C in these drinks quickly becomes negligible.[33] Drinking spruce water, as directed by Native Americans, would have prevented and cured scurvy. By contrast, spruce beer did not, although it combined British love of beer with prevailing medical knowledge. As a result, even though officers followed medical advice proffered by Lind and Pringle on how to prevent scurvy, the remedies available to them while on winter command in North America were of little help.

THE SIEGE OF QUEBEC, 1759–1760

One such terrible winter was that of 1759–60, when the British were only months away from securing control of New France. In September 1759, British forces won the battle of the Plains of Abraham and occupied Quebec. Arriving at the end of June, British forces under James Wolfe had laid siege and bombarded the city, until open battle on the Plains was fought on 13 September. The French surrender was formally signed on 18 September 1759. In traditional Canadian history, this battle marks the country's beginnings, and represents the start of both British rule and the uneasy Anglo-French relations in that country. As exhibited in Benjamin West's famous painting of General Wolfe's heroic death at the moment that British victory was announced, it is considered the climactic battle of the North American campaigns, if not of the entire war.

An examination of the 1760 siege of Quebec, which followed the British victory on the Plains of Abraham (September 1759), corrects and complements traditional as well as recent accounts of the famous battle between Generals Montcalm and Wolfe. Conventional military histories concentrate on the two commanders in their final battle. With both commanders dying soon after victory was declared, these narratives fail to appreciate the precariousness of subsequent British control. They also ignore the role of subordinate officers, soldiers, and civilians, and of imperial structures so necessary to achieving and maintaining British military control.[34] Recent "new" military histories question the effectiveness and significance of the two generals while examining the infrastructure and the social context of warfare.[35] Nevertheless, while the battle's significance for subsequent North American history is undoubted, historians have generally neglected its British framework and wider imperial contexts.

At the end of September 1759, the British had possession of the fort and town of Quebec, but were surrounded by French forces. French troops were positioned along the Jacques-Cartier River and up into Montreal. The inhabitants of Quebec were French, and not friendly to the British stationed in their city. After all, British forces had spent the previous few months burning down their houses and destroying their crops. At that point, James Murray was appointed brigadier general and commander of British forces at Quebec. His garrison consisted of twelve regiments, totaling roughly 7,300 men. Murray was directed to maintain Britain's control of Quebec and, if possible, the surrounding area. The French were sure to attempt an attack with the spring thaw, if not sooner.

Although Murray had an impressive number of men compared to French forces stationed nearby, he was alone in the midst of hostile forces. French civilians were glad to assist French forces and Native Americans, who for the most part were loosely allied with the French and were eager to kill British troops who left the main body and ventured into the forests. By the end of November, the British fleet had left North America, to keep free from the ice of the Saint Lawrence River. Murray and his forces were completely isolated from access to additional supplies, troops, or communication from Britain until the Saint Lawrence reopened in May.

In Murray's journal, which was kept for official purposes, problems in the garrison began soon after its establishment in late September. The troops kept busy at first repairing the quarters and preparing for winter, as well as for enemy attacks. By mid-November, Murray remarked on "a very unusual Desertion" among his forces, as well as problems with drunkenness and theft in the garrison.[36] By 15 January 1760, Murray had had to fix the price of grain, bread, and meat sold by Canadians so that it was affordable for the garrison, as well as for the inhabitants of Quebec. He soon seized cattle and corn from Quebecers, upon realizing that they had been supplying French troops, while his own forces were suffering food shortages. The soldiers also suffered on the four-mile trek to fetch wood and drag it back to the fort through snow, as they did not have sufficient clothing for the climate, resulting in frostbite.[37] Troops wore any additional clothing they could find to protect them from the cold, albeit with limited effect. Captain Knox remarked:

> Our guards, on the grand parade, make a most grotesque appearance in their different dresses; and our inventions to guard us against the extreme rigour of this climate are various beyond imagination: the uniformity, as well as nicety, of the clean, methodical soldier, is buried in the rough fur-wrought garb of the frozen Laplander; and we rather resemble a masquerade than a body of regular troops. . . . Yet, notwithstanding all our precautions, several men and Officers have suffered by the intenseness of the cold, being frost-bitten in their faces, hands, feet, and other parts least to be suspected.[38]

Captain Knox first mentions problems with disease in the garrison in December. Only 4,138 soldiers of the original 7,300 were listed as fit for duty on December's monthly return, with 2,077 soldiers sick in the garrison or at the general hospital, equivalent to a sick rate of 28 percent.[39] In January 1760, Knox recorded in his journal:

> The men grow more unhealthy as the winter advances, and scarce a day passes without two or three funerals; though several do recover, yet the hospitals still continue full: it is, indeed, melancholy to see such havock among our brave fellows, and their daily sufferings distress the Officers beyond expression.[40]

The records for January agree with Knox's impression, as 96 men were listed as having died (from nonbattle causes) during that month, with a sick rate of 25 percent.[41]

It is in February that Murray first mentions the sickness of the troops causing problems for the rest of the garrison. Servants of officers and prisoners were ordered to help with garrison duties, and orders specified that this was "on account of the weakness of the regiment, through sickness, and the great severity of duty."[42] Ninety-two men died in February, and barely 4,000 were fit for duty by the end of the month, with a continuing sick rate of 28 percent.[43] By March, Murray had to cancel his plans to attack a nearby French holding because of a lack of healthy men to carry out the attack. It is hardly surprising that sickness was disrupting strategy and regular duties: the return of 24 March has only 3,513 men fit for duty, with a sick rate of 36 percent and 166 dead during that month alone.[44]

Murray recognized that, despite his efforts, his troops' health was getting worse:

> The Sickness still on the Increase, notwithstanding every measure was taken to prevent it spreading, and the Cause being Manifestly the Scurvy, gave order this day about the method of Boiling and preparing the Salt Pork, it being Impossible to procure fresh Provisions, or Vegetables.[45]

By the end of March, the ground had at least softened enough for Murray to order his men to bury the hundreds of dead soldiers, whose bodies had accumulated over the winter. Such a sight was surely demoralizing, even to men used to seeing the gore of a battlefield. After all, only 58 British soldiers had been killed during the battle in September on the Plains of Abraham. In comparison, from the end of November 1759 to the end of March 1760, 460 soldiers had died, their bodies piled and waiting for the spring thaw.

Spring and relief for the garrison did not arrive in April. Instead, April was the sickliest month of all. It opened with attempts by French forces to surprise and burn various British outposts. In response, Murray organized defensive works. This was difficult, partly because the continued cold weather meant he could not drive fortifications very deep into the ground, and also because the troops were so sickly he was "obliged to use them with the utmost tenderness."[46] By 25 April, Murray bewailed the health of his troops, as an additional 200 men had fallen sick in just the previous week. During April, 149 men died of disease, while none were wounded or killed in skirmishes; a mere 2,612 men were left fit for duty.[47]

This sickness had serious consequences for the garrison. Colonel Malcolm Fraser of the Seventy-Eighth Regiment, or Fraser's Highlanders, recorded in his journal on 25 April, "Great havock amongst the garrison occasioned by the scurvy etc; this is the more alarming as the General seems certain the French are coming to attack the place, and will he says, be here in a very few days."[48] On 27 April, Murray received word that the French had landed at Point au Tremble, and were making their way toward his garrison. Thanks to the information gained from a French soldier found shipwrecked on an ice floe, Murray had sufficient time to decide how to respond to the French attack. In his journal, he explains that because of the sickness in the garrison, he did not have enough men to guard Quebec against the advancing French. He decided instead to risk an open battle, hoping that his numerically inferior, but more experienced troops, would repeat their success of the previous autumn.[49]

On 28 April, French and British forces met again, this time in reversed positions, in what is known as the battle of Sainte-Foy or the battle of Quebec. The British were now guarding Quebec against French attack. As in the previous battle, the defending party was soon chased into the town, and the French won control of the Plains of Abraham. John Johnson, the clerk of the Fifty-Eighth Regiment, described the battle as one between "starved, scorbutic skeletons" on the British side and the French "army of all healthy, strong, young men." He blamed the disastrous British retreat on "the weakness of the men, either through wounds, scurvey, sickness, or real want of the common necessaries of support."[50] The British remained holed up behind the town walls, while the French established their siege on the Plains. Within the town, Murray anxiously counted his stock of ammunition, and recruited the sick to make wadding and fill sandbags. The siege continued for many days, each side battering the other with its small store of ammunition, while repairing the daily damage each night.

Both the French and the British eagerly watched the Saint Lawrence for the sight of a ship bringing reinforcements. On 9 May, a British vessel finally arrived, followed by three more on 15 May. With British victory assured by the arrival of supplies, the French pulled out of Quebec on 16 May, to continue the battle in Montreal. Contemporaries were not yet convinced that British control was secure. The French officer Anne-Joseph-Hippolyte de Maurès de Malartic reported to the Chevalier de Lévis, near the end of May 1760:

> I do not think Mr. Murray is in any state capable of more undertakings; he has no more than fifteen to sixteen hundred men fit for service; many still have the scurvy. He told me yesterday, in all confidence, that he longed for all of this to finish; that he does not like this country; that almost all of his men were ill and no longer recognizable.[51]

Similarly, less than two weeks later the governor general of New France, Pierre de Rigaud de Vaudreuil de Cavignial, Marquis de Vaudreuil, noted that British troops in various forts and throughout New England were reduced by sickness and that the "garrison at Quebec cannot hide the depths of its misery," bolstering his anticipation of French military success.[52] Yet, by 13 July 1760, Murray wrote to the commander in chief, Jeffrey Amherst, that he was leaving for Montreal the next day with 2,200 men, and that he "had the happiness to inform you, Sir, that since the weather has been warm our Sick have recovered surprisingly."[53] With the surrender of New France signed on 8 September 1760, Murray wrote to his superior officer, "The troops under my command are greatly recovr'd, and will be very comfortably quartr'd this winter, in comparison of the last, I can almost venture to assure you, that we shall entirely get the better of the scurvey."[54]

MEDICINE IN THE GARRISON AND THE ARMED FORCES

It was just after suffering defeat at the hands of the French, at the end of April 1760, that Murray wrote to Amherst to explain what had happened at the battle of Sainte-Foy, referring to "the most inveterate Scurvy."[55] This disease, Murray claimed, had devastated his garrison stationed in Quebec and was partly to blame for British failure. Explaining the British defeat to William Pitt in a letter that was published in the *Gentleman's Magazine* of May 1760, Murray wrote:

> The Excessive coldness of the Climate, and constant living upon salt provisions, without any vegetables, introduced the scurvy among the Troops, which, getting the better of every precaution of the Officer, and every remedy of the Surgeon, became as universal as it was inveterate, in so much, that before the end of April one thousand were dead, and above two thousand of what remained, totally unfit for any service.[56]

The use of the term "inveterate"—obstinate and deep-seated—suggests that various methods of prevention and treatment were tried. Indeed, as in previous land campaigns during the war, the garrison employed methods suggested by Lind and Pringle.

Murray wrote in his journal that the hospital of the Quebec garrison used spruce beer as an antiscorbutic, and in early April he ordered spruce beer "to be given to all the Men as a Preservative against that fatal Disease."[57] Dr. Russel, the garrison's surgeon, directed wine to be given to the troops in March. As another antiscorbutic recommended by Lind, vinegar was regularly administered to the troops at Quebec. Orders from February doubled the daily amount issued to troops, as officials insisted, "Nothing is better for the scurvy, which is the cause of the disorders in the army."[58] In March, officers were reminded to ensure that the vinegar was thawed before being issued.[59] Ginger, presumably classified as a hot antiscorbutic, was also regularly administered, to be mixed with water and drunk daily.[60] The diet of salted meat was also modified in accordance with theories of digestion and putrefaction. It was ordered that no men be allowed to eat the salt pork without steeping it in water for at least "twenty hours, changing the water three times, scraping and washing the salt off at each time that the water is removed."[61]

Medical officials acknowledged that these measures were unsuccessful. Letters written by regimental surgeons and physicians in the North American campaign demonstrate that they were clearly distressed and perplexed by the rates of scurvy. Both Lind and Pringle relied on this extensive correspondence with military and naval medical officers to inform their theories of disease. For Lind, the incidence of scurvy in the garrison at Quebec was important enough that he included an excerpt from Murray's letter on the garrison's defeat in the third edition of his famous treatise.[62] Even more significant, in this 1772 edition of his treatise, Lind challenged his own previous theory that scurvy was a disease of putrefaction. He based his dissatisfaction on numerous dissections that he had since performed, his recent observations made on scurvy sufferers at Haslar Hospital, and the rate of scurvy in the garrison at Quebec:

> It was remarkable, that the dreadful mortality from the scurvy at *Quebec*, in the year 1759, happened during so severe a frost, that the dead bodies could not be buried for a considerable time, until the thaw came on; there being no possibility till then of digging their graves; and at that time all animal substances were kept perfectly free from corruption, by being exposed to the air. It is certain that diseases commonly deemed putrid, seldom occur in winter, or during so severe a frost.[63]

Lind regretfully concluded:

> The term *putrid*, respecting animal and vegetable substances, is not indeed, in my opinion, sufficiently defined and restricted, so as to serve as a solid basis or foundation of any theory for explaining the symptoms of the scurvy. The idea of the scurvy proceeding from animal putrefaction, may, and hath misled physicians to propose and administer medicines for it, altogether ineffectual.[64]

The data from the garrison at Quebec were crucial to Lind's reconsideration of his theory of scurvy. Although no material survives regarding Lind's medical network, Pringle's ten volumes of medical correspondence and notes (held at the Royal College of Physicians of Edinburgh) demonstrate the extent to which this leading European physician relied on the observations and experiences of military medical men stationed abroad, as well as indicating the vibrant nature of British military medicine during the mid-eighteenth century. Pringle wrote to numerous military medical men, surgeons as well as physicians, soliciting their opinions and observations on disease and medicine. Among his correspondents stationed with the army in America were surgeons Dr. [Richard] Huck, Mr. [John] Adair, Mr. Russel (possibly the surgeon at the garrison at Quebec), and Mr. Ramsay, and the physician Dr. [George] Munro, in addition to other surgeons, apothecaries, and physicians stationed in Europe, the West Indies, Senegal, and India and on board naval vessels throughout the mid-eighteenth century.

When writing to his correspondents, Pringle not only requested general observations, but also posed specific questions regarding the efficacy of debated treatments (such as bleeding for yellow fever) and theories of disease (such as whether they were endemic or contagious, and how they acted in different climates). He asked his correspondents to evaluate published medical works to see whether their firsthand experiences accorded with what well-known treatises claimed. For example, Dr. Cuthbert noted that his experience with scurvy at the Navy Hospital at Portsmouth agreed with "Dr Lind's idea of the nature of the disease."[65] Pringle also recorded that Dr. Huck's "opportunity of seeing a great number of cases of the yellow fever among our Troops in general confirms Dr Hilary's practice," explicitly referring to "Dr Hilary's book" (William Hillary's *Observations on the Changes of the Air . . . in the Island of Barbadoes*, published in 1759).[66] Pringle put much stock in the observations of his correspondents, often writing additional notes in the margins upon having discussed theories and treatments further after the initial correspondence.

Claims to experience and observation were a common rhetorical device among eighteenth-century writings, but in the case of Lind and Pringle, it is evident that they relied on the network of British military medicine in order to empirically inform their theories of disease and treatment. As a result, the firsthand experience of even lowly military surgeons was solicited and assiduously collected, meaning that military medical men stationed in the colonies were considered experts, providing reliable observations and informed medical judgments. Moreover, empirical practices such as dissection, still relatively uncommon in the metropole, could be instituted with greater ease in colonial military medicine: stationed in the West Indies, a Dr. Temple casually wrote to Pringle that he "had seen several bodies opened, in all which he had found evident marks of inflammation" as further support for his theory of yellow fever.[67] As Mark Harrison has demonstrated, "Imperial wars, territorial annexation, and colonial trade made a deep impact upon British medicine, providing a major stimulus to the emergence of what was known as 'rational' or 'scientific' medicine," in part through access to first-hand observations and cadavers for postmortem investigations.[68] Although not effective according to modern-day biomedicine, military surgeons—such as those at Quebec—were clearly instituting and evaluating the leading advances and innovations in British medicine. Moreover, British military medicine during the Seven Years' War provided an active network of correspondence, and one in which colonial experience helped shape medicine in the metropole.

Little is known about the majority of the medical men serving with the army. Few records exist on the background and ambitions of these hundreds of individuals.[69] All medical men, including regimental surgeons and mates, would have undergone an examination by the College of Surgeons before being admitted to serve, though this did not mean they possessed formal medical qualifications. Early modern European civilian medicine has been characterized by a tripartite division, with university-trained and theory-laden physicians at the top of the hierarchy, manual and apprentice-trained surgeons in the middle, and apothecaries responsible for drugs and some general medical knowledge at the bottom. These last were notably wealthy in eighteenth-century Britain, as Adam Smith observed, but low in social status. Beyond these were the many irregular practitioners, who often combined medical arts with other trades and skills. With the decline of regulatory bodies such as the College of Physicians, and with patients choosing from a variety of practitioners, historians have noted that the tripartite division in this period could be more theoretical than practical. Roy Porter and W. F. Bynum, in particular for the eighteenth century, have pointed out that medical provision and use were more fluid, and more likely more consumer-driven, than this division portrays.[70] Military medicine supports this flexibility, for divisions between physicians and surgeons were not always clear in practice, although close attention was paid to rank, particularly for the purposes of half pay.

Pringle's correspondents demonstrate this professional fluidity: many of those named above were surgeons, and Pringle drew on physicians and apothecaries as well. Even within these official designations, medical backgrounds and appointments in the armed forces varied beyond what are usually described as "surgeons" and "physicians." George Monro, appointed surgeon to the hospitals in North America from 1757, was then appointed assistant physician to the hospital for the expedition to Martinique in 1761, with John Adair, the hospital director, noting that Monro "has not only had a regular Education, & the Degree of Doctor in Physick, but has given many proofs of his Knowledge and Abilitys in Physick both in the Hospital and in the Army."[71] Likewise, Richard Huck, surgeon to the hospitals in North America, held an MD from St. Andrew's University. Huck's service illustrates the scope and span of responsibilities and opportunities of a military medical practitioner stationed in the colonies: he was a regular correspondent not only of Pringle but also of John Campbell, fourth Earl of Loudoun and commander in chief of North America in 1756–58, providing letters with the most gossip and military details of campaigns in North America and the West Indies of those that survive in the Loudoun Papers.[72]

The distinction between surgeon and physician was most likely not strictly adhered to in military contexts because it held little practical consequence for treatment during campaigns.[73] Regimental surgeons, for example, were responsible for treating all medical concerns of rank-and-file men, whether surgical or disease related. Rather than categorizing military medicine according to the tripartite model of civilian medicine, military medical historians have identified the key division as that between regimental medicine and the hospitals. Whereas the day-to-day concerns of most troops were dealt with by the lowly surgeon (and occasionally an accompanying mate) within the regiment, seriously ill troops were sent to a permanent general hospital, staffed by more eminent and well-paid physicians, surgeons, and apothecaries, assisted by nurses.[74] Those at the top of the military medical hierarchy held degrees from leading European universities, published medical treatises, and were also part of a vibrant civilian medical network, demonstrating that military experience was no drawback to social and medical advancement more broadly, as discussed in more detail in chapter 3.

Regimental medical experience was thus deemed by contemporaries as useful in the development of medical expertise, challenging the modern assumption that general care in the army was poor. Active observation, experimentation, and evaluation of medical theories stemmed from regimental practice and shaped regimental care, while also influencing metropolitan medical theory and orthodoxy through correspondence between regimental surgeons and scientific luminaries in Britain. Responsible for the health of hundreds of men, regimental medical men quickly gained much medical experience dealing with both disease and battle injuries. Because of this, and because service in the army exempted such men from the licensing restrictions of the Colleges of Physicians and Surgeons, medical service in the army was a common option for ambitious but poor medical men, especially those who had studied at the Scottish universities.[75] This was borne out in the American colonies, as John Morgan—later to become one of the most influential physicians in America—served as a lowly provincial regimental surgeon during the Seven Years' War.[76] Indeed, Paul E. Kopperman suggests that regimental surgeons had more education than often presumed, particularly when compared with the majority of medical practitioners found in eighteenth-century civilian society.[77] As one regimental surgeon of the War of Austrian Succession noted,

> Our Regim[en]tal Surgeons from the beginning are generally well educated. . . . We have a weekly Club w[h]ere all are welcome to come, the chief Subject of conversation relates to our own business; it being a standing rule with us, that if any thing remarkable happen'd during the last weeks practice, it's to be made publick for the good of the Society; by this means we know the practice of the whole army during the Camp[aig]n, & in winter quarters that of the Garrison, where we have an opportunity of attending the hospital.[78]

As Tabitha Marshall has cogently demonstrated, historians have been misled into reading late eighteenth-century calls for reform as accurate descriptions of the state of British regimental medicine during the eighteenth century.[79] Following contemporary medical practices and theory, medical care in the garrison at Quebec was clearly part of a broader practice of innovation, observation, and medical expertise within the British armed forces. Moreover, the experience of scurvy and the observed failure of Lind's recommended remedies did not remain confined to the colonies, but instead were part of a transatlantic network of correspondence, and used to refine Lind's own theories on the disease.

IRREGULARS AND DISEASE

Within the British garrison, the rates of sickness during the winter suggest something more than just a challenge to Lind's theory of scurvy. British regulars suffered the least from scurvy, compared with the two regiments under Murray's command that can be classed as "irregulars": the Highland regiment and provincial Rangers. From November 1759 to April 1760, British regular forces at Quebec had a morbidity rate beginning at 22 percent and peaking at 32 percent in March and April. Fraser's Highland regiment, by contrast, had rates of sickness from 41 to 73 percent. This was not the only campaign on which Highland regiments were sicklier than regular

British troops; when on campaign in the West Indies in 1759 and in 1762, officers and soldiers remarked on how quickly and easily the Scottish soldiers became ill. A Scottish soldier in North America commented at the end of the war that the Highlanders, "although brave in action, shrink under, and get sick, when obliged to perform excessive fatigues."[80]

Highland regiments, established by the Crown to take advantage of the bravery and martial tradition of Scottish Highlanders, had first been used in the late seventeenth century in order to maintain peace in the wild Highlands, acting against the Macdonalds at Glencoe. The Scottish regiments first fought outside of Britain in 1739, and were famously praised for their brave conduct in Flanders during the 1740s. It was not until the Seven Years' War that Highland regiments were widely used and posted abroad in the large numbers that became characteristic in the nineteenth century. This was partly due to the failed Jacobite rebellion in 1745. After the '45, young Scots were encouraged by British governmental policy to join Highland regiments, and at the same time, in the aftermath of the rebellion, men found themselves with few other options.[81] Fraser's regiment, for example, was led by the son of Lord Lovat, who was executed in 1747 for his role in the rebellion. Fraser himself had fought in the rebellion against British forces at the head of the Fraser clan, but surrendered, to be pardoned in 1750. During the Seven Years' War, he proved himself so worthy in his British military service, this time fighting against the French, that he had much of his family's forfeited estates returned to him a decade earlier than previously decreed.[82]

Highland regiments were distinctive during the Seven Years' War, and not only because of their fighting spirit, but also because of their dress. Soldiers wore traditional Highland garb, otherwise banned by post-rebellion decree in 1747. Their differences were not always popular with the English.[83] A soldier petitioned Lord Barrington in 1757 to be changed from his current appointment in a Highland regiment. He explained:

> A Highland Company is not my choice, because I am no Highlander, and these Battalions are at best looked on as Irregulars and destined to remain in America even when the War is at an end, besides these, there are other circumstances I must not name attending the Highland corps which increase my objections to continue amongst them.[84]

The Highlanders' distinctive dress seems also to have led to their higher rates of sickness, especially in the North American climate. During the siege at Quebec, the soldiers noted that the Highlanders suffered the most from cold, and explained their sickliness by their uniforms. Malcolm Fraser wrote in his journal during the Quebec siege: "The garrison in general are but indifferently cloathed, but our regiment in particular is in a pityful situation having no breeches, and the Philibeg [kilt] is not all calculated for this terrible climate. Colonel Fraser is doing all in his power to provide trousers for them."[85] The French nuns in the Ursuline convent in Quebec not only helped nurse the sick soldiers, but also knit stockings for the inadequately clothed Highlanders during the siege.[86]

The other irregular regiment at Quebec with a noticeably higher rate of sickness than the British regulars in 1759–60 was that composed of American-born provincials: Captain Hazzan's Rangers (companies designed for wilderness warfare and trained to be sent out on scouting parties).[87] Even during regular campaigns, it was no secret that provincials were sick far more often than British regulars, as both provincials and British officials commented on the number of provincials struck down by diseases in North American military camps.[88]

Surgeons and physicians stationed in North America also noticed these tendencies among provincials. Dr. Richard Huck reported that provincial troops were remarkably sicklier than British regulars. He ascribed this provincial weakness to their laziness and prearmy lifestyle, telling Pringle that the provincials were spoiled by their previous habits of living in luxury:

> I don't know how to account for this extraordinary sickness among the provincials more than the regulars. Tho their diet was the same, yet the last probably messd more regularly. . . . At home (particularly the Connecticut people) they live in a kind of ease and affluence that renders them incapable of bearing hardships without risquing their health. They cannot stir in a morning without their tea or chocolate, and bear sleeping upon the ground very ill in place of a feather-bed. I do not know if it is owing to the pampered manner in which they are brought up, but they certainly have not the strength and stamina of Europeans. One may generally know a country born man after two or three days sickness by his face.[89]

Dr. Kirkpatrick, also a British physician in North America, concurred with Huck and added:

> Those who come from Europe are longer lived than the natives. This remark seems to extend to all the British Colonies in America; for Ma-

jor Rutherford who had lived many years in New York, made the same remark viz, that the constitution of those who are born in that settlement is seldom so good as of those who come from England; and that neither the people of New York nor of New England can bear so much fatigue nor sickness as those who come from Great Britain.[90]

According to Lind and Pringle, disease, and especially scurvy, affected some types of individual more than others. Specifically, Lind believed that a melancholic temperament and "laziness and indolence of disposition, and from thence a neglect of using proper exercise, or a sedentary and inactive life," were contributing factors in one's susceptibility to scurvy, as a person who was depressed, lazy, and inactive had a lack of firmness in the body and in digestion.[91] A letter to the *Gentleman's Magazine* in September 1756 asserted that scurvy was not so prevalent in the merchant marine as compared with the Royal Navy, the reason being that in the navy, sailors could avoid exercise and hard labor, instead indulging in "an idle, lazy life at sea."[92] The letter concluded, "Till such or other means are fallen upon to discourage indolence and lazyness, we may ever expect to hear, that large rates in particular are harrassed with the scurvy, when all trading vessels keep constantly healthy."[93] As Amherst had noted in his journal, exercise and a diet of fresh provisions were necessary for maintaining the health of British garrisons in North America. It was particularly important for provincial troops in British garrisons to have this healthy regimen, as Amherst observed a tendency of provincial troops to avoid work and eat too much fried pork.[94]

The sickliness of provincial soldiers was commented on not only by British officials. Provincials themselves noted that they were sicklier than their British counterparts. Captain Samuel Jenks, from Massachusetts, recorded in his diary three months after the beginning of his 1760 campaign: "The provincials begin to be very sickly. Two of our battalion died yesterday, and several officers and soldiers are very sick in our reg[iment]. I desire to bless God I am enabled to go forward with the army, & have not missed one tour of duty yet."[95] Less than three weeks later he wrote: "The men in camp begin to die very fast, and its very sickly, there is about 1,200 men of the provincials now return'd unfit for duty, and great many more taken sick almost every day."[96] A day later he continued: "There is not above a third part of the men now in camp that are fit for duty, and dies more or less every day."[97]

That foreign British troops were healthier than the native-born provincial soldiers is unusual. In the other colonial theaters of the Seven Years'

War, British regulars suffered from foreign climates and diseases to which they were not accustomed, as examined in more detail in chapters 2 and 5 on West Indian and East Indian campaigns, respectively. It is significant, in this respect, that apart from scurvy, the diseases afflicting soldiers were not products of the North American climate. According to the diary of Captain Jenks, the provincials were suffering from flux, fevers, and smallpox. Flux, referring to dysentery or diarrheal diseases, and contagious fevers such as typhus, were common complaints in unsanitary and crowded conditions, such as those that prevailed in army camps. Smallpox in particular, because of its highly contagious nature, quickly spread within the confines of an encamped army.[98] British regular soldiers suffered less from such maladies, first, because they were more likely to have been recruited from urban centers in Britain where such crowd diseases were prevalent, and, second, because they had already been used to living in army camps before arriving in North America.[99]

Provincial soldiers, including those from New England towns, were not used to the close quarters of camps. In military camps, soldiers ate, slept, exercised, and used latrines in unsanitary conditions conducive to the spread of disease. Captain Jenks reflected, "I could not help thinking what lodging I have exchanged for this, which is not half so good or convenient as we generally provide for our swine at home."[100] It was not simply the inconvenience of rough conditions that bothered Jenks. On two occasions he notes that he went for a walk "to get clear of the smell of the camps."[101]

SMALLPOX AND THE AMERICAN COLONIES

Among these crowd diseases, smallpox was especially feared by provincial soldiers, and also appeared to target provincial soldiers more than British regulars. On 14 September 1760, Captain Jenks recorded: "Our men break out very fast with the smallpox. I am greatly afraid it will spread in the army, altho' all the care we have taken to prevent it."[102] From Massachusetts, Sergeant David Holden noted, "Men carried out of camp with the small pox more or less every day."[103] Officials reported smallpox among troops from the outbreak of the war, spreading from an epidemic beginning in French Canada in 1755. Late in 1756, the commander in chief, the Earl of Loudoun, reported to the Duke of Cumberland, from New York:

> I have hitherto forgot to Acquaint Your Royal Highness, that the *Small Pox* is spread over, I think, the whole of this Country, except *New En-*

gland, from where I have not heard of it yet: It is at *Albany*, It is *here*, and it is at *Philadelphia*, and among the *Six Nations*; they got it from the *French*, at *Niagara*; and the French in *Canada*, had it all last Year; when it first broke out, it made a very great Alarm in the Country, but now that is over, except among the New England Men.[104]

Provincials were understandably terrified of catching the disease. Writing at midcentury, physician Richard Brocklesby (1722–97) reported, "Small-Pox is reckoned deservedly amongst the most dangerous diseases that are commonly to be met with throughout all Europe."[105] Those lucky enough to survive could be left with blindness, skin infections, infertility, and a horrifically ravaged appearance. Incubation lasts from ten to twelve days, after which sufferers experience back, muscle, and head pains, high fever, and the characteristic rash. In severe cases, the rash becomes confluent, causing septic skin infections and massive hemorrhages of the skin, lungs, and other organs. Two main kinds of smallpox are widely recognized: *Variola major*, with a mortality rate of approximately 25 percent, and *Variola minor*, with a mortality rate of approximately 1 percent. The severity of smallpox appears to have changed over time: most medical historians agree that smallpox became much more fatal sometime during the sixteenth century, and eighteenth-century contemporaries recognized that there could be a "good" kind and a "bad" kind, most likely corresponding to *minor* and *major*.[106]

There is no cure for smallpox, but one attack provides lifelong immunity. As a result, inoculation, in which infectious material is purposefully administered in order to cause what is hoped to be a mild attack, was used to confer immunity on an individual. The practice, in various forms, originated in Asia, and gained notoriety and finally acceptance in Britain during the eighteenth century. The operation was risky and dangerous at best, practiced only in the immediate threat of a smallpox epidemic. Not only could an inoculated individual end up suffering from a severe or fatal form of the disease, but also once inoculated the patient was a source of infection. Inoculated patients were carefully sequestered for the duration of the disease and its incubation, and were advised to follow a diet and bleeding regimen before and after the procedure.[107]

Smallpox is spread by airborne droplets through the respiratory tract, and is thus easily spread within living quarters, as well as carried in a sufferer's clothing, possessions, and bedding. The disease was contagious in crowded and unsanitary living situations, such as urban centers. During the time of the Seven Years' War, smallpox was endemic in London: the

Bills of Mortality show deaths from smallpox every year, with epidemics peaking every two to three years. In eighteenth-century British towns with a medium level and density of population, such as Penrith in Cumbria, demographic historians have demonstrated that smallpox epidemics occurred in regular five-year cycles, predominantly affecting children.[108] Smallpox was thus a constant presence in eighteenth-century British urban life. Apart from adult rural immigrants, therefore, adult populations in urban centers were immune to the disease, having most likely survived a smallpox attack during childhood.

As a result, many if not most British Army recruits would have been immune to smallpox.[109] Studies of the British Army suggest that most men came from lower-class, laboring, and low-skilled backgrounds, and especially from urban centers such as London, when other work could not be found. In order to successfully recruit, sergeants established themselves in manufacturing towns, places with population density sufficiently high to maintain endemic levels of smallpox.[110] In his military medical treatise based on observations recorded during the Seven Years' War, Richard Brocklesby explained, "In the army, at the beginning of the late war, I found two out of nine soldiers in the marching regiments, who, by living remote from the metropolis in country quarters, had till then escaped this disease."[111]

Like rural Britons, American-born provincial soldiers were less likely to have suffered from smallpox before joining regiments in the 1750s and 1760s. Not only was the population density insufficient to maintain smallpox in the major urban centers (including New York and Boston, which were more sparsely populated than British towns), but quarantine measures imposed on incoming ships ensured that outbreaks were unusual. Although the American colonies had suffered from epidemics in the 1720s, prompting Cotton Mather to encourage inoculation (and igniting religious controversy over the practice), most populous centers avoided outbreaks for up to twenty years at a time.[112] As a result, provincials born during those periods would be vulnerable as adults to smallpox, and greatly feared its incidence; the disease was even a factor in encouraging the establishment of universities in the American colonies so that provincials would not risk smallpox when sent to Britain to pursue their studies.[113]

With the onset of war and the arrival of troops from Europe, smallpox broke out in the American colonies. In the French colonies, French officials recognized that the disease was imported from Europe. M. de Doreil wrote to Paris in October 1757: "Upon the troubles of war has supervened an epidemic disease which has been introduced by the ships that brought the soldiers. It has already committed great ravages, and apprehensions are entertained for the consequences."[114] With the movement of troops, the disease quickly spread. When surrendered British soldiers were attacked by Native Americans allied with the French at Fort William Henry in August 1757, officials claimed that items stolen from the British had spread smallpox among the Native Americans.[115] Montcalm, the French commander, recorded in November 1757: "Smallpox, which in Canada is considered a common disease appearing every twenty years, has wrought havoc this year, since it began two years ago. It was spread by the Acadians and English taken at [Fort] William Henry."[116]

The disease also influenced Native American military strategy. Based on his examination of variation in annual rates of Amerindians allied with the French, D. Peter MacLeod argues that smallpox was integral to war strategy. These fluctuations do not directly correspond to the success or failure of French military ventures, but rather to the incidence of smallpox.[117] French officials were aware of these consequences, and tried to obviate them in various ways. On occasion, they even told their Amerindian allies that it was the British who were responsible for spreading the disease, a tactic of blame that was hardly new, and one that would again be used during the American War of Independence.[118] Montcalm recognized the diplomatic and strategic ill-effects of smallpox, and wrote in his journal early in 1758, "The Indians have lost many from smallpox, which is frustrating: they will not want to fight alongside us, and it will cost the King so much to pay for funerals and other ceremonies, that officers at the outposts will have good opportunity to work on their *Memoirs*."[119]

The effects of smallpox were similarly felt among provincials. As immunity to smallpox is not genetic, and as there is no perceptible difference between the genetic immunity of Europeans and Native Americans, American-born Europeans in the eighteenth century were just as susceptible to the ravages of the disease as Native Americans.[120] With provincial soldiers living and fighting side by side with British soldiers and then returning to their homes when winter brought campaigns to an end, smallpox first attacked provincial troops and was then spread throughout the colonies.

British officials noticed the high rates of smallpox among the provincials, and were aware of its harmful logistical effects. Loudoun described the course of the disease to Cumberland in the spring of 1757:

> We have the Small Pox raging among the troops that are embarked, and among the Ranging Companys—Mr. Webb has it among the Troops, the Independent Companys, and the New York Provincials; but the kind is

> good and very few die, but I expect it will go over the whole continent. The Terror People have for it in this country is inexpressable, altho' that is a good deal diminished from the care we have taken, both of the People that are infected with it and to prevent its spreading.[121]

During the siege of Louisbourg in 1758, Captain John Knox recorded in his journal, "The troops have suffered considerably by sickness; but, though I am told so, I find, upon inquiry, the loss has been mostly among the Rangers and New England artificers, to whom the small-pox has proved fatal."[122] Robert Rogers, the provincial Ranger leader, likewise reported that many Rangers had died from smallpox during 1757.[123] Both Loudoun and Amherst wrote on the topic of smallpox, not only to officials in Britain, but also to the governors of the American colonies, who were understandably concerned about outbreaks of the disease. Amherst made what appears to be a reference to inoculating provincial soldiers when he wrote to Lieutenant Governor De Lancey in 1758 pleading for more troops and arms, assuring him, "Such of Your Men as have not had the small pox and are afraid of it, shall be so disposed of, that they need be under no apprehensions."[124]

No other references to inoculation being conducted in North America during the war survive. As inoculating thousands of individuals (including caring for the infectious and helpless patients for weeks afterward) would require large-scale organization and resources, the lack of any accounts or hospital preparations concerning inoculation indicates that no such operation took place. Along with the high rates of smallpox that provincials suffered throughout the war, this suggests that Amherst's proposition was never implemented as a central directive.[125] Ad hoc and individual inoculations were likely carried out, organized at the regimental level by surgeons and officers who could ensure consent and care, but no evidence suggests widespread or standardized inoculation throughout the British armed forces during the time of the Seven Years' War.[126]

It is unlikely that the provincials who feared smallpox would have been happier being inoculated, as many were as scared of inoculation as of smallpox itself (since unlike vaccination, inoculation transmits the actual disease in its full strength). Even in British urban centers where smallpox was endemic, inoculation schemes caused alarm during this period: at Winchester in 1758, and again in 1763, apothecaries and surgeons publicly declared a boycott of inoculations "in order to put an entire stop to the distemper spreading again."[127] In parts of the American colonies, inoculation was even more controversial and feared. In her study of smallpox in Washington's army during the American War of Independence, Ann

Becker notes, "Mistrust of the procedure [of inoculation], combined with religious scruples, resulted in strong opposition to inoculation in the city of Boston, and indeed, in much of New England during the Revolutionary period."[128] As a result, widespread inoculation among the 30,000 troops scattered throughout North America during the campaign would have caused more problems than it offered solutions. As every inoculated soldier would have been infectious and unable to care for himself for a few weeks at least, general inoculation would have crippled the British forces, killed a portion of soldiers inoculated, and spread smallpox among camp followers and into nearby settlements. Moreover, it would have exacerbated existing provincial resentment of British military demands, if not motivating outright provincial refusals and mutinies.

During the American War of Independence, British forces and the Continental Army instituted nominally "voluntary" inoculation. Such measures could be implemented in part because the acceptance of inoculation was more widely spread by the third quarter of the eighteenth century, and because smallpox presented a more immediate and widespread danger during the American war.[129] The absence of centralized, large-scale inoculation among British forces during the Seven Years' War should not be considered a sign of either a lack of consideration for troop welfare or a lack of medical improvement on the part of British authorities. Inoculation should not be considered as progress, but—just as contemporaries saw it—as a debatable, novel, and dangerous operation, one that would not have been welcomed had it been implemented centrally, particularly by imperial military officials. Medical practices such as inoculation need to be understood within their social contexts, just as diseases such as smallpox were understood by contemporaries as a particular threat to provincials, even if this was not always the case.[130]

Reinforcing the idea that widespread inoculation would have been resisted by provincials, provincial soldiers were reluctant to serve with the British Army because of smallpox, just as in the case of Native American French allies. In June 1758, James Abercromby reported to Pitt, "I have left two Additional Companies of Lord John Murray's with four Companies of Provincials, computed at 100 each, to garrison Fort Edward, and one Company of the Royal Americans, for the Duty in Albany, as no Provincials wou'd venture to serve there, on Account of the Small Pox."[131] Smallpox had appeared in Albany as early as October 1756, when Amherst wrote to the governor of New Hampshire. Amherst pledged that he would "take every step in my power" to prevent the disease spreading through the province, as well as asking Governor Wentworth to help ensure that the provincial troops did not disembark at Albany. Amherst ended his letter insisting, "I do assure you no care shall be wanting on my part to prevent this misfortune from spreading."[132] Amherst knew well the danger smallpox posed to his campaign. In November 1756 he wrote to Governor Hopkin at Albany expressing hope that the smallpox would abate with the arrival of winter. He also noted that rumors of it breaking out among troops had caused "both the New England Troops and the Indians [to] leave us and go home."[133] Provincials even used the disease as an excuse for desertion, one writing to Amherst explaining:

> On hearing that the small pox is in many places between Pitt and New York which disorder I never had, and shou'd I take the Infection at this advanced age it wou'd probably prove fatal and in such an Event a Wife and nine Children would be robed of their principal support. This Circumstance I relyed on your Excellencys goodness to Excuse my attending in New York with the Vouchors for the Cherokee Expedition [in] 1760.[134]

For Amherst, a commander already constantly beset by troop shortages, provincial reluctance to serve because of smallpox fears was yet another aggravation foisted on him by the uncooperative and ill-tempered inhabitants of the American colonies.

Illness and temperament were inextricably linked in eighteenth-century medical theory. This is clearly demonstrated in the debates, still raging during the eighteenth century, regarding the effect of the New World environment on physical and moral characteristics of plants, animals, and humans.[135] Character and constitution were thus relevant to one's susceptibility to disease and its resulting virulence. Brocklesby theorized that the bad habits of a military life meant that smallpox was more virulent within an army than among a civilian population: "A greater relaxation of all sobriety and temperance is supposed to prevail, in all military life, than among other orders of men. It is therefore natural to conclude, that such a disease as the small-pox is more destructive, in every army in England, than any other acute disease."[136] Like scurvy, smallpox was believed to affect a certain type of person more so than another. And, like scurvy, smallpox affected provincials far more often than it did British-born regular soldiers. Smallpox was thus another problem associated with undisciplined provincial troops, which meant that disease was seen as symptomatic of other reasons for troop shortages among provincials, such as laziness, lack of motivation, and being pampered. Writing from New York,

Governor De Lancey explained to Pitt in 1759, "There is a great Backwardness in the Men of this Province to inlist arising from the sickness and deaths the last year, occasioned by the great fatigues [that] the troops in the pay of this Province underwent."[137]

Relying on the already established linkage between disease and laziness or a weak constitution, medical officials stationed in North America posited that provincials were sicklier because they were naturally less disciplined and energetic than British troops. In choosing such an explanation, officials resorted to theories that were already common outside of medicine. Jeffrey Amherst found himself frustrated by this natural disposition of provincial troops, complaining in his journals not only about their physical sickness, but that they deserted far more easily and were distracted by thoughts of home. In his entry of 14 November 1759, he griped, "The Provincials have got home in their heads & nothing can stop them or make them do an Hours work tho' the whole Country depended on it so I must sen[d] them all away."[138] In his letters to political officials in Britain, Amherst frequently repeated such sentiments. Describing the provincial Rangers, Amherst wrote, "I am sorry to say I do not give the least Credit to any Ranger Reports, from all I have seen of them, they are the most Careless, Negligent, Ignorant Corps I ever saw, and if they are not beat on all Occasions I really cannot find out the reason why."[139] By late 1761, Amherst concluded despondently that the "disregard of orders, and studying of their own ease, rather than the good of the service, has been too often just grounds for complaint against some of the provincial officers, and all their men."[140]

Such tirades against the indolent nature of provincials, and their refusal to submit to British authority and discipline, prove interesting both in themselves and because they appear to herald the future of British-American relations, which were to dissolve into open war in less than fifteen years. This is not to suggest that later hostilities in the American provinces stemmed directly from campaigns during the Seven Years' War. The route from one war to another was hardly straightforward. Yet the tensions caused by the raising and quartering of large numbers of troops during the war, and their continued presence after the war, intensified provincial antagonism over the role of the army in the American colonies.[141] And in their shared experience of warfare and disease, constitutional and moral differences between American-born and British-born soldiers became both apparent and a cause for mutual frustration. As is so often the case, disease highlighted social distinctions, and by so doing, further accentuated them. Disease, in conjunction with contemporary medical assumptions, reified and cemented preexisting stereotypes in the minds of

British officials in America, who served as the main point of contact between the British state and its American constituents.

The difference in disease rates between provincials and regulars was not simply theoretical: because most British soldiers were recruited from urban centers and passed through cantonments before arriving in the American colonies, these men had already experienced the crowd diseases common to army camps and hence were largely immune to afflictions such as smallpox. Colonial American settlements, on the other hand, did not have the population density to sustain such diseases. Also, American-born soldiers who fought alongside or as part of British regiments during the Seven Years' War generally came from different social backgrounds and joined for different motivations than their British counterparts. Although not all British soldiers represented the dregs of urban society, they did come from lowly backgrounds and mostly had no other opportunities waiting for them after their lengthy military service.[142] By contrast, many American-born soldiers, especially the New England provincial regiments, signed up for a few years of military service at most, and usually expected to return home every winter. Many provincial recruits came from land-owning families, and most anticipated settling on their own farmland within a few years: their military service was but a temporary adventure.[143] The hardships of army life and its accompanying physical afflictions made these differences very apparent.

The effects of disease did not end with the conclusion of the war. Outbreaks of smallpox in North America throughout the 1760s were correctly associated with provincial soldiers returning from the war.[144] Benjamin Gale wrote in a letter to John Huxham, published in the *Philosophical Transactions* of 1765:

> During the late war, the small pox was brought into divers towns, in this and the other colonies, by the return of our soldiers (employed in His Majesty's service, in the pay of the New England colonies) for winter quarters, and by seamen employed in our navigation to the British islands in the West Indies, where the small pox was universally prevalent, which produced an universal concern among the inhabitants, lest the same should become general, and spread through this and the other colonies in New England.[145]

Smallpox famously erupted again during the American War of Independence.[146] British measures regarding smallpox have been portrayed by historians of the American war as callous and deadly, including alleged spreading of smallpox among vulnerable provincials.[147] A detailed examination of British responses to smallpox among American provincials during the Seven Years' War provides a longer context in which to evaluate British imperial governance, one in which British officials were aware of the fear of the disease as well as the political and diplomatic benefits of accusations of its purposeful spread. During the Seven Years' War, officials were neither willing nor able to implement centralized and unpopular measures such as mandatory inoculation. Instead, British authorities showed themselves sensitive and responsive to provincial attitudes regarding smallpox. This was consistent with British practices of negotiating with colonial populations and assemblies regarding recruitment and provisioning.[148] Inoculation among provincials illustrates how the nonimplementation of medical practices could be more beneficial than its reverse, for in this case it encouraged the continued support of colonial populations. Responses to disease demonstrate that British officials were frustrated by and attentive to colonial circumstances, learning how to adapt to novel physical and social conditions. Disease highlighted and exacerbated tensions between groups of people: British regulars and provincial troops, British imperial authorities and American colonists, Europeans and Native Americans, armies and civilians. Such antagonisms had a demonstrable physical basis. Yet medical care and measures such as quarantine represented possible relief for such tensions.

But medical care did not guarantee good health. As the returns of the garrison during the siege of Quebec demonstrate all too well, diseases such as scurvy were part of North American life, and with warfare, diseases such as smallpox spread among soldiers and civilians alike. In the American colonies, scurvy in particular continued to disrupt British imperial governance because of constant supply problems.[149] Although contemporary preventatives and cures such as spruce beer did little to alleviate high rates of sickness, their application demonstrates not only that officials were cognizant of the consequences of disease during campaigns, but that they felt responsible for maintaining the health of rank-and-file soldiers. This responsibility was shouldered by officials who lived and worked with the soldiers, such as Murray, as well as by those, like Amherst, who were more concerned with the broad strategy of campaigns. The imperial fiscal-military state not only mobilized men, but—for both humanitarian and strategic practical reasons—also cared for their health and welfare, applying the expertise of medical men.

The implementation and evaluation of specific measures devolved to officials far away from the seat of British government and British medicine. Regimental and hospital surgeons, acting as experts on behalf of the British state, implemented contemporary medical theory, while also observing and recording results. In the process they shaped the nature of eighteenth-century medical practice more broadly. Regimental medicine—which cared for the day-to-day welfare of rank-and-file men in the armed forces—was not a parochial appendage to medical science, but instead helped forge medical expertise, acting as a site for medical observation, research, and innovation. The fact that these measures were unsuccessful in the short term does not deny their long-term significance: although scurvy and smallpox were not prevented, the structures of observation and evaluation at the local level meant that colonial medicine was developing into its own area of expertise, while medical theories were constantly refined and tested, practices that underpinned eighteenth-century medical development more broadly.

British responses to scurvy demonstrate a sophisticated attempt to adapt to the foreign North American environment, following the advice of renowned experts of the time. In the development of these new methods, officials relied on observations of physical phenomena to inform military strategy, but also used them to mold and justify intellectual, medical, and political opinions. By the same token, observations garnered during campaigns contributed to a developing sense of difference and identity. While it is true, as Linda Colley has argued, that war contributed to the development of British identity during the eighteenth century, in this case, the experience of war and disease contributed to a developing sense of provincial distinctiveness.[150] The problems of disease, particularly among American colonial populations, were demonstrated even more forcibly in the sickly West Indian campaigns, as will be shown in chapter 2.

CHAPTER TWO

The Black Vomit and the Provincial Press: The Campaigns in the West Indies

The spectacular role of disease in West Indian campaigns has long been recognized. This medical observation led British military and naval officials to advocate a strategy of haste, attacking the enemy before disease killed too many troops. The disastrous Cartagena campaign of 1741 was an infamous example of the problem presented by disease to British operations in the West Indies. It was sickness, rather than wounds or battle fatalities, that forced the British to depart from Cartagena. By that time, the original force of over 11,000 was reduced to 2,200 British regulars and 900 provincial Americans fit for duty. According to one officer, the force lost more than a third of its strength over three weeks at Cartagena Harbor: "Every body was taken alike; they call the distemper a Bilious fever; it kills in five days; if the Patient lives longer, 'tis only to die in greater Agonies, of what they then call the black vomit."[1] Officers, soldiers, and sailors knew that the West Indies was a sickly and deathly location, and for this reason troops often attempted to desert upon hearing that they were to be deployed there. During preparations for the Cartagena campaign, Lord Cathcart commented to Lord Harrington, "Considering the Nature of the Service the troops are going upon, the loss that way [desertion] is not to be reckoned very considerable," with even two regimental surgeons deserting before the transports sailed.[2]

The horrors encountered by British troops fighting in the West Indies during the eighteenth century have been aptly documented by naval, military, and medical historians. Black vomit, feverish agonies, and sudden death are all symptoms of yellow fever, a disease endemic in the West Indies during the eighteenth century.[3] Given that yellow fever fatally struck only large groups of newcomers, the disease seemed to offer French and Spanish garrisons a natural defense against besiegers. John R. McNeill, a historian specializing in the role of disease in Caribbean geopolitics, explains: "Without continual and reliable assistance from tropical disease, Spain would have lost its Caribbean holdings to Britain. . . . The Spanish won their New World empire in the sixteenth century with decisive help from Eurasian diseases; they kept it in the eighteenth with the help of African ones."[4]

In West Indian campaigns of the Seven Years' War, British forces struggled against what one military captain called "a climate more fatal than the enemy."[5] Although the British were ultimately victorious, first against French-held islands and then in 1762 capturing the prized Spanish colonial port of Havana, the course of disease shows the long-term cost of colonial expeditions. In part, this was the result of British attempts to adapt to the demands of West Indian campaigns. Building on experiences from the 1740s, British officials generously resourced Caribbean campaigns, following contemporary medical and military advice. This included the recruitment of additional troops from the American colonies, who were thought to be better adapted to the West Indian climate. Yet when these troops fell ill, and when American colonial newspapers reported the details of grisly sickness and deaths, what was a British military victory had the potential to be portrayed as a failure of imperial governance.

This chapter examines the role of and responses to disease during the 1759 campaigns against French-held Martinique and Guadeloupe and the 1762 campaign against Spanish-held Cuba. Contextualized by contemporary and modern medical understanding of tropical disease, this chapter shows how the British campaign against Martinique in 1759 failed because of debilitating disease among British troops, while, under the resourceful leadership of John Barrington, the British successfully took Guadeloupe a few months later by adapting to their precarious situation. With more forces, especially those recruited from North America, Martinique was finally taken in 1761 under Major General Robert Monckton and Rear Admiral George Rodney, just a few months before the much-celebrated successful campaign against Havana in 1762 under the direction of Lieutenant General the Earl of Albemarle and Admiral George Pocock. Although officials were aware of the dangers of disease in the West Indian climate and followed the advice of medical authorities concerning hot climates, little could be done to prevent high rates of morbidity and mortality. The analysis here thus serves as a reminder that rates of disease are not always an accurate way to assess medical care and adaptation to foreign environments, whether physical or cultural. The chapter concludes with an examination of the reports of disease in colonial American newspapers, tracing the role that disease played in the emerging colonial public sphere and its nascent imperial frustrations. In this respect, the reporting of disease had as central a role as disease itself in imperial concerns. In the broader context of imperial-colonial relations, disease in West Indian campaigns demonstrates the difficulties of colonial warfare and its potential for straining relations between Britain and its colonies.

This analysis builds on existing scholarship that explains British military successes during the Seven Years' War through adaptation to the West Indian environment. British victories of the 1750s and 1760s are often contrasted with British failures during the 1740s, showing that British officials learned from previous West Indian campaigns by improving resource provision during the Seven Years' War. The naval historian Richard Harding has examined in detail the difficulties inherent in West Indian amphibious campaigns, specifically the dangerous waters and climate, and the operational difficulties when directing combined naval and military operations at such a distance from London. Whereas the British campaigns of the 1740s, and particularly Cartagena in 1741, were a spectacular and much-publicized failure, Harding concludes that those of the 1750s and 1760s were successful because of better leadership and the greater mobilization of resources.[6] Likewise, David Syrett argues that British preparations for Havana exceeded Cartagena in terms of logistics and resources, resulting in success at Havana.[7]

The analysis here focuses on the role of disease in this British adaptation to West Indian campaigning. Although historians have long recognized the role disease played in the Caribbean, their analyses have tended to focus on the failure of contemporary medicine to prevent disease, often highlighting notorious eighteenth-century practices such as bloodletting and purging. In contrast, this chapter details the more mundane—but more effective—medical measures that allowed British forces to remain operational for longer stretches: fresh provisions, additional medical personnel, and increased and targeted recruitment of troops. Historians often overlook such measures because—not being drugs or vaccines—they are not classified by modern biomedicine as medicine. Yet, for contemporaries, diet and nursing were not only central to early modern medical care, but could also be exorbitantly expensive. Their implementation thus demonstrates the willingness of British officials to expend significant energy and resources and follow the advice of experts to care for troops in warm climates. Moreover, the experience of the war contributed to the development of a new type of expertise in the service of Britain's expanding empire, that of tropical medicine.

The 1762 Havana campaign, specifically, underscores the ways in which contemporary medical theory about warm climates influenced military strategy, in the form of recruitment of North American troops. Troop welfare was also a concern of the burgeoning colonial public sphere. Reports and anxieties about the sickliness of provincial troops were discussed in colonial assemblies and published in colonial newspapers, showing that disease was a political issue as well as a military problem. Thus, although British officials were able to adapt to the West Indian environment for long enough to achieve impressive military victories, disease and reports of disease demonstrated not only the linkages between different theaters of war, but also the complexity and precariousness of British imperial command.

THE WEST INDIES AND THE BLACK VOMIT

During the eighteenth century, islands in the West Indies were acknowledged as sources of tremendous wealth, responsible for most of Britain's colonial and commercial income within its mercantile system.[8] Providing sugar and its by-products rum and molasses, as well as cocoa, spices, dyes, and cotton, West Indian planters dominated Britain's merchant community, and were powerful in Parliament as well as in financial circles. Pitt's ally William Beckford was only one such notable example, rising quickly through the ranks of city politics to be elected as one of the city members of Parliament in 1754.[9] Yet the islands were not simply significant colonial resources. Strategically, they provided trained sailors and were important as bases from which to protect British trade from Spanish and French privateers. Hence, they were integral to British naval and mercantile aspirations. N. A. M. Rodger estimates that French privateers took 1,400 British merchant ships in the West Indies during the Seven Years' War, adversely affecting not only British colonial trade, but also shipping in the American colonies and basic provisioning of the British West Indian islands. Depredations could be stopped only by the capture of French bases such as Martinique.[10] The islands were thus bulwarks against French power and commerce, and supplied colonial trade and the needs of the navy without being seen as part of a territorial empire.[11]

The debate surrounding which colonial possessions should be returned to France during the early 1760s clearly articulates how contemporaries viewed the West Indies. While the retention of Canada was most commonly advocated in terms of security for the American colonies, it was the key position of the sugar islands to commerce and naval operations in the

Atlantic that was offered as proof of their value, along with their wealth. Guadeloupe especially was singled out for the abundance of its exports; in 1761 its annual produce sent to British markets was above £600,000, comparing favorably to those of Canada, the American colonies, and Minorca.[12] Pamphleteers also emphasized the strong bond between West Indian planters and Britain. The West Indian "Sugar-Gentlemen" were known as part of the London, Liverpool, and Bristol merchant communities, and as active members of Parliament. Compared with the American colonies, pamphleteers argued, the West Indian climate was cause for a closer and less troubled relationship with Britain. As the climate of the West Indies differed from that of Britain, the islands grew different crops and so did not compete with British produce. The hot and moist climate also meant that "the Inhabitants of the *West Indian* Islands never consider themselves at home there; they send their Children to the Mother Country for Education; they themselves make many Trips to the Mother Country to recover their Health or enjoy their Fortunes."[13] Yet the inhospitable climate of the West Indies was also an argument against the islands' retention. While a tropical environment was necessary to grow their specific produce, it was also the cause of great sickness. One pamphleteer argued on the authority of none other than Aristotle and Hippocrates "that *Moist and Heat are the Causes of Putrefaction*: and consequently, those Climates, where Moist and Heat prevail, as in the *Sugar-Islands* and *Louisiana*, may destroy a great many Settlers."[14] The islands' tropical climate, therefore, was the source of their wealth and strategic significance, the basis for their inhabitants' closer connection with the metropole, and the reason why the islands were difficult to obtain and maintain.[15]

In eighteenth-century medical thought, the infamous sickliness of the West Indies was inseparably linked to its climate. With more continents open to settlement and more campaigns in far-flung climates, the diseases common in these areas had become of increasing general concern since the mid-eighteenth century. James Lind's best-selling tropical medical advice book, *An Essay on Diseases Incidental to Europeans in Hot Climates*, proposed to assuage such concerns. First published in 1768, and translated into German, Dutch, and French, it remained popular throughout the nineteenth century. Lind described his book as a kind of sequel to his *Essay on the Most Effectual Means of Preserving the Health of Seamen, in the Royal Navy* (1757), as it instructed readers on how to preserve their health once they had safely arrived in foreign lands. Much of its evidence derived from the experience of the Seven Years' War, but this seminal book on medicine in hot, or tropical, climates also demonstrates the significance of the war in other ways. According to Lind, the war had highlighted the problem of "the great mortality in hot climates," demonstrating that "sickly or unhealthy settlements require a constant supply of people, and of course drain their mother-country of an incredible number of its inhabitants, and some of those too its most useful individuals."[16] Focused on preserving the health of overseas regiments and settlers (and not those traveling simply for pleasure), Lind noted that the war had increased British involvement in such foreign locations. His work, full of practical and helpful advice, was thus both the product and consequence of the Seven Years' War. As the first work to systematically and convincingly group diseases and medicines of all hot and foreign climates together, Lind's book established the field of tropical medicine, an approach that—for better or worse—would come to underpin modern European imperial endeavors.[17]

Dedicated to the secretary of the Admiralty and self-described as a useful book in the service of a growing empire, Lind's *Hot Climates* argues its expertise in a number of ways. Although he notes that foreign climates often differ in degree, rather than in kind, from European environments, Lind repeatedly stresses that exact knowledge was needed to preserve the lives of Europeans posted abroad. He concludes his overview of his book by affirming that "an inexperience of foreign countries, and an ignorance of the true causes of their sickness, prove as fatal to Europeans" as the unhealthy climates themselves.[18] Even the great father of English medicine, Thomas Sydenham, could not be relied on for guidance, according to Lind, since "Dr Sydenham's judicious practice was local," confined to temperate England; indeed, only to part of London.[19] Instead, Lind repeatedly claims that what is required is medical advice that incorporates an understanding of the nature of foreign climates. As a result, Lind's guidance is supported by observations and reports provided by those with firsthand experience of such warm climates, such as surgeons, apothecaries, and physicians who were stationed abroad with the armed forces during the war. His network of empirical observation thus provided the authoritative expertise for the burgeoning field of tropical medicine. Criticizing overreliance on systems, the eighteenth-century nemesis of enlightened science, Lind repeatedly explains how his medical directions had been gathered, tried, and tested throughout various stations overseas, "where they have been experienced and approved as the most successful methods of treating fevers, not only in our men of war, but in many of our settlements."[20] As a result, Lind decisively concludes that "the diseases of strangers [foreigners] in different climates bear every where a great similitude to each other."[21]

According to Lind, the origin of the debilitation that struck Europeans upon moving to hot climates was the new climate itself: "Men who thus exchange their nature for a distant climate, may be considered as affected in a manner somewhat analogous to that of plants, removed into a foreign soil; where the utmost care and attention are required, to keep them in health, and inure them to their new situation; since, thus transplanted, some change and alteration must happen in the constitutions of both."[22] As his choice of simile makes clear, Lind was optimistic that a proper location and moderation in diet, alcohol, and exercise could prevent the fevers and fluxes (diarrheal disorders) often fatal to newly arrived Europeans. As the state of health arose from a careful balance of the body and its functions, maintained through a continuous cycle of repletion and evacuation, the extreme heat and moisture of foreign, warm climates could upset this delicate cycle, thereby accelerating putrefaction, and result in disease. Excessive sweating, for example, indicated the body's attempt to adapt to the new climate, and could disrupt the body's natural balance. Lind claimed that by carefully following his advice, Europeans could acclimatize to foreign climates, just as a newcomer's decreased sweating demonstrated his seasoning to the warm environment. Key among Lind's recommendations was the avoidance of hard labor, particularly in the sun, along with the avoidance of a diet difficult to digest, the drinking of spirits, and debauchery in general.[23] Once a person had survived the initial period of acclimatization and resided in a hot climate for a sufficient amount of time, the "merchant, farmer, or soldier, thus constitutionally naturalized to the country, becomes more useful, and his services may be more depended upon there, than ten new arrived unseasoned Europeans."[24]

Building on theories of putrefaction articulated by Pringle, Lind saw the problem of disease in foreign environments as stemming from the nature of warm climates to encourage putrefaction. Diseases of hot climates were thus essentially the same, and yellow fever, recognized by Lind as the most fatal to Europeans in the West Indies, was no different from other tropical diseases. Contemporaries saw yellow fever as an obvious product of moving to the hot climate, as newcomers were frequently seized by it, even though no one around them was sick. Pringle's network of observers in the West Indies confirmed this medical theory: among others, both the naval surgeon Mr. Little and the army surgeon Mr. Ballantyne, stationed in Jamaica, agreed that yellow fever struck those newly arriving in the West Indies. As Dr. Munro, stationed at Antigua, explained, he "never knew a native, or old inhabitant [in the West Indies], have the yellow fever, & most of the practitioners in town, who have greater opportunities than I have had, have told me the same thing," adding that it was common among European sailors.[25] Similarly, William Hillary, a physician in Barbados, characterized yellow fever as a disease that struck newcomers to the West Indies, "especially those who come from a colder, or more temperate climate, to this much warmer," and who were immoderate in alcohol and exercise.[26] Moreover, he held that the disease was indigenous to the West Indies and nearby American colonies, because of the region's distinctive climate. Richard Huck, physician to the general hospital during the Havana campaign, praised Hillary's book on yellow fever upon his return to Britain. Not only were Hillary's methods followed by the British Army during the campaign, but Huck reported, "Other practitioners whom he met with established in those parts conceded in recommending Dr. Hillary's book, as the best upon that distemper."[27]

In the twentieth century scientists were able to identify and follow the progress of the yellow fever virus. Yellow fever indeed attacks the liver, producing its eponymic jaundice. It is now established that one attack gives an individual lifelong immunity. As yellow fever in children has mild and often unnoticed symptoms, populations in areas with endemic yellow fever can become imperceptibly immune. Its presence is discernible only when nonimmune new adults arrive, who are attacked with the violent symptoms of the virus: high fever, delirium, black vomit, bleeding from various parts of the body, and frequently death within a few days. In 1900, scientists established that the *Aedes aegypti* mosquito transmits yellow fever, which explains why the fever is endemic to tropical areas. Since *Aedes aegypti* thrives in tropical regions and prefers breeding in areas of stagnant water, Lind's and Hillary's observation that the fever is confined to tropical areas is vindicated.[28] Their conclusion that the disease was limited to European newcomers arriving in a tropical climate is also understandable.

Modern medicine has not yet found a specific treatment for yellow fever, although methods such as dialysis can help with problems such as kidney failure. The only effective medicine is a preventative vaccine. In eighteenth-century medicine, although Hillary and Lind both recommended various forms of treatment, Lind was clear that the best practice was to avoid getting seriously ill when arriving in the West Indies. Fresh provisions, as part of a diet easy to digest (particularly in contrast to military rations), were always a wise choice, if possible, alongside avoiding immoderate drinking and exertion, and settling in dry, ventilated environments. Relying on already acclimatized troops was also one of the few successful measures available to contemporary officials. As Lind and others had observed, rates of sickness and mortality were significantly reduced after roughly a year in the Caribbean.[29] Since yellow fever could not be entirely prevented, the most that officials could do was try to lessen its ill effects by recruiting troops accustomed to the climate (particularly for laboring tasks), choosing drained settlements, and ensuring regular and abundant supplies of fresh provisions and medical care. In the Seven Years' War, this was generally accomplished, even though it strained British logistical capabilities.

MARTINIQUE AND GUADELOUPE, 1759

Under the general direction of William Pitt, British forces set out for the West Indies in November 1758 to take French-held Martinique and Guadeloupe. This campaign was meant to damage French fighting ability and trade, but it was also considered with anticipated French peace negotiations in mind. Specifically, Britain required territorial bargaining chips in the Caribbean in order to retain gains such as Louisbourg or to trade for losses such as Minorca.[30] Under the military command of Major General Peregrine Hopson, close to 5,000 British soldiers sailed from England in the autumn of 1758, to be joined by some detachments resident in the Leeward Islands and a few hundred slaves from West Indian islands to act as laborers during the campaign. Commodore John Moore headed naval forces, with ten men-of-war, six frigates, four bomb ketches, various sloops, a hospital ship, and at least sixty transports.[31]

The forces arrived in Barbados early in January 1759 and sailed for Martinique a week later. In his journal, published in 1762, Captain Richard Gardiner notes that, upon sailing from Barbados on 13 January 1759, "the Troops unaccustomed to the Climate, suffered greatly from *Fevers*, from the *Flux*, the *Scurvy* from the Use of Salt Provisions, and from an accidental *Evil*, the *Small-Pox*, which broke out amongst the *Transports*."[32] On 16 January 1759, British ships fired on the French posts along the coast of Martinique, and the following day troops landed at Port Royal to attack the French plantations, stores, and villages. According to the unpublished journal of Guy Durant, who served as deputy paymaster during the expedition, British troops were forced by fatigue and heat to retreat.[33] Just a few days later, the British forces sailed to Guadeloupe, and stationed themselves at Basseterre.

From Basseterre, Hopson related to Pitt the details of his precarious situation. He explained that more than 1,500 troops were ill, "occasioned by the very great heat and fatigue that [they] undergo which is unavoidable. . . . This great Number of sick embarrasses me so much that it is yet impossible for me to determine whether to attack the retreat of the Enemy here, or to embark the whole, or a Part of my Force, and Land them on the side of this Island called Capsterre."[34] Hopson soon fell sick as well, as did the paymaster, Durant, and increasing numbers of men. Army memoranda indicate that regimental hospitals were overcrowded and having difficulties dealing with the ever-increasing number of patients. In response, more surgeons and mates were ordered, sick soldiers from regimental hospitals were sent directly to the physician, more supplies including fresh provisions were given to the sick, and those with infectious disorders were separated from other patients.[35] On 27 February 1759, the commander, Hopson, died of a fever and flux.

As Hopson's successor, Major General John Barrington convened a council of war upon taking command in order to review his position. Army returns of 28 February 1759, just two months after their arrival in the West Indies, indicate only 2,796 soldiers fit for duty. This number—just over half the original force—was insufficient to maintain constant guard in addition to normal camp duties, let alone form detachments. The second point discussed at the council was the health of the troops, upon which military physician Thomas Brooke advised, "If we continue longer the whole Army may be soon rendered unfit for Service." Barrington and his officers concluded that their position was untenable, and unanimously decided to decamp to Fort Louis, on the other side of Guadeloupe.[36]

Writing to Pitt a few days after the council of war, Barrington acquainted the minister with his new command, and explained the difficulties that he now faced. It is clear that Barrington was critical of Hopson's leadership, declaring that he would put an end to the army's inactivity. Indeed, Barrington believed that Hopson's lack of decisive action was responsible for the sickness among the forces.[37] Listing the number of invalids and describing the defensive layout of Guadeloupe, Barrington justified the decision to move to the other side of the island on the basis of health considerations and the advice of medical "Faculty."[38] As in the council of war, expert medical opinion as well as present and anticipated levels of sickness among the troops were considered essential to the planning and justifying of strategy.

Major General Barrington was much more frank about both Hopson and his present situation in his letters to his brother, William Wildman (Viscount) Barrington, then secretary at war in London. Major General Barrington informed his brother that the army was so weak that if the French knew the number of sick they would surely attack and easily overrun the British forces. He criticized Hopson's apathy, from which he claimed much of the present sickness resulted, while also critiquing Hopson's lack of care concerning the general welfare of the troops. Significantly, Barrington had resisted the urge to intervene when under Hopson's command because of political considerations, but finally could no longer restrain himself when he saw the troops' suffering:

> When I saw the army starving and the Hospitals neglected it was no longer time to think of personal pique I offerd to take both under my Care and I hope the army have had no reason to complain of anything since but the unavoidable distresses that must Ever Accompany this Climate.[39]

As this was a private letter, not so much between a commander and a secretary at war as between two brothers describing personal frustrations and fatigue, Major General Barrington's admission that he intervened to improve the medical care and provisions of the troops reveals the tension between his commitment to the welfare of the troops and his regard for seniority and rank. Barrington carried his thoughts into action: the additional surgeon's mates appointed, even before Hopson's death, are listed as mates "employed under Barrington."[40] Taken while he was second in command, this action demonstrates sincere care for the welfare of troops.

Sickness created similar problems and reveals similar consideration by commanders in the navy. On 6 March 1759, Commodore John Moore wrote to Pitt that because of sickness and his inability to press men, his ships were far short of their complement. Writing to the Admiralty on the same day, Moore reiterated that he could not recruit more seamen from where he was stationed, as seamen were already in demand among the convoys necessary to protect the trade of the islands: "Few of the Transports have now hands to weight their Anchors, & the Squadron is so divided & weak that, we are not in a Condition to give them much Assistance; Twenty Men a day fall down in Fluxes on board some of the Ships."[41] As a consequence, the navy could not offer its complement of seamen and marines to help the British soldiers during the expedition and was exclusively occupied with convoy duty and blockading enemy provisions. Yet, with fortunate results for the campaign, it appears there was no friction between the naval and military forces even in the midst of sickness, unlike during the Cartagena expedition.

Despite Major General Barrington's concern for the health of his troops, the sickness never entirely abated. Yet he clearly did take steps to improve conditions for his troops, and it is no coincidence that British forces were more successful under his leadership than under that of his predecessor. Along with ordering additional medical personnel, Barrington sought fresh provisions for his men and worked with naval officials to arrange for the transportation of supplies from nearby islands, as well as ensuring that his men were settled in a healthy locale, all of which were expensive but medically sound practices. From early in March, Barrington ordered fresh provisions from North America, specifically live cattle and sheep to replace salted meat "for the sake of the Mens health," anticipating Pitt's own orders to the army and navy to obtain fresh provisions for "the Preservation of the Healthy, and to the Recovery of the Sick."[42] Despite the reluctance of British West Indian islands to supply slaves and laborers to the expedition, the General Assembly at Barbados passed a motion to provide British troops with fresh provisions. Barrington received bullocks, goats, fowls, geese, and ducks, as well as over 200 sheep and 300 "turkies" by mid-April.[43]

Better health and success against Guadeloupe were not achieved solely by means of fresh provisions, but also by a change in strategy. Specifically, Barrington adapted to Guadeloupe's geography and to the small number of forces he now had under his command. Instead of pushing for open battle or one large attack, Barrington ordered various small detachments to attack along the coast, relying on British naval capabilities. This nullified the numeric superiority of French forces as troops were dispersed among various coastal points, which at the same time made full use of the Royal Navy.[44] As a result, the defenders formally surrendered 1 May 1759, unaware that French reinforcements were to arrive later that day.

Writing to his brother on 9 May 1759, Barrington asserted his relief and surprise at victory, as he had thought that the expedition was sure to fail. He expressed similar sentiments in his formal announcement of British success to Pitt.[45] Over the two months from the first arrival of British troops in the West Indies until Hopson's death in late February, sickness had almost halved the available land force and had similarly struck down the Royal Navy. Given that sickness was sure to increase with every day still in the West Indies, Barrington's pessimism is understandable. Yet victory was achieved by adapting to the conditions in which he found himself during March and April of 1759. This shift involved Barrington's consideration of medical advice when deciding on strategy in the council of war, along with appointing five new medical personnel and ordering fresh—and expensive—provisions from nearby markets. As demonstrated in his criticisms of Hopson, Barrington believed the welfare of troops to be of utmost importance to a commander's twin duties: caring for the men in his charge and completing the mission assigned to him. As the campaign's outcome demonstrated, such considerations were indeed integral to military success.

Officials in Britain and the British public were delighted with the capture of such wealthy islands. Brigadier Crump, the newly appointed governor, estimated that Guadeloupe could provide 80,000 hogsheads of sugar a year, "which is more than equivalent to Barbados and all our Leeward Islands."[46] Despite this, Crump complained about the continuing sickness of the British garrison. Of a garrison of 1,000, since Barrington's departure three months prior, 8 officers and 577 troops had died from disease. Although Crump was trying to improve this situation, specifically by making use of a French physician experienced in the local climate, he was a realist about his chances and, therefore, also requested additional reinforcements.[47] Until Guadeloupe and Martinique were returned to the French at the end of the war in 1763, there were just over 1,000 British soldiers garrisoned on Guadeloupe, at a cost of over £60,000 each year.[48] In return, Crump estimated an annual revenue of at least £100,000 from duties imposed on exports. This amount would increase according to Crump: crops and buildings were being repaired, and commerce was sure to flourish under responsible British governance, especially compared with what Crump called the "violence and oppressions" of previous French rule. British liberty and commercial prosperity were linked in victory against French absolutist ambition.[49]

HAVANA, 1762: DISEASES OF HOT CLIMATES AND THE RECRUITMENT OF PROVINCIALS

Regarded as even more valuable than the French islands, Spanish-held Havana was often described as the pearl of the West Indies and the key to the Caribbean. Rich in resources and Spanish imperial wealth (the British captured goods and currency worth £3 million), it was also the strategic linchpin of Spanish America, serving as the home port for Spain's American fleet. Considered invincible, Havana had successfully fended off foreign attacks since 1555, when the defensive fortress El Morro had been built.[50] As with other bases in the West Indies, the city's defenses worked in tandem with the climate's sickliness: a besieging force was certain to fall sick from the diseases that attacked newcomers before it penetrated the fortifications.[51]

This first campaign against Spain in the Seven Years' War was no exception: British forces suffered from rates of disease reaching 60 percent during the siege of Havana. As a result, historians have been critical of the campaign, even though it was ultimately successful. In his classic history of the Seven Years' War, Julian Corbett blames the new ministry's delay and Albemarle's hesitance for the high rates of disease, while Christian Buchet likewise faults Albemarle's tentativeness.[52] David Syrett agrees that time was of the essence at Havana, "for if the Spanish could hold the fortress, it would be only a matter of time before yellow fever forced the British to withdraw from Cuba," as they had at Cartagena.[53] In their definitive history of British naval medicine, C. Lloyd and J. L. S. Coulter claim that the Havana expedition "was almost a repetition of the Cartagena disaster, except that on this occasion the city was taken."[54] Similarly, Allan J. Kuethe concludes that the Spanish did not adequately prepare their defenses at Cuba because of their reliance on disease: "Except for the outcome, the events at Havana during the summer of 1762 closely resembled the Battle of Cartagena."[55] More recently, in his study of the role of disease in the Caribbean between 1620 and 1914, J. R. McNeill concludes that between Cartagena and Havana, the only difference "was a few days. . . . Had yellow fever come sooner at Havana, [the Spanish governor] Prado would have been a hero, Pocock and Albemarle disgraced.'"[56] The British campaign against Havana is thus evaluated in comparison with the well-publicized British failure at Cartagena twenty-one years earlier. The high rates of sickness in both are used to demonstrate that British officials neglected the welfare of their troops, thus jeopardizing not only the men's lives but also the mission itself.

With returns in October 1762 reporting less than 900 troops fit for duty out of a total of 7,225, it is indeed surprising that the British took Havana from its defenders instead of reembarking, as they had done at Cartagena. Moreover, little evidence of successful preventative measures exists. Instead, officials concluded that high rates of disease and mortality were simply expected when on campaign in that part of the world. By the end of his campaign in 1762, the head of the land forces, George Keppel, third Earl of Albemarle, concluded that one should anticipate one-third of a force unfit for service at all times, and simply recruit accordingly.[57] His view echoed that of General Barrington, who also concluded that officials should bring a force two-thirds above the actual manpower required when campaigning in the West Indies.[58]

Yet, as at Martinique and Guadeloupe, measures taken for the welfare of troops reflected contemporary theories of disease. It was contemporary medical theory that encouraged the recruitment of men who were "seasoned" to the climate: those from the West Indies and the American colonies. In terms of strategy, this proved successful: with the help of American reinforcements, the British took Havana. This strategy proved problematic in the longer term, however. While historians have documented high rates of sickness during the siege, British troops fell fastest from disease *after* they had won possession of the fort, continuing to suffer from disease throughout 1762 and 1763, which weakened later British campaigns, as well as encouraging hostility among American colonials toward service in the British army.

By the time of the Havana siege, the last of the key French posts in New France had fallen to British forces (Montreal, September 1760). In January 1761, British forces won control of Pondicherry, the last major French holding in India. In March of 1761, French officials had tendered the opening of peace negotiations with British officials. Both countries were financially and militarily exhausted after five years of formal warfare. Yet British and French officials could not agree on peace terms. By mid-August, France and Spain had arrived at their own agreement, the Family Compact. News of the agreement, and so of Spain's effective entrance into hostilities, did not reach London until September 1761. Although Pitt blamed his resignation in October on the reluctance of British officials to act immediately against Spain, plans for action followed soon enough after Britain's declaration of war against Spain on 4 January 1762. Isaac Barré reported to Amherst from London in February 1762: "The declaration of the Spanish war dragg'd thro' the Streets more like a funeral than a triumph. We are drain'd of money & our resources are mostly stopp'd."[59]

Orders for the raising of 4,000 troops were sent on 13 January 1762 to the commander in chief in North America, Jeffery Amherst.[60] Orders to Monckton, then finishing his successful siege of French Martinique, were sent in early February, informing him that the majority of his forces must join the expedition against Havana in April, whether or not his present siege was successful.[61] Albemarle's instructions to "make the most vigorous attack" on Havana, alongside naval forces commanded by Pocock, are dated 18 February 1762.[62] Throughout January and February, troops, provisions, and ships assembled at Spithead. On 5 March 1762, the force sailed to the West Indies.

Meanwhile, in North America, the raising of troops proved difficult. Not only did Amherst not receive his orders until 1 April, but he was also becoming increasingly frustrated with the dilatory provincial assemblies. Raising troops in America for service elsewhere was uncommon; the last expedition in which this had occurred was the disastrous expedition to Cartagena in 1741. On that campaign, sickness so overwhelmed the troops that they were forced to return home without prize money, and without many of their comrades. Yet these were not the only reasons for dissatisfaction among provincial troops. They were regarded as undisciplined and inexperienced, and hence assigned to the strenuous and unglorified tasks of carrying stores and laboring, rather than fighting. Provincial officers found their ranks of commission ignored by British officers and, thus, were regularly passed over for promotion. With British ships undermanned due to sickness, provincial soldiers were pressed into naval service, where they found themselves separated from their units and their officers, and complained of brutal usage.[63]

British officials were no happier with the provincials during and after Cartagena. Because of provincials' increasing sickliness and ill discipline, General Wentworth had specifically asked Newcastle in 1741 for European recruits to complete his regiments, as he had "too good reason to think that they [provincials] are not very much to be depended upon."[64] Admiral Charles Knowles reported, "From the first sight of the American troops they were despised, and as many of them were *Irish*, (suspected Papists) were never employed till now; but as Sickness encreased amongst the others (and hourly Attacks expected from the Enemy) it was thought expedient to have them ashore."[65]

For these reasons, historian Douglas Edward Leach has argued that the experience of Cartagena encouraged the development of a "self-conscious Americanism," and for Albert Harkness, Jr., the expedition marks the first use of "American" "in the sense in which we define it."[66] Although other historians such as Richard Harding have challenged the extent to which these antagonisms were the result of friction between provincials and British regulars, rather than between the army and navy, provincial discontent over the campaign certainly existed.[67] In 1740, army officer William Blakeney ominously warned Newcastle that "from the highest to the lowest, the Inhabitants of these Provinces seem to set a great value on themselves, and think a regard is due to them, especially in the assistance they are able to give the Mother Country on such occasions; and, as they are a growing Power, should they be disappointed in what is promised them and which they expect, future Occasions of the like Nature may suffer for it."[68]

In Whitehall's orders to Amherst for the 1762 campaign, the secretary of state for the Southern Department, Charles Wyndham, second Earl of Egremont, tried to obviate these problems:

> Give the Provincials the strongest assurances of their being set down at New York, as soon as the Campaign shall be over, and that, during

> the Expedition, they shall be treated, in all respects, on the same Footing, and with the same indulgence, as His Majesty's Regular Troops, and, in order not to fail in this very desirable point, it is also left to your discretion to offer any farther douceurs [gifts or gratuities] to those troops.[69]

Albemarle was also instructed to "take especial care, that they [the provincials] be treated with all such proper Attention and Humanity, that they may not return home disgusted with the Service, but on the contrary, may be induced readily and chearfully to act in conjunction with our Regular Forces on any future Occasions."[70]

Even with these considerations, the provincial assemblies were reluctant to raise the requested 2,000 troops. Governor John Wentworth of New Hampshire wrote to Amherst, complaining, "I shall meet with little difficulty, neither would there be any opposition in levying the 143 men, if I could assure the men that they were to serve in regiments, at Halifax, Quebec, or Montreal, but the people in general entertain terrible thoughts of serving in the West Indies."[71] Similarly in May, Amherst received a letter from Governor Cadwallader Colden of New York explaining why recruitment was so slow. Members of the New York Provincial Assembly had informed Colden that rumor had it that the destination of the expedition was the West Indies and that provincials would be enlisted to join the regular troops. If, suggested Colden, Amherst were to state that the provincial troops "are to be Employed on the Continent of North America only, & that they shall be Returned to the Province, as soon as the Service is over, without being Compelled into the Regular Troops, the Numbers required of this Province may soon be Compleated."[72] Amherst replied to Governor Colden that he had already explained for what duration and how the provincials were to be employed in relation to the regular troops, and that their destination must remain a secret.[73] Other provinces had still not provided the necessary recruits by the end of May, forcing Amherst to remind governors that if the requested number was not raised, they would be drafted from provincial militias.[74] Finally, in June 1762, two divisions of troops sailed from America, with 1,910 provincial troops and 1,844 regular troops on board, along with over 100 recovered troops from Monckton's successful expedition to Martinique.[75]

If provincial troops were regarded as less disciplined than regulars from Europe, and if they required more assurances and paid *douceurs* to be enlisted, why were officials so insistent on raising them for the Havana expedition? And more specifically, why had Egremont asked Amherst to raise "an equal number of regulars and provincials, or, if that is impracticable, as great a proportion of the latter as can be procured?'[76] In part, this was because of general manning considerations, which meant that as many troops as could be raised were to be used for such an expedition, particularly after the campaign against the French in North America had concluded. Significantly, however, the climate and concerns of disease played a large role as well in the recruiting preferences of military administrators. As Lind pointed out, in the West Indies, one acclimatized soldier or laborer was worth as much as ten unseasoned and newly arrived Europeans.[77]

For West Indian campaign administrators, this meant that British regular troops should be accompanied by men accustomed to the climate. Black regiments from Jamaica were requested for the Havana campaign, and when this demand proved difficult to fill, Albemarle asked simply for "men from Jamaica accustomed to a hot Climate."[78] He also requested troops from North America. Although one might not think that the West Indies had the same climate as that of the mainland American colonies, there were similarities: not only did cities such as Philadelphia suffer from yellow fever outbreaks, but Lind had observed that South Carolina, Georgia, and Florida had the same diseases and climate as the West Indies.[79] The 4,000 troops ordered to be raised by Amherst, and especially the 2,000 provincials, were therefore welcome additions to the men on campaign at Havana. Pocock waited impatiently for the troops from North America while stationed in Havana, noting that their "arrival at this time would be very acceptable and necessary, to shorten and ease our Work, as the season of the Year is not favourable to the Health of Europeans."[80] General Barrington's experience in 1759 agreed with this sentiment, as the General wrote to Lord Barrington while stationed at Guadeloupe, "I must now finish this long letter with one piece of advice to ministers that when ever they have a mind to make Conquests in this part of the world that they should raise the troops for them here as I am fully Convinced Europeans Can not stand this Climate at any season of the year."[81] The recruitment of North Americans for the Havana campaign, then, reflected expert medical advice, as well as that of military and naval administrators with experience in West Indian campaigns.

HAVANA, 1762: THE SIEGE AND ITS AFTERMATH

Because news from Europe traveled by ship across the Atlantic, reports of Britain's declaration of war reached Cuba long after its formal announcement on 4 January 1762. Havana governor Juan de Prado had received instructions to improve the fortifications of Havana only on 17 February 1762. As the British fleet was still assembling at Spithead on this date, Prado had ample time to complete his mission. In a letter of 13 May 1762, Prado blames sickness, specifically a "pox similar to Matlazagua," for his slow progress.[82] While *Matlazagua* is not a common Spanish term for yellow fever in the eighteenth century, Mexicans did call an outbreak of fever in 1736 *Malazahuatl.* The disease was characterized by high fever, jaundice, bleeding from the eyes, ears, and mouth, and high rates of mortality, with death often occurring seven days after its onset—all known symptoms of yellow fever.[83] When court-martialed for having lost Havana to the British, Prado explained that the fortifications were not improved as ordered because laborers from Mexico had infected the city with yellow fever, causing general confusion as well as killing his chief engineer and many of his workers.[84]

At this stage, yellow fever was proving lucky for the British, who assembled at Barbados in April and then sailed through the treacherous Old Bahama Channel for complete surprise. Prado and his officials were not prepared for a full-scale attack. Since the British fleet had intercepted the ships carrying news from Spain on June 2, Prado heard only rumors that the British might attack Havana.[85] When British ships sailed into view of the city on 6 June, they were initially dismissed as a convoy from Jamaica. By the next day, however, Prado realized his mistake as troops landed at the Bacuranao River, near Cojimar. On 8 June, women and children were evacuated from the city of Havana, while the Spanish forces and the local militia attempted to ready themselves for an assault.

The city of Havana was protected by a narrow and curved channel winding into a well-fortified harbor. Not only had the Spanish sunk three of their ships in the harbor to block access to British ships, but the entrance was guarded by two well-positioned forts: El Morro and San Salvador de la Punta fortress (La Punta). In the first stage of the attack, the British established their camp by Cojimar, investing the fort La Cabaña and clearing roads to allow the transport of supplies for artillery batteries that needed to be built. When the British took La Cabaña on 11 June, construction began on the main batteries in front of El Morro. On the west side of the harbor, a small detachment under Colonel William Howe was established at the Chorrera River, from which fresh water was supplied to the troops.

Judging from returns of 16 June 1762, the army was in relatively good health. Howe had just over 2,000 rank-and-file troops under his command, with 2,029 fit for duty, 8 sick, and 1 wounded.[86] For all the armed forces,

Albemarle listed a total of 10,714 rank and file. Of these, 7,553 were fit for duty, with 554 sick in camp, 504 sick in hospital, and 1,001 sick on board ship. Only 3 had been killed since the previous return, 6 were wounded, and 28 were dead (noncombat fatalities).[87] Yet Albemarle expressed concern over the health of the troops, most notably regarding cases of drunkenness and what he considered its root cause, ill discipline. Albemarle gave orders reminding his officers to curb excessive drinking and maintain discipline among their troops, as otherwise sickness would result.[88]

Work on the batteries continued until lack of sand and water began to trouble the troops at the end of June.[89] On 30 June the batteries were finally complete and began firing, yet they soon caught fire, which could not immediately be put out because of the scarcity of water and sand. A new battery had to be built at a greater distance from El Morro. With the siege now gravely set back and even shorter of supplies, troops began to fall sick. With only 400 fit for duty of its original 2,500, the small detachment stationed at Guanabacoa was forced to join the main army on 17 July.[90] Albemarle reported to Egremont in a letter of the same date that soldiers from North America not having yet arrived, he was lacking troops and ammunition, and had sent to Jamaica with a request for both.[91] Although he makes no mention of it, the returns of 17 July 1762 show Albemarle's force considerably weakened. Out of a total of 11,203, only 5,353 were fit for duty, with a staggering 4,236 sick in the camp, and a further 807 sick elsewhere, presumably in a general hospital.[92] In Howe's camp, the return for 18 July 1762 shows roughly the same proportion, with 1,006 fit for duty and 890 sick, out of a total of 2,001 rank and file.[93]

A Scottish soldier, who had also been present at the Martinique siege, described the situation:

> The fatigues on shore were excessive, the bad water brought on disorders, which were mortal, you would see the men's tongues hanging out parched like a mad dog's, a dollar was frequently given for a quart of water. In short by dead, wounded and sick the army were reduced to two reliefs, and it was supposed that we should be obliged to re-embark without taking the place.[94]

In his published description of the campaign, Lind noted jaundice, as well as reports of fluxes and intermitting fevers.[95] With yellow fever having struck the town of Havana just months before, and with the description of jaundice and quick deaths, it seems evident that much of the sickness was due to yellow fever. Yet, the description of bad water and fluxes also suggests that dysentery was afflicting the men, along with intermitting fevers, a symptom indicative of malaria.

Despite the sickness, the work on the batteries continued. Occasional sorties by the Spanish troops were repulsed, although a British officer complained that "notwithstanding the heat of the climate the Spaniards run confounded fast."[96] Relief for the overworked troops was expected when transports from North America finally arrived at the end of July, after being waylaid by bad navigation and French ships. Landing on 27 and 28 July, just under 4,000 new troops were quickly put to work to complete the mining. As a soldier reported, "The arrival of the American reinforcements has with very great reason cheered our drooping spirits."[97] On 30 July, land mines were sprung in advance of a successful British assault. On 31 July, Albemarle declared that from then on, no sick were to be sent to the general hospital, suggesting that this hospital had no more room for the sick. Regimental hospitals continued operating, and were to receive their supplies from the deputy director.[98]

With El Morro under their control, British troops were more confident that they would soon possess the city of Havana. While building their batteries for the city, the soldiers now relied on help from seamen in various laboring tasks.[99] Yet even with the additional help of provincial troops, the chief engineer reported that a shortage of tools slowed construction on the batteries.[100] Yet the main factor that plagued the British operations was, again, disease. Sickness levels still increased, and, despite their supposed seasoning to the climate, North American troops soon joined the ranks of the sick.[101] Likewise, a naval return for 7 August 1762 shows 1,876 rank and file sick out of 5,459.[102]

On 10 August 1762, the batteries against the city of Havana were complete. Albemarle offered terms of capitulation to Governor Prado, but notwithstanding Prado's large number of sick, wounded, and dead from the daily bombardment, he refused the offer of surrender.[103] The British began firing on the city on 11 August. By two o'clock that afternoon, Prado asked for a suspension of fire in order to negotiate terms of surrender. On 14 August 1762, terms were formally agreed on and signed, and the siege was over. In his entry for this day, Prado estimates the Spanish loss of life from the siege at 2,910 troops, plus 800 or 900 slaves.[104] The British return dated 13 August 1762 lists a (rank-and-file) total of 260 battle fatalities, 576 wounded, 51 dead from wounds, and 632 dead from sickness, for a total of 943 dead since British forces had arrived in Cuba.[105]

Even with only 657 soldiers dead from sickness, Albemarle's army was far from well upon taking possession of the city of Havana. An officer's published account of the siege recalls that the men were less impressed at the time of their victory with the thousands of pounds gained in prize money than with the "fresh provisions, rest, and shelter, for the many thousands poor sick wretches we had in our camp and hospital-ships, all mouldering away for want of nourishment when their disorders had left them. Our battalion is so weak that we have not above 150 men fit for duty."[106] Albemarle confessed in a letter to Egremont that although the terms of capitulation were very good for the British, he might have agreed to worse, as he "wanted to get into the town at any rate, the army was so very sickly."[107] A return from 16 August 1762 shows that only 4,203 rank and file were fit for duty out of a total 10,804, with 5,232 sick (the remaining 1,369 listed as absent, on command, or taken prisoner by the enemy).[108]

By this date, the British had entered the city, and found the large number of Spanish sick and wounded lying in convents, churches, and private homes.[109] As mentioned in chapter 1, the Highland regiments were known to succumb to illness during campaigns, and as one contemporary remarked, this was the case "particularly in such a climate" as that of the West Indies.[110] Although the siege was over, the worst of the sickness had only just begun. All three Highland regiments arrived in Cuba from North America at the end of July. In those few intervening weeks, 235 men had died, and out of the 1,823 rank and file embarked, only 101 were fit for duty by mid-August. Among these troops, 1,631 were counted sick, with worse to come.[111]

Albemarle wrote Amherst a letter to accompany the Highland regiments, announcing the success of the siege, but also explaining that the regiments were being sent to a "northern climate in hopes that the change of air may recover them."[112] Amherst saw the Highland regiments in New York on 5 September 1762.[113] He wrote to John Calcraft and George Townshend on their condition, describing them as "such Feeble, Worn out Objects in General, as I never before Saw."[114] On 18 September, Amherst sent John Adair, director of the general hospital, to examine the Highlanders. In his report, Adair described them as "being reduced to the lowest State with dangerous Fevers, and Fluxes; Many of whom are too far gone to be recovered, . . . there is not, in my Opinion of the whole Brigade Thirty Men fit for Service."[115] Adair proved correct in his observations, as he recorded on 25 October that 198 men from the four regiments had died in hospital over the previous month.[116]

In Havana, meanwhile, the troops were not doing much better than the Highlanders in New York. A return of 21 September 1762 shows that out of a total 8,725 rank and file, only 1,032 were fit for duty, with 6,206 listed as sick and the remainder absent, on command, or taken prisoner.[117] On 7 October, Albemarle wrote to Egremont, reporting:

> Our sickness instead of diminishing increases daily notwithstanding the great care and attention that is paid to the sick. We have Buried upwards of 3,000 men since the capitulation, and I am sorry to say there are many Men in the Hospitals who are so exhausted by Fatigue and the heat of the Climate that it is not thought they will recover. I have scarce a Relief for the necessary guards of the garrison, and in many parts of the Country the Militia and Peasants are still in Arms for want of Troops showing themselves amongst them.[118]

The total of all those killed, dead, and wounded from 7 June to 4 October 1762 shows that Albemarle was hardly exaggerating. The return from the day before the capitulation (13 August) listed 988 dead; the 4 October return reported 4,295 total fatalities (3,788 from sickness).[119] By 11 October, Albemarle's original force of 11,203 was reduced to 880 fit for duty and 5,713 sick (see table 2.1).[120]

TABLE 2.1. Returns of rank-and-file British forces at Havana under Albemarle, 1762

Date	Total	**Fit for duty**	Sick (all categories)	Dead of all causes (since previous return)	Other
17 July	11,203	**5,353**	5,043		807
13 August				988 (since 7 June)	
16 August	10,804	**4,203**	5,232	191	1,369
21 September	8,725	**1,032**	6,206		1,487
4 October				4,295 (since 13 August)	
11 October	7,225	**880**	5,713		632

Note: A complete set of returns does not survive. The few surviving have varying categories, including "fit for duty," "total," and variations on "sick" (e.g., "sick in camp," "sick in hospital," "sick onboard"), in addition to other categories, such as "absent," "missing," "on command," "on furlough," and "prisoners with the enemy." The category "dead" includes those listed dead from "sickness" or "wounds," and those "killed" (i.e., in combat), but not those "missing" or "deserted." See figure 3.1, return from Havana. For more on British returns, see chapter 3.

Sources: TNA, CO 117/1, fols. 94–95; SRO, HA 67/969/E8 (17 July 1762); TNA, CO 117/1, fols. 107–8 (13 Aug. 1762); TNA, WO 34/55, fol. 193 (16 Aug. 1762); SRO, HA 67/969/E25 (21 Sept. 1762); SRO, HA 67/969/E17 (4 Oct. 1762); SRO, HA 67/969/E7 (11 Oct. 1762).

This was no comfortable state for an army trying to hold a city in the midst of an enemy island. As Albemarle explained to Amherst, he could not possibly return the full complement of provincial troops to him just yet, as he had barely enough to maintain a garrison.[121] As the town still held over 1,000 recovering Spanish soldiers and sailors, Albemarle was justly anxious. Thomas Mante, assistant engineer, recalled in his published account, "In this situation, the utmost vigilance was necessary to prevent quarrels between the conquerors and the conquered, and keep the latter in awe."[122] The British were not completely successful at keeping the Spanish in awe, as an unknown soldier reported in his diary on 4 November that officers had uncovered a Spanish plot "to rise and put us all to death, as our garrison was so much weakened by sickness."[123] A few months later, in January 1763, news reached the British garrison of a peace treaty between France, Spain, and Britain. By June, Spanish ships had arrived informing the British garrison that they were to vacate Havana, which they did early in July 1763.

The news that Havana, long considered by the Spanish to be impregnable, had fallen to the British influenced peace negotiations between the two countries and engendered enthusiasm in Britain and great concern in Spain. For Spanish officials, the loss of Havana made reform a matter of urgency, with many advocating a British model for colonial commercial renewal.[124] At the end of September 1762, Newcastle reported to Lord Hardwicke that peace "is at *some distance* and probably would not have been brought about at all, if this great event of the Havannah had not happened."[125] News of the British victory was greeted with jubilation in Britain, with newspapers such as the *Gazette* and the *London Chronicle* reprinting detailed accounts of the siege, including the terms of surrender. Returns from 13 August were also reprinted, but not with the total number of troops, and not with the numbers sick; only the number of troops killed, wounded, and dead, divided by regiment, were listed in newspapers.[126] In the chief engineer's journal of the siege, reprinted in most newspapers, no mention of sickness appears. In Albemarle's letters announcing British victory, also widely reprinted, disease was not mentioned. Albemarle has only one sentence on problems encountered, tersely concluding, "The difficulties the officers and soldiers have met with, and the fatigues they have so chearfully and resolutely gone through, are not to be described."[127] The *Gentlemen's Magazine* and the *Annual Register* also expressed their happiness with the conduct of the siege, the sickness simply demonstrating the superior ability of British tars to withstand adversity. As the *Annual Register* of 1762 explained,

> Several dropped down dead with heat, thirst, and fatigue. But such was the resolution of our people, such the happy and perfect unanimity which subsisted between the land and the sea services, that no difficulties, no hardships, slackened for a moment the operations against this important, strong, and well-defended place.[128]

Throughout the course of the campaign, hardly any news on the progress of the siege appeared in English newspapers. Although readers were remarkably well informed about the nature and destination of a Cuban attack that was meant to remain secret, from June until late September very little news on Havana was reported.[129] What was reported in London newspapers took the form of optimistic rumors. By the end of June 1762, the *London Evening-Post* reported that merchants and troops in the West Indies "expected soon some very agreeable news from the Havannah."[130] In late July, the *London Evening-Post* printed a letter dated 1 June, from Antigua. It contains one of the very few references to sickness and the problems it might cause British troops, though the author is on the whole sanguine, stating, "I make no doubt of [Albemarle and Pocock] being masters of the Havana in a month more: nothing in the West Indies can stand against such an army and such a fleet."[131] The *General Evening-Post* also printed a letter in late July, dated 24 May 1762 from Jamaica, in which the author hoped by his next letter to inform his readers that Havana was taken.[132] By the middle of September, the *London Evening-Post* wrongly informed its readers that Havana had surrendered to British troops on 24 July.[133] After the reports of victory and the details of capitulation in late September and early October, no more news on the British troops stationed at Havana appeared in London newspapers.[134]

In the American colonies, one finds more remarks on the conduct of the campaign, and so, more on the hardships suffered by the troops. In part, this was because news of the siege could more easily reach American colonial newspapers while it was still being conducted. As a result, the accounts of the siege were not overshadowed by the spoils of victory. By 2 August 1762, the *Boston Evening-Post* reported, "There were great desertions from both sides; that it began to be sickly in our camp; and that we had lost a great many soldiers in killed and wounded since they landed."[135] The same issue also contained a letter dated 14 July, claiming that 2,200 men were dead from sickness and fighting. At the end of August, newspapers from Boston and New York printed a letter from Captain McAuley reporting, "Many of our troops were sick, owing to the fatigues and dews, but few died, and even those that were taken down soon recovered."[136] The *Boston Gazette* reported in early September "a considerable sickness" among provincials on Cuba.[137] Colonial American newspapers were first to announce the taking of Havana on 13 September 1762, and many sermons and entertainments celebrated the victory.

American colonists were also better informed on the sickness among the regiments because large groups of troops were sent to the colonies to recover, along with some Spanish soldiers and Governor Prado. The *New-York Gazette*, *New-York Mercury*, *Boston Gazette*, and *Boston Evening-Post* all reported on the arrival of the first ships carrying troops from Havana. In the issue of 20 September 1762, the *Boston Gazette* commented that these troops—the sickly Highland regiments—had left the Havana "merely because they were by sickness rendered incapable of duty."[138]

Throughout October, November, and December of 1762, colonial newspapers continued to report on the health of the troops stationed in Havana, including quite accurate reports on the low number of men fit for duty in the garrison. In early November, the *Boston Gazette* published a letter stating that the Spanish had 6,000 active soldiers upon their surrender, "and we were not able to bring more than half that number fit for duty."[139] This letter was printed alongside reports from London that the British peace treaty proposed to return Havana to Spain, even before it was known whether it had been taken. In early December, provincial newspapers reported, "The British troops at the Havannah and its dependencies, fit for duty, is said not to exceed 8 or 900 men."[140]

On 25 December 1762, the *Providence Gazette* stated the following, without further commentary, "From Hebron, in Connecticut, we have an account, that out of 18 soldiers which went from that town, in the expedition to the Havana, 15 are dead, two are sick at New-York, and one is returned."[141] John Watts, a merchant in New York, was less circumspect on the state of the returning troops in his various business letters. He closed his letter to William Baker with the remarks, "We have nothing new to tell you, the poor remains of our Provincials are dropping in from the Havanna, 'tis melancholy to behold the Effects of that ill conducted destructive expedition, that has been an advantage to no body but a few of the Leaders."[142]

Rumors about the shocking state of the troops in Havana freely circulated in the American colonies, and the few letters sent by provincial soldiers to their relatives in the American colonies only increased fears. General Gage, stationed in Montreal, complained to Amherst in November 1762:

> Your acc[oun]ts of the Havannah troops are dreadful indeed, every Post brings the News of fresh Deaths by the means of private Letters; which causes worse effects on People's Imaginations, than if they had a Regular List of all who are really dead; Every Person who has a Friend or Relation there, concludes him no longer in the Land of the Living unless he actually hears from Him, which has been the Case of very few.[143]

The American colonial press has long been regarded as playing a crucial role in shaping American public opinion just before and during the American War of Independence, developing into an outlet for political debate from the Stamp Act crisis of 1765. Newspaper historian David Copeland claims that this role coalesced earlier, during the Seven Years' War. According to his analysis, it was the experience of wartime reporting, including shaping public opinion against what they portrayed as French aggression and Indian cruelties, that formed American colonial newspapers into a coherent group that urged political action and framed public debate. Over the period 1754–63, American newspapers "developed into a unified medium that established a collective consciousness that made newspapers a powerful force in the colonies during the Stamp Act crisis."[144] While Copeland is careful to note that this consciousness was not yet critical of British or imperial governance, historians of eighteenth-century newspapers have demonstrated how they—as part of the public sphere—were more often than not subversive of authority. Colonial newspapers needed to look no further than the British press for an example.[145] Moreover, Copeland demonstrates that colonial papers were sophisticated and adept at molding public opinion by the close of the Seven Years' War, which suggests that reports on the Havana campaign may have been purposefully reproaching British imperial authority.

The returning troops also brought their diseases with them, making the grimness of the Havana campaign inescapable not only to those following accounts of the war, but to all inhabitants, especially in major port cities. Governor Colden of New York expressed to Amherst his apprehension about the contagious diseases troops would be bringing back from the West Indies. While Amherst assured him all regulations concerning quarantine and medical examinations would be followed, he also chided the governor, "Whatever their Ailments may be, I hope the people of this country will join with me, in thinking that due care Should be taken of them [troops from the West Indies], and that no Idle reports of timorous people should prevent their receiving the Necessary help for their Recovery."[146]

Even though care was taken to keep the troops in army hospitals, an outbreak of yellow fever in Philadelphia in the fall of 1762 was thought to have started with sailors recently arrived from the West Indian campaign.[147] These diseases continued to incapacitate the North American troops for some time, and thereby disrupted operations in mainland North America. Although British officials had envisaged a campaign into Louisiana with the troops from Havana, this was canceled as Albemarle and Amherst insisted that the troops were in no condition to fight again.

More pressing still in North America in 1763 was the situation of the Amerindian campaign, or Pontiac's War. With people fleeing towns and their homes out of fear for their lives during the fighting, Amherst was hard-pressed to find as many troops as possible. Before the outbreak of native hostilities, Amherst was already desperate to economize and save on the number of men. Reviewing his regiments in 1763, he despairingly commented on one, "A vast diminution for a regiment and all the men at Crown Point are recruits raised since the regiment came from the Havana, and some of the officers as well as the men have yet frequent relapses of their disorder."[148] The sickness at Havana not only reduced the number of troops available for later campaigns in North America, but it also made the army itself weaker, with soldiers frequently continuing to suffer from illnesses. This seriously affected the army's response to the Indian uprising, and at various points jeopardized British success.[149]

Although American newspapers may have been critical of British West Indian campaigns, American concerns about service in the British army and about the threats posed to civilians by the presence of sick British troops were not necessarily signs of American hostility toward Britain.[150] The patriotic celebrations upon the news of Havana's reduction demonstrate that provincials still clearly considered themselves as a province of the great mother country. As Harding has pointed out, American Revolutionary rhetoric that harkened back to injustices committed against provincial troops in previous campaigns had more to do with concerns of the 1770s and 1780s than actually remembered wrongs. Yet, as both Harding and Leach suggest, the period of the Seven Years' War intensified tensions within American society about the British Army, as large numbers of troops were quickly raised, employed, and deployed within the provinces.[151] In the case of Havana, North America's close proximity to the West Indies led to the recruitment of North American troops as a possible way to limit the impact of the unhealthy tropical climate. The close proximity also meant that those in the colonies were not shielded from the horrors attending a siege in the West Indies. Although provincial assemblies were slow to recruit for most campaigns, the marked hostility to recruitment for the Havana campaign along with the absence of colonial criticism over disease rates at Quebec in 1759–60 suggests that provincials—like British regulars—found Caribbean expeditions particularly distasteful.

While the conduct of the American colonies during the Seven Years' War influenced the nature and course of metropolitan assertions of authority in the 1760s and 1770s, the reverse is also true. Although the war encouraged colonial anxieties about metropolitan power, American contributions to the war effort also "heightened [colonial] expectations for a larger—and more equivalent—role within the Empire."[152] British public opinion downplayed American contributions during the war and focused instead on the provinces' illegal trade with the French and on the role of British military and naval intervention in ensuring successful campaigns. Indeed, P. J. Marshall argues that "British opinion seems to have interpreted the American response to the war not as generous contributions by dutiful fellow subjects but as generally pusillanimous attempts to evade what was necessary for their own survival."[153] The disjuncture between colonists' convictions regarding their wartime sacrifices and the opinion of the British public and imperial officials was itself a product of the difference in the reporting on campaigns, especially those in the sickly West Indies. Historians have rightly stressed the relative freedom and vibrancy of the English press at midcentury, especially concerning foreign affairs and military and naval campaigns.[154] Yet a brief survey of American colonial reporting on West Indian campaigns compared with the London press shows the complications of newspaper reporting during imperial warfare. While it is true that the British press freely reported military and naval setbacks, the recounting of the toll and cost of a victory could be more damaging than defeat.

There is nothing to suggest that such omissions were the result of official censorship (as discussed in chapter 3), rather than simply the difference between reporting of campaigns happening some thousands of miles away across the span of an ocean and that of campaigns happening nearby. Yet contemporaries clearly made the connection between disease among troops and officials' leadership and command, as Major General Barrington had done. In his memoirs of the campaigns in the West Indies during 1759, Captain of Marines Richard Gardiner criticized Moore's leadership on various points concerning naval tactics, but especially castigated him for neglecting the health and care of the sick sailors under his command. Gardiner cited Moore's harsh cruelty to an individual seaman sick with scurvy, and more broadly blamed Moore for encouraging sickness and death among the fleet through his thoughtless actions, further relating Moore's ill regard to the good of the service and the nation, asking rhetorically "how many brave and gallant Englishmen might yet have lived to do their Country Service," had Moore provided proper medical care and attention.[155]

Such criticisms illustrate that officials were aware of, and responsive to, the difficulties posed by the West Indian climate during campaigns. In 1759 and again in 1762, imperial authorities recruited West Indian locals as laborers, in line with the most advanced medical knowledge of the day. Although hampered by the resistance of colonial officials, in both the Caribbean and North American colonies, British campaigns made use of troops that they believed were more seasoned to the environment. While on campaign, troops were not simply left to suffer. Instead, officials generally procured fresh provisions and additional medical care, attempting to lessen the ill effects of an unhealthy climate as much as was possible. Major General Barrington's correspondence is evidence of his concern for his troops' health and his efforts to prevent and ameliorate sickness. His victory was understood in contrast to the failure under Hopson's leadership: concern for the welfare of troops coincided with military victory. Measures taken at Havana, including the recruitment of provincial troops, followed contemporary medical advice. These were costly measures, not only in terms of money spent, but also in terms of relations with the American colonies, with serious implications for military operations in mainland North America.

Yet overall, such actions could do little to lessen rates of disease in the West Indies. Rates decreased only when troops were stationed in that climate for at least a year, which involved an initial period of great morbidity and mortality.[156] As a result, campaigns in the West Indies were inevitably accompanied by very considerable rates of sickness and death and, consequently, by difficulties that exacerbated tensions in already precarious colonial-imperial relations. Evaluations of British command at Cartagena and Havana are thus most insightful when they consider what measures were available to contemporaries, examining in detail what measures were taken, instead of focusing on their efficacy in preventing or curing disease. At Cartagena, for example, the problems with scurvy were the result of administrative problems, not medical ignorance—problems that Barrington carefully avoided in Havana.[157] When evaluating responses to yellow fever, one should remember that no helpful medical treatment was known at the time; the only efficacious responses would have been prevention through mosquito control and vaccination. These two methods remain beyond the reach of much of the world's population even today. Recent publications on global health indicate that yellow fever is still a problem because of this very reason.[158] It is not that vaccinations are ineffective; rather, the challenge is establishing regular vaccinations in areas where basic infrastructure is lacking. Since effective medicine requires knowledge of social context, so should historical analyses of medicine. Accounts that focus on treatments such as bleeding and purging for eighteenth-century yellow-fever sufferers neglect the resourcing of fresh provisions, the use of locals accustomed to the climate, the insistence on moderation in exercise and diet, and the stationing of troops away from marshy environments. These practices were not only fundamental to eighteenth-century medical theory, but also provide insight into the nature and scope of care for eighteenth-century forces.

It is unclear whether British forces experienced notably different levels of medical care than did French or Spanish forces. Detailed histories of medicine during their campaigns have yet to be written, although general histories suggest that financial impediments resulted in poorer provisioning for Spanish and French forces.[159] Moreover, drawing comparisons is difficult given that circumstances varied, resulting in divergent rates of disease. Particularly in the West Indies, as Paul Kopperman has pointed out, rates of sickness were more indicative of circumstance, such as the season and the length of time troops had spent there, than the state of medical care.[160] Christian Buchet's detailed comparison of French and British rates of sickness in the Caribbean over the late seventeenth and early eighteenth centuries shows that British ships had higher rates of disease, most likely the result of longer transatlantic voyages.

By the time of the Seven Years' War, British officials had responded to this problem, putting in place strategies that allowed the navy to improve sanitary and logistical methods.[161] Similarly, British forces during Caribbean campaigns faced different challenges than did their adversaries: as attackers, with few troops stationed in the West Indies, British troops confronted the medical problem of newcomers to a foreign climate, whereas the besieged counted on the advantage of seasoned troops. Compared with the French and Spanish, British officials relied less on local militias, sending over an impressive number of regular troops. This resulted in a qualitative advantage for the British during campaigns, but it also resulted in higher rates of sickness among those unseasoned British regular troops. Tracing the details of medical care demonstrates that British officials were willing to expend significant resources on the health of the armed forces, informed by contemporary medical knowledge. Yet, overall, rates of troop health were determined more by the season and the type of troops, than by the extent of care provided.

Eighteenth-century medical care thus worked within the constraints of military tactics and strategy. As the British campaigns of 1759 and 1762 demonstrate, this consisted of trying to batter defensive forces before disease incapacitated too many unseasoned troops, supplemented by as many seasoned forces as could be willingly supplied. While attacks on Guadeloupe and Martinique took place in the healthy season, Havana was besieged during the unhealthy season. George Anson, first lord of the Admiralty and experienced in the problems of Caribbean campaigns, had expedited preparations at an impressive pace, but given the demand for immediate action against Spain, British forces still had to endure campaigning over the wet season. Although medical advice could not prevent campaigns during the unhealthy season or avoid the use of unseasoned troops altogether, the use of seasoned troops, fresh provisions, and other aspects of medical care contributed to the ability of British forces to sustain their attacks long enough to secure victories, in contrast to Cartagena in 1740.

Armed with their experience of the Seven Years' War, British medical men argued that diseases and medicine in warm climates were distinctive, as demonstrated through empirical observations. Those trained in its methods were experts, able to serve the expanding British Empire through their specific knowledge of what would become known as tropical medicine. The Seven Years' War was central to this development, lending "great urgency to medical investigations" into the nature of disease in warm climates, and resulting in a proliferation of writings that defined nontemperate and non-European areas as a coherent and distinctive disease environment.[162] This was a practical enterprise, focused on maintaining the health and thus the might of imperial projects. As historians of colonial medicine have pointed out, it was by no means a humanitarian or even always a neutral endeavor; tropical medicine has also been described as "the scientific stepchild of colonial domination and control," grouping and pathologizing entire climates and peoples as part of the theory and practice of European imperialism.[163]

During the period of the Seven Years' War, officials translated contemporary expert medical advice into military policy, conserving enough manpower to allow military victory over the French and the Spanish in the West Indies. The experts did not think it impossible. While British officials decided that victory was worth the attendant rates of sickness and death, the general public was not necessarily in agreement. Thus, the Havana campaign was more popular in Britain, where details of its sickliness were obscured, than in the American colonies. Such obscurity in coverage could not be maintained on campaigns close to home; as the next chapter demonstrates, reporting of disease in the war's European campaigns was a significant political problem for the British public, as it was for the American public during the Caribbean campaigns.

CHAPTER THREE

Flux, Fever, and Politics: The European Theater of War

Although British involvement with European Continental campaigns during the Seven Years' War has received less historiographical attention than colonial campaigns, British forces and British finances were integral to Continental warfare. British-allied victories such as those at Minden (1759) and Wilhelmsthal (1762) ensured that Prussia kept Silesia and that Hanover was free from Austrian and French control by the close of the war.[1] The number of British regulars sent to fight in Germany was on par with those sent to America, while British money funded more troops in Germany than it did in North America and the West Indies combined.[2] Moreover, mid-eighteenth-century wartime policy has long been recognized as a key factor in the development of political debate and of the enhanced role of public opinion in Britain.[3] The extent of British activity on the Continent was vigorously debated in the House of Commons and in the public sphere, remaining a focus for partisan debates and popular concerns throughout the war. Public debate was not only relevant to political officials: military officers were also vulnerable to the sway of public opinion. As William Hotham advised his brother, an army captain, "A Philosopher may say he cares not for popular clamour, but it is a wrong maxim for military people to be of that opinion."[4]

Disease during Continental campaigns was linked to public and partisan concerns over responsible policy and expenditure. Although rates of disease did not reach the extraordinary levels of the Caribbean campaigns, disease was similarly used to publicize and criticize campaigns on the Continent. When reports of high disease rates circulated, members of Parliament castigated the government for mismanagement and used disease as a partisan issue with which to attack unpopular foreign policy. Not only were officials concerned with the health and welfare of troops, but disease as a political issue was integral to debates concerning the planning and the conduct of European campaigns. This chapter's analysis of disease not only provides insight into the nature of eighteenth-century British political debates in Parliament and the public sphere, but also demonstrates that Europe was considered a foreign and insalubrious environment, similar to the Atlantic colonies. As a result, health concerns in Germany were politically fraught, even more so than those regarding the West Indies.

This chapter examines "regular" diseases of eighteenth-century armies: fevers and diarrheal diseases. Often called crowd diseases, these illnesses inevitably accompanied armies on campaign and then spread to nearby civilian populations. As their name suggests, these army diseases were similar to those found in crowded, urban areas during the eighteenth century, especially institutions such as jails and hospitals. Frequently linked explicitly to broader programs of social reform, much of British and European eighteenth-century medicine focused on improving the health of the general population, implementing preventative measures in urban and institutional settings as well as providing hospitals and dispensaries on an unprecedented scale.

As this chapter demonstrates, the experience of disease on campaign played a significant role in eighteenth-century medical developments more broadly. As in colonial campaigns, military medical practitioners on the Continent made use of extensive firsthand observations of crowd diseases and utilized the distinctive structure of military medicine to develop new methods of medical research. At midcentury, British military medicine was not in competition with civilian medicine, but instead was part of it, reinforcing and providing further opportunities for its new approaches. This is shown most tangibly in the careers of practitioners, who applied methods learned in military or naval contexts to civilian projects after the war, or who refined an interest in the health of lower orders that had been initiated while treating soldiers and sailors. The medical expertise developed during campaigns was thus not necessarily a challenge to metropolitan knowledge, as was the case in colonial environments, but often buttressed domestic initiatives, thereby contributing to the development of eighteenth-century medical professionalism and authority.

This chapter opens with an overview of the nature of disease during European campaigns, tracing how provisioning and logistical difficulties contributed to crowd diseases such as typhus fever and dysentery. The details of camp regulations and sanitation illustrate the measures taken by contemporaries to try to reduce the incidence of disease. Key to medical care during Continental campaigns, the nature of military hospital medicine is then examined, placed within the context of eighteenth-century civilian hospital medicine. The chapter concludes by examining the relationship between disease and public opinion, outlining contemporary ideas about the health of the general population and the use of disease to criticize military and political leadership. During the Seven Years' War, reports on rates of disease and recovery were used to criticize and reform military hospitals during the Continental campaigns. By the same token, quantitative reports on the health of British armed forces demonstrate the extent to which disease was a political and public concern during this period.

THE CONTINENTAL CAMPAIGN: MILITARY PROVISIONING AND CROWD DISEASES

Although hostilities between France and Britain were apparent from 1754 in North America, the situation in Europe was not so clear. Prussia and France had signed a treaty in 1741 concerning attacks on Hanover, but this was subject to renewal in 1756. Early in 1756, Britain signed the Convention of Westminster with Prussia, a carefully worded defensive treaty. In response, Russia allied with Austria, and in turn Austria and France signed the Treaty of Versailles on 1 May 1756.[5] Meanwhile, French forces prepared for an attack on British-held Minorca, as well as on Britain itself. The army in Britain was so short of troops that Hanover and Hesse-Kassel were asked to render aid, each sending over half of their available battalions to defend Britain against French troops.[6]

Despite their help in scaring off a potential French invasion, the German troops serving in Britain were remarkably unpopular. Along with Braddock's defeat at Fort Duquesne and the loss of Minorca, government officials were castigated in the press and in pamphlets for having mishandled the opening of the war and depending on foreign troops. In a pamphlet published in 1755, John Shebbeare warned that reliance on foreign mercenaries and British involvement in Continental affairs in general, and in the Electorate of Hanover specifically, demonstrated the military and moral weakness of Britain. Paying German states for their soldiers, not raising a proper British force, and abandoning the American colonies, "the legal child of *England*," for the "bastard and unnatural State" of Hanover meant the ruin, financial and moral, of the British nation.[7]

When the theft of a handkerchief from a Kent shop by a Hanoverian soldier in September 1756 was publicized, it became a focus for outrage and criticism of German troops and Britain's relationship with Germany.[8]

Whereas complaints about the German troops stopped when they were sent back to Germany on Pitt's entry to office in November 1756, tirades against British involvement in Germany were not so quick to end.

As a result of widespread opposition to Britain's involvement in a Continental campaign, no British troops were sent to Europe in 1756 or 1757. Instead, the Treasury funded roughly 50,000 Hanoverian, Hessian, and Brunswick soldiers to protect Hanover and aid Prussia.[9] Moreover, in March 1757, the Duke of Cumberland was appointed commander of the German-allied army in western Europe (to be replaced by Ferdinand of Brunswick in November 1757), while King Frederick II commanded the mostly Prussian army in central Europe.[10]

Conditions were less than ideal for these field armies even in the early stages of the war. Forage for horses and supplies for the soldiers soon ran short, causing marauding, which in turn led to indiscipline, sickness, and desertion. Andrew Mitchell, the British minister to Prussia, reported on 28 April 1757, "About seventy Horses of our Cuirassieres have died this Day in the road, the Forage is scarce, and our marches are fatiguing."[11] Cumberland admitted that it was lack of provisions that kept the armies from fighting, and not a lack of men or faulty strategy. He wrote to Mitchell at the beginning of May 1757, "Every thing is extremely quiet in these Parts & the Distresses of Provision & Forage seem to be at present a very strong Barrier between the two armies."[12]

Civilians in the German countries also suffered, as the armies consumed all they could find. George Cressener, the British minister to Cologne, reported at the end of May 1757 from Cologne, "Every sort of Provision and Forage grows so scarce and dear here, all over the Electorate, and the two Dutchys, that many Persons are dead for want, and the Inhabitants in general are in great misery, having neither bread for themselves, nor Forage for their Cattle."[13] With the interruption of war, harvests often failed, and, worse, the thousands of troops took whatever provisions they could find, often leaving famine and disease in their wake. Officials recognized the havoc they wrought among civilian populations, yet could find no alternatives. As Captain James Webb wrote about the state of British troops in Hanover and Brunswick, "Is it not a cruel necessity to be obliged to pillage these poor miserable people after what they suffer'd from us last year; there is but little corn on the ground and that little we must take, though the remaining inhabitants must starve."[14]

Opposing armies were not immune to such shortages either. British military officials carefully described the state of the French, Austrian, and imperial armies to their superiors. Colonel Joseph Yorke informed Cumberland in early June 1757 that the French Army was "embarass'd in their operations by the want of Forage."[15] The anonymous source of British intelligence that regularly reported to Cumberland from the front lines of the French Army also kept the commander in chief informed on French rates of sickness. In June, it suggested that the French army was preparing for a battle, as a hospital in Wesel had been opened with 5,000 beds, adding as well, "There are already many soldiers ill, and around fifty wounded as a result of various skirmishes."[16]

After Pitt agreed to send 8,000 British troops to Westphalia in 1758 under the Duke of Marlborough, the British Army formally entered warfare on the Continent, and British officials became responsible for coordinating provisions to these soldiers as well. To supply British troops in the field, contractors and magazine keepers were paid by British paymasters and overseen by commissariats. Contractors were responsible for supplying forage and provisions, which were then delivered to magazines scattered throughout campaign territory, each magazine overseen by a magazine keeper. Troops were to give receipts to the keepers for what provisions they used, and the receipts were in turn paid by the Commissary of Accounts.[17] In times of war, when the movement of troops was unpredictable and scarcity of provisions was all too common, the system often broke down.

Henry Hulton, who went to Germany as the agent for the British Commissariat of Accounts in March 1761, reported that he found various problems and abuses upon his arrival; not only disorder, but even "collusions and frauds," which caused shortages of provisions and, consequently, pillaging.[18] While such accusations are credible, historians have generally concluded that it was not so much corruption as understaffing and inefficient administrative structures that caused problems.[19] As shall be discussed in further detail, criticism of the Commissariat, and of the welfare of the British forces in Germany in general, was tied to political concerns during the course of the war. As a result, contemporary complaints against and vindications of the supply system were in part motivated and informed by partisan politics. Yet these concerns were also military and strategic. If soldiers were not properly provided for, they would not be able to fulfill their military duties and would also tend toward ill discipline and disobedience, ravaging the countryside and civilians for their own purposes and, thereby, denying the army the goodwill and cooperation of local populations.[20]

During campaigns, ensuring a regular supply of provisions was important not only to feed soldiers and to keep them under formal authority, but also to prevent diseases. Hungry soldiers would pillage, which led to diseases through overeating and through the loss of camp discipline. As General George Townshend remarked during his 1762 campaign in Portugal, a lack of provisions was "ye source of sickness mutiny & desertion."[21] As well, maintaining camp discipline, and specifically orders regarding sanitation, was directly related to preventing outbreaks of disease such as dysentery.

Lieutenant Colonel James Oughton, from the First Battalion of the Thirty-Seventh Regiment of Foot, sailed from Britain on 17 July 1758. In his journal, he recorded the state of the army and its provisions, as well as his impressions of the various German towns in which he stayed. Because of food shortages and the danger of soldiers marauding if no supplies were provided, markets had to be carefully controlled by military officials. Stationed outside of Munster, Oughton noted: "The Inhabitants being threatened with Military Execution brought in a little provision and the prices were regulated. But no Bullocks being brought orders were given to send out parties & bring them in by force."[22] By mid-August, Oughton complained about incessant rains and muddy roads, as well as lack of supplies, marauding, and the sickness that inevitably accompanied such conditions.

Oughton also included in his diary Prince Ferdinand's orders for camp hygiene. These instruct the troops not only to maintain a clean camp, but also to move regiments onto dry ground and to establish another hospital for the British at the rear of the camp. On 6 September 1758, the orders first mention a specific disease, "Fluxes," as a problem for the soldiers.[23] According to Donald Munro (1728–1802), who served as physician to the hospital for British forces in Germany during the war, the sickness was dysentery, which began soon after the army went into the field, and continued when the army went into its quarters over the winter.[24] Dysentery, which sickened British soldiers throughout their service in Germany, was believed to be related to the conditions of army camps. Contrary to what other physicians had previously argued, Munro believed it was not caused by fruit, but by the hard labor of soldiers in the heat and from the effects of putrefying matter found in abundance in army camps.[25]

Camp orders given to British troops while in Germany concerned safeguarding troop health by attempting to prevent the causes articulated by Munro. According to the various military treatises published during the eighteenth century for officers and rank-and-file troops, army camps were meant to be orderly places. Humphrey Bland's military treatise, the fifth edition of which was published in 1743, specified that it was the duty of the quartermasters and the camp colormen to precede the army to their camp, and to

> make their Necessary Houses, and to get them finish'd, if possible, by the time the Regiments arrive, that the Camp may be kept Sweet and Clean; for which Reason the Centries must have Strict Orders not to suffer anyone to ease himself any where else. . . . The Quarter-Masters and their Serjeants are to see that the Streets are Swept clean every Morning, and that the butchers and Sutlers bury their Garbidge and Filth every Day; and that all dead Horses are immediately Burned, that the Air may be kept from Infection.[26]

Similarly, camp orders from the Warbough Camp on 16 October 1760 stated, "Great Attention to cleanliness in Camp & particular care to be taken, that all dead Horses, and the Entrails of Beasts are buried deep in the Earth, that new Necessarys be made every two days, and the Old ones fill'd up, and in general that the Camp be kept sweet and clean as possible."[27] According to one British soldier's description, the traditional "Necessarys" used in British army camps during the Seven Years' War were dug-out pits at the back of the camp, away from the tents, which could be easily filled over with dirt every few days. They consisted of "a long hole cut in the ground, with a pole fixed upon two forked ones, on which the men sit."[28]

By early 1761, orders on cleanliness specifically tied poor hygiene to the raging sickness.[29] These were accompanied by directions that officers ensure their men receive "good food" and vinegar, that drinking water was boiled "or at least it may be suffer'd to stand a few hours in order to have time to get clear," and to keep the sick in isolated, well-ventilated, noncrowded, clean, and fumigated hospital houses.[30] Especially during the summer, cleanliness was thought to be integral to a well-regulated army camp. Daily orders frequently noted that "during the Excessive hot weather every commanding officer is to take the greatest care that Cleanliness is kept in camp—and the general officers commanding corps will severely punish all those who disobey this order."[31] Orders from military officials repeatedly stressed the importance of discipline and cleanliness in camp to avoid what was often termed "disorder." By this term officers and medical staff referred both to disease as disorder within an individual and to the lack of discipline in camp, which was directly related to an outbreak of disease in individuals. Discipline, by maintaining order and cleanliness in camp and keeping individuals well regulated, was thus crucial in preventing disease.

Dysentery and diarrheal diseases ("flux") are common to crowded populations living in unsanitary and transitory circumstances. Soldiers based in army camps frequently suffered from such complaints, notably even during World War I. John Pringle described dysentery as "the constant and fatal epidemic of [military] camps."[32] The disease's origin is an infected individual or animal, which carries the viral, bacterial, or parasitic pathogen and usually passes it on via infected stools: infected matter, often carried by flies, is transmitted to drink or food that is ingested by susceptible individuals. Because of the symptoms of diarrhea and vomiting, one infected individual can easily contaminate his or her surroundings, and especially a camp's water supply, thereby quickly spreading the disease. As a result, a clean water supply, sewage removal, and general sanitation measures are the best preventatives against such outbreaks, not only by separating refuse from food and water, but also by preventing flies from multiplying.[33] The orders given by military commanders concerning the regulation of camp sanitation, especially those relating to the camp toilet pits, the boiling of water, and the burying of garbage, were thus consistent with both eighteenth-century and twenty-first-century medical standards.

The other disease that plagued and debilitated the British troops serving in Germany during the war, as well as armies on campaign in general, was typhus. Although typhus is unheard of in Western countries today, throughout the eighteenth century typhus epidemics were frequent, producing fever, debility, and mortality rates ranging from 10 to 70 percent.[34] Caused by the microorganism *Rickettsia prowazekii*, the disease is transmitted between humans by body lice. A louse ingests the blood of an infected human through a bite, and then spreads the microorganism either through the skin by an individual's scratching of a louse bite, or by the person inhaling dried *rickettsiae* from louse feces. Typhus epidemics can start from an animal reservoir, through the inhalation of dried forms of the organism present in clothes and similar materials, or from a previously infected individual who suffers a relapse of the disease from nutritional deprivation or the onset of other diseases.[35] Body lice are almost nonexistent today in developed Western countries, but they are commonplace in areas where people do not frequently wash or change their clothes. As they live in the seams of clothing and require the warm habitat of a human's normal temperature, body lice will not live in unworn clothing, and will leave a feverish or dead individual. As a result, these lice are common where people live in a cold climate and huddle together for warmth while infrequently changing their clothes.[36]

Because of these factors, typhus is common in times of hardship, such as famines, and in crowded conditions, such as urban slums or poorly administered institutions. Its eighteenth-century names reinforce this association: it was known as hospital or jail fever, as well as ship or (army) camp fever. Typhus has also long been associated with war. This is not only because warfare leaves civilian populations without proper fuel, clothing, and sanitary structures, but also because typhus arises in the crowded and unsanitary conditions of military camps, and is thereby spread from troops to the civilian populations. The resulting degree of contagiousness and mortality can be high.[37] Lack of provisions for soldiers while on campaign in Europe, therefore, not only meant that the men would go hungry; shortages of food and fuel among both civilian populations and in army camps suggested that typhus would soon strike.

Although diagnosing a disease from a distance of two and a half centuries is a precarious practice, the symptoms and methods of transmission of what eighteenth-century practitioners called hospital, jail, ship, camp, malignant, and petechial fever, as well as the stable nature of the virus, evince that these diseases are known today as epidemic typhus.[38] As Richard Brocklesby, physician to the British Army serving in Germany, reported, according to the medical registers kept at military hospitals during the war, preventing fevers ought to be of the utmost importance to the army as "full eight times the number of men have been lost in this manner, of late, more than fell immediately by their wounds, or in battle."[39] Such observations were common among military medical practitioners. Frederick Hoffmann (physician to Frederick of Prussia) recorded that Dr. George Barnstorff, physician to the Duke of Hanover and an experienced military physician, claimed, "Setting aside wounds, which are the trophies of war, all the diseases of camps are . . . reduced to two heads, a malignant fever, and a dysentery; all the rest being only the harbingers or followers of these two."[40]

According to eighteenth-century medical thought, fevers and fluxes were not necessarily distinct diseases. The appearance of one could give rise to the other. Dr. Robert Knox, physician to the British Army in Germany, wrote to John Pringle after the war describing the circumstances that gave rise to the fevers and fluxes of the army while near Munster in 1760–61. Knox's account is worth recording in full, as it neatly summarizes the common description of fevers and fluxes while on campaign, and the all-too-common consequences attending these diseases:

> The predisposing causes to this disease and the Fevers and Fluxes of this campaign may be collected from the following. . . . There was a great scarcity of good Water, as the men were often obliged to use water from stagnant Ponds or Pools, where the Horses water'd, which made it exceedingly muddy and impure. Diarrhoas and a few Dysenterys appeared first in their Camp with some remitting Fevers from the Middle of July. From the 31st of July until October the Army Encamped on the Dymel near Warburg, where there was no opportunity of changing the encampment, nor sufficient Hospital Room for the Regimental or General Hospitals. It was likewise impossible to have sufficient quantity of straw, or conveniences for keeping the Tents or Hospitals well aired, and Clean, upon account of the Rains and wet Ground; as it was the most rainy season from the beginning of August until the end of November, that I ever saw in Europe. Those Fluxes, Putrid, and Remitting fevers became very Epidemic, in so much that the Populous villages of Corbecke, Hohenwaple and Brendorf were almost totally depopulated. The Town of Warburg lost above one half of its inhabitants, and the Army at the same time was very sickly, but did not lose so many men in proportion, to the inhabitants, in they were better supplyed with Provisions, and Medical assistance when sick, yet I cannot help taking notice of this Circumstance, that there was 3 Regiments of Infantry, 900 Men each compleat in the Spring, were at one time reduced to not above 60 Men a Regt able to do duty, and the [illeg] Regt had not above 35 Private men on the Hess expedition, in the Winter [17]60, [17]61.[41]

The locations in which fluxes most frequently gave rise to fever, as Knox reported, were hospitals. Donald Munro also noted that fever often appeared in patients who were brought into a military hospital, and further observed that in the military hospitals during the German campaigns "Fluxes are liable to be complicated with other Disorders, as well as with the malignant Fever."[42] This association between hospitals and fever was by no means new; as mentioned above, one of the names for typhus in this period was hospital fever. John Pringle had pointed out that it was a disease not of military camps so much as of the hospitals in military camps, and wrote in the preface to his *Observations on the Diseases of the Army*, "Among the chief causes of sickness and death in an army, the Reader will little expect that I should rank, what is intended for its health and preservation, the Hospitals themselves."[43] During his service in Germany as physician to the British troops in the 1740s, Pringle had observed how easily a fever epidemic arose when a hospital was filled to overflowing by patients suffering from the flux.[44]

Hospital fever was thus thought to arise from corrupt air, produced by crowded living situations or from putrefying matter. According to eighteenth-century medical theory, humans constantly exhaled matter, in breathing and through the pores. In normal circumstances, this effluvium was not harmful. Once confined, however, such a substance could quickly become a kind of poison, occasioning disease in those who inhaled it, by respiration or through their pores.[45] While the exact details of how this air was rendered noxious remained uncertain, it was generally believed that animal respiration rendered the air unfit for further respiration, as demonstrated by experiments with diving bells, patients in confined spaces, and putrefying animal matter.[46] For these reasons John Arbuthnot thought it important that cities, prisons, and hospitals be built so as "to give a thorough Passage to the Air."[47]

HOSPITAL MEDICINE

Air, then, was rendered injurious not only by normal human effluvium, but also by the decay and putrefaction of animals. As common fevers, gangrenous wounds, and especially dysentery were associated with putrefaction, disease and infections were thus not only a result of noisome air, but could also produce such air. As a result, fevers originated in military hospitals both because they were frequently crowded, and because the sick and wounded had especially dangerous effluvia. For these reasons, Brocklesby and Munro included various detailed observations on and recommendations for military hospitals in their works on the British Army during the Seven Years' War, as Pringle had done after the War of Austrian Succession (1740–48). They agreed that as diseases of all sorts ran the danger of degenerating into a hospital fever if the wards were crowded, it was through the proper management of a hospital that military medical practitioners could prevent disease. Munro explained, "There is no Part of the Service that requires more to be regarded than the Choice of proper Places for Hospitals, and the right Management of them, on which the Health and Strength of an Army often depends."[48] Brocklesby concurred that "numbers of brave men are annually lost in the hospitals, for want of order and proper subordination among the Physical Officers."[49]

The physicians recommended that buildings chosen as the sites for the main general hospitals, usually situated in towns away from the main areas of fighting, should be large, airy structures that allowed the division of patients into wards according to their disorder and whether it was infectious. Even more important, practitioners had to take special care that hospitals did not become crowded. Munro suggested that this could be done by using various types of hospitals, especially those that could move with the army: the temporary regimental hospitals, which were usually a house or tent procured by the regimental surgeon for a few men, were complemented by flying hospitals at the rear of a camp.[50] Campaign orders demonstrate that such small hospitals were regularly established, usually directing attention to choosing a healthy location and other measures to prevent pernicious air.[51]

In camps during the war, regimental surgeons reported every two weeks to the inspector general of British infirmaries on the state of their patients.[52] The seriously ill soldiers were either sent by wagons to the larger and more permanent general hospitals, or billeted in private houses to avoid crowding in the hospitals. Particular care had to be taken of recovering or convalescent soldiers, as they could cause overcrowding in hospitals or relapse into illness. They were also routinely suspected of malingering.[53] Munro and the commanding officers were not unreasonable in worrying about convalescent soldiers; it was reported that the town of Grabenstein had been "pillaged by several sick that are there."[54] In his military treatise, Humphrey Bland also warned of the dangers of a military hospital if soldiers remained too long:

> For it often happens, when they stay too long after they are Recover'd, that they Relapse and Die. . . . But the least Evil that can happen by their remaining too long in the Hospital, is, that they will thereby contract a slothful, lazy, idle Habit, and turn, according to the Military Phrase, *Malingerors*.[55]

Military hospitals were thus rather dangerous places, as they could give rise to epidemic fevers if not properly managed, as well as encouraging poor discipline and bad habits in soldiers.

For medical officials, by contrast, hospitals provided useful medical experience and authority. Compared with regimental medicine, as outlined in chapter 1, military physicians and the staff of military general hospitals had reputable medical qualifications, were paid better, and enjoyed greater respect from military officials.[56] Richard Brocklesby studied at Edinburgh's esteemed medical school before receiving his MD from Leiden, along with honorary degrees from Dublin and Cambridge, while Donald Munro obtained his MD from the University of Edinburgh. Although these medical men could not compare in prestige and wealth to the most popular physicians, who catered to the rich and powerful in English urban centers, the examples of Munro and Brocklesby demonstrate that military physicians were part of a successful and respected medical circle.[57] Each had had a private practice in London before serving with the army; among Brocklesby's patients were Samuel Johnson and John Wilkes.[58] Brocklesby was an early participant in the Society of Physicians and a fellow of both the Royal College of Physicians and the Royal Society.[59] He was also the only committee member of the Society for the Encouragement of the British Troops in Germany and North America who did not have either an aristocratic title or military office.[60] Munro became a fellow of the Royal Society in 1766, was physician to St. George's Hospital in London from 1758 until 1786, and was one of the first hospital physicians in London to give courses relating to the medical arts.[61]

Both Munro and Brocklesby commonly received correspondence from other military practitioners concerning their medical practice, similar to Pringle, as discussed in chapter 1. Brocklesby included a letter from a military physician based in Senegal in his *Oeconomical and Medical Observations*, and Munro was listed as the recipient of letters on diseases in warm climates, read at a meeting of the College of Physicians in 1771, and published in 1778. His published works included references to his correspondence with the surgeons Francis Russel and Richard Huck on campaign in North America.[62]

Experience in military and civilian hospitals shaped the medical development of these physicians. They were responsible for large groups of men, all of whom were under their command and, apart from officers, of lower rank. Medical practice in a hospital was far different from the medical practice of those physicians catering to urban, wealthy elites. John Pringle was explicit about the opportunity provided by the experience of hospital medicine, particularly during military campaigns. During his time in Flanders during the 1740s, he wrote to Andrew Mitchell (a fellow Scot of almost the same age) that "nothing does way so much to any man's Genius as an Hospital to mine."[63] He further elaborated on how the experience of campaigning helped to shape his medical understanding and knowledge: "I have double pleasure now in reading medical books, because I can turn theory into practice, confirm from experience my former expectations or at least be sure they have not be[en] in just."[64]

Helped by mates and female nurses (usually specified as a "sober woman that has no child to carry with her"), hospital physicians had control over the diet and daily regimen of their patients.[65] The three types of diet—full, middle, and low, with a few substitutions for medical purposes—were streamlined to cope with the feeding of large numbers of patients, and boards displayed a patient's regiment, name, diet, and medicine.[66] As military physicians had large numbers of patients under their command and labored in circumstances that seemed ideal for comparisons, they experimented with methods of medical care. Similar to Pringle, Brocklesby felt that such experimentation added to the authority of his medical recommendations: "Thus I generally endeavoured (having patients enough for this intention) to make proper trials, at different times, of every likely method of cure." He thanked the hospital mates for giving his experimental ideas "a candid trial in many instances."[67]

Such practices were similar to those of other medical physicians serving in infirmaries back in Britain. Although most British civilian hospitals were charitable institutions, headed by governors and funded by subscribers, the nature of their medical practice was similar to British military hospitals, as they catered to the selected poor.[68] In civilian hospital practice, the use of streamlined diets and regimens reinforced the medical and social authority that medical practitioners had over their patients. As Mary Fissell demonstrates in her study of the Bristol Infirmary, hospital medicine was not only very different from the traditional patient-driven medical marketplace, but it also helped change the nature of medical practice and medical authority generally over the course of the eighteenth century. As she describes this change, "Patients were deskilled, denied interpretative authority over their own bodies as their interpretative roles in illness were contested by surgeons."[69] By the same token, the authority of the medical men attached to these institutions was substantially raised, as they were invested with medical expertise as well as social status.

Susan C. Lawrence agrees that the nature of the medical practitioners' authority was greatly influenced by hospitals, claiming that the medical authority of the modern medical profession was constructed through these institutions during the eighteenth and early nineteenth centuries.[70] Hospital practitioners and the medicine they advanced did not challenge the status quo, but rather should be classified as "safe" science. By their activities in a medical community that conducted itself through societies, journals, and teaching, they strove to establish their respectability and their authority as gentlemen and as practitioners. Although military medical practitioners used new approaches such as quantitative evidence to help drive medical innovations, these were not necessarily a challenge to traditional civilian medicine, but rather helped to inform its methodology.[71]

Munro and Brocklesby were clearly part of the medical elite community, and rather than challenging this circle, were comfortable using their military medical experience to join this professional elite. Although both had backgrounds that officially excluded them from Oxbridge and, thereby, should have made it difficult for them to practice medicine in London, neither suffered such professional repercussions. Brocklesby, a Quaker, established his practice in London with a degree from Leiden, and Munro practiced in London with his Edinburgh MD. Their service with the army was in no way incompatible with their civilian medical careers; it was in fact an important and valued component of their medical résumé and experience. They both also returned to military medicine after establishing their private practices; Munro served during the American War of Independence, and Brocklesby became physician general to the Ordnance in 1794.[72] This suggests that divisions between civilian and military physicians, present during the late eighteenth and early nineteenth centuries, were not yet apparent during the 1750s and 1760s.[73] Instead, not only were Dissenting physicians able to establish practices in London before serving with the army and, therefore, did not use military medicine as a last resort, but respectable medical men also easily moved between civilian and military practice, indicating no major division between these areas. The experience of military medicine during the Seven Years' War was not only key to the British campaign in Germany, but was also a coherent part of the development of medical professionalism, in terms of both expertise and social status.

POLITICS AND MANPOWER

British hospitals were not only sites of medical innovation and developing expertise during the war; they also became the focus of claims of mismanagement. The secretary at war, Viscount Barrington, wrote to the Marquis of Granby, commander in chief of the British contingent in Germany, early in 1761, "I have for some time had the mortification to hear various reports, to the disadvantage of the Hospital department in the Army under your Lordship's command." He demanded to know why those who sickened had not recovered, and what he could do about it, such as by providing more hospital supplies, more or better hospital personnel, or other remedies.[74]

Barrington's interest in the reports of high morbidity and mortality, and in low recovery rates in British hospitals, challenges the commonly accepted view that political officials were little concerned with wartime rates of disease in the army. Hamish Little, for example, claims with respect to eighteenth-century European warfare in general, and the Seven Years' War in particular, that the suffering of wounded and sick soldiers was widespread, partly because of "limited or erroneous medical knowledge" and partly because of "ruthless economies." He continues, "It seems to have been generally recognized that it was cheaper to recruit a new soldier than to attempt to cure or to rehabilitate a sick or injured one."[75] The standard histories of the Army Medical Department, as well as the standard military histories of the army in Germany, echo Little's judgment, if they mention the role of disease and medical care at all during this period.[76]

In recent years historians of medicine have examined military medicine in increasing detail and have established that hospital care for soldiers was a sophisticated and fundamental part of military activities.[77] Nevertheless, the broad military medical reform programs of the late eighteenth and early nineteenth centuries, especially the Parliamentary Enquiries and the formation of the Army Medical Board in 1793, have still misled many historians to assume that officials, and especially political officials, took no notice of troop welfare before these reform movements, except as it regarded economy.[78] Examining the papers of political authorities demonstrates, however, that they were interested in the medical care provided to troops and, significantly, that disease and the welfare of troops were part of reports and political debates on the conduct of the war.

Barrington was clearly prepared to invest more resources in the British hospital to improve the health of British soldiers. A few days after he had written to Granby, Barrington met with and was advised by the Hospital Board to obtain additional wagons for the transportation of sick men to the general hospitals and to establish more and better-furnished accommodation for convalescent soldiers. These recommendations Barrington conveyed to Granby on 9 January 1761, instructing immediate implementation.[79] The physician general Clifton Wintringham and the hospital surgeon Philip Burlton, stationed in Germany with the British Army, wrote to Barrington a few weeks later, upon Barrington's orders, providing their own summary of the problems attending the British hospitals in Germany. In their report, Wintringham and Burlton denied that the hospitals had serious problems, alluding to the hospital rates of discharge to disprove the allegation that very few soldiers had rejoined the army.[80] They did, however, admit the "well known & a melancholy truth confirm'd by the experience of all Ages, that the British Troops soon after their removal into this Climate, become very sickly, & that many of them die."[81] Yet they defended the reputation of the medical services by blaming the provisioning and staffing of the hospital for the men's distresses.[82]

Barrington was not satisfied with this explanation. Although he does not seem to have responded directly to Wintringham and Burlton, he wrote to Granby, clearly exasperated. Barrington's response reveals that there was no doubt in his mind that suggestions from the medical practitioners would be seriously considered, if not immediately implemented. He considered himself a responsible and responsive statesman, one who would not only remedy any problem concerning hospitals as soon as it arose, but also had the good of the service in mind, and not just the furthering of his own personal ends:

> Surely no Complaints as to these defects reached your Lordship, for it does not appear they were remedied on your side [of] the Water & certainly were not represented on this. The least intimation to me would have produced an immediate recall of whoever was thought insufficient for his Office, and the utmost care & diligence would have been used in sending over such as both *in number and qualifications*, would have been sufficient for the Service required of them. . . . My utmost diligence shall be exerted to forward whatever you deem expedient for this most useful and compassionate part of the Service. . . . All those employed in that branch were recommended by the Hospital Board here, and were never protected by me farther than they appeared deserving.[83]

Barrington's correspondence is notable for two reasons. First, it shows that he felt compelled to respond to the rates of sickness and reports from officers concerning the state of the troops. Not only did reports excite his concern, but he also solicited advice on possible solutions from medical men, both those on the Hospital Board and those serving with the troops in Germany. He then implemented their recommendations on personnel and supplies, both of which required spending substantial sums of money. His correspondence suggests not that he was goaded into such action, but rather that he initiated improvements and preempted Cabinet decisions.[84] His sense that he was directly responsible for the state of the armed forces is evident in his correspondence. Barrington was particularly annoyed by any suggestion that he might have placed unsuitable men in the service of the army for reasons of personal preferment. Similarly, Barrington appears to have done his utmost to prevent the sale of posts, specifically those of regimental surgeons.[85] In Barrington's view of the medical corps in the army, men advanced through merit, rather than through political connections or wealth.

Second, Barrington's correspondence demonstrates that he was well aware of the state of British troops. In a letter of February 1761 to Thomas Pelham-Holles, Duke of Newcastle and minister of finances from 1757 to 1762, regarding the raising of more troops, Barrington used army returns to establish that out of the 19,609 British soldiers in Germany, 5,596—29 percent—were sick.[86] Barrington candidly noted to Newcastle that "the usual computation is, that two thirds of the sick will recover, so as to serve again next Campaign," the remaining one-third added to those wanting to complete regiments to full strength, taking account of those who would die before campaigning recommenced.[87] Barrington's letters reveal that obtaining and processing knowledge of rates of sickness, rates of recovery, and their impact on forces available to fight was an integral and crucial part of his common duties as a secretary at war.

Knowledge about rates of health and sickness among troops was gathered through what officials called "returns." Although military commanders often described the state of troops under their commend in their official correspondence, most frequently they cited numerical information on troops' effectiveness by making reference to what the returns stated, while also sending such returns back to central authorities. Military returns had been in use since at least the early eighteenth century, when George I used them to establish the state of British land forces upon his accession.[88] During the Seven Years' War, returns were collected on a monthly and sometimes also weekly basis, and could be filled out on preprinted standardized forms. By 1758, the publisher J. Millan advertised blank forms for "Returns Weekly, Monthly, and General" available for sale, along with other military and naval-related texts.[89] Returns were thus not a development of the Seven Years' War, though it appears that their regularity, particularly concerning regiments stationed overseas, coalesced in this period. Although a "return" or a "monthly return" could refer to any sort of regular numerical account, by the later eighteenth century "monthly return" appears in published texts almost exclusively with reference to military matters, and most notably when Parliament demanded detailed and accurate reports of troop strength.[90]

Returns differed from muster rolls, although one could be used to complete missing information in the other. Musters and their accompanying rolls or reports were designed to establish the exact funds due to an officer for his troops. This was accomplished through a review carried out by a civilian official, who then reported directly to the Crown, itemizing every officer and man. Muster rolls were thus the basis for the financial administration of each troop unit, including baggage, clothing, and weapons. As a result, muster rolls usually consisted of long lists of names of troops, along with dates of enlistment. Under George I and continuing under George II, reforms were instituted that attempted to regularize musters, including ending the practice of false or inaccurate musters that had traditionally been used to compensate officers and companies for unreliable or delayed pay, along with other contingencies. After the reform of mustering orders in 1747, musters were to take place at the more realistic and lesser frequency of twice a year, although even this was not achieved during the Seven Years' War, and particularly when troops were stationed overseas.[91] Reviews of troops, which were likewise made more regular under George I, were concerned with establishing discipline among them, inspecting a corps for drill uniformity.[92] Musters and reviews were thus infrequently conducted—usually from once to twice a year—and their accompanying reports took the form of detailed lists or qualitative descriptions.

By contrast, monthly and weekly returns provided a brief and numerical overview of the troop strength of units, broken down by regiment, usually taking up a half page to one large page at most. As a result, personal characteristics about troops, such as names or ages, were left out. Returns were predominantly quantitative, providing numbers of men under category headings. During the Seven Years' War, the usual categories for rank-and-file troops were fit for duty, sick in camp (or garrison or barracks), sick in hospital, and then variations on categories, such as absent, on command, on guard, recruiting, and prisoner with the enemy. Also often included were categories such as killed, wounded, missing, and dead (referring to death from nonbattle causes). Returns thus provided tabular and easily digestible quantitative information on the current state of manpower (see fig. 3.1).

Officials, both civil and military, were aware of the usefulness of returns. According to a House of Commons committee investigating the state of the army and marines in 1746, muster rolls were deemed "of no use at all" in determining the strength of regiments, whereas returns were requested, as these documents were "from whence only the Number of real effective Men can possibly be known."[93] Moreover, military officials paid close attention to returns, remarking on and inquiring into discrepancies. When Lieutenant General George Townshend sent in inconsistent returns

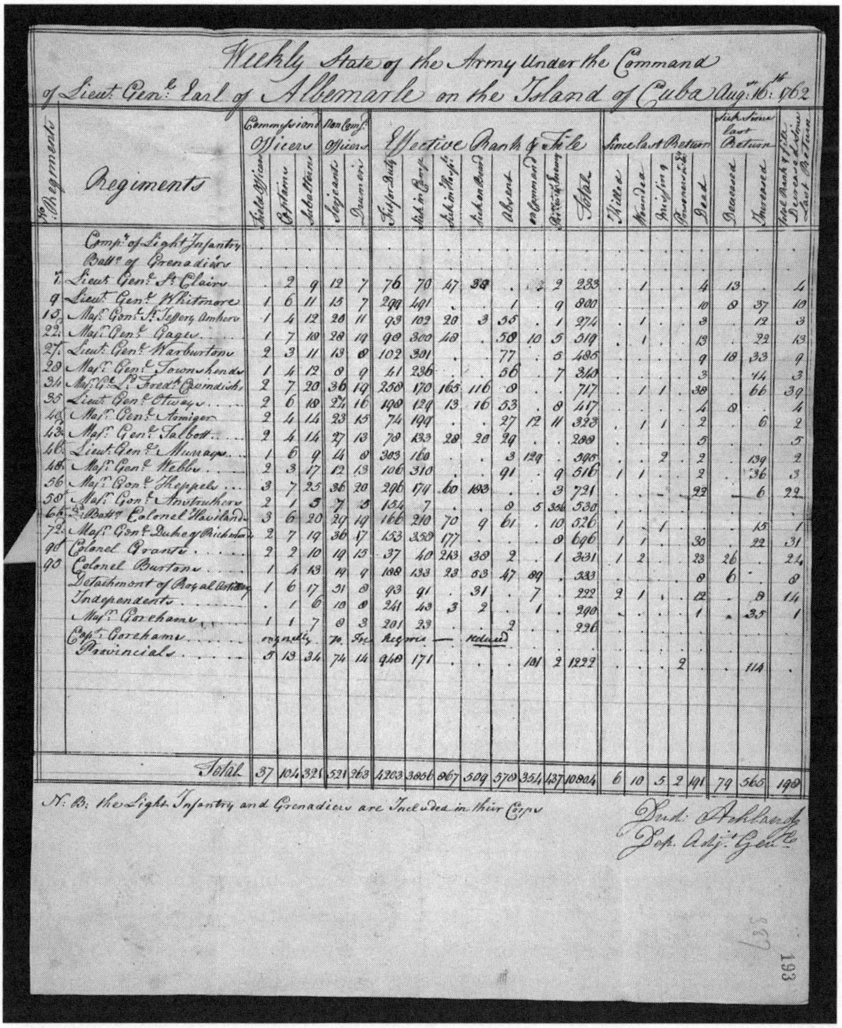

Weekly State of the Army Under the Command of Lieut. Genl. Earl of Albemarle on the Island of Cuba Aug. 16th 1762

No. Regiments	Regiments	Commissioned Officers: Field Officers	Captains	Subalterns	Non Comd. Officers: Serjeants	Drummers	Effective Rank & File: Fit for Duty	Sick in Camp	Sick in Hospital	Sick on Board	Absent	on Command	Prisoners with Enemy	Total	Since last Return: Killed	Wounded	Missing	Prisoners	Dead	Sick Since last Return: Deceased	Increased	Total Rank & File Decreased since Last Return
	Compy. of Light Infantry	.	.	.	.	.	.	.	.	.	.	.	.	.	.	.	.	.	.	.	.	.
	Battn. of Grenadiers	.	.	.	.	.	.	.	.	.	.	.	.	.	.	.	.	.	.	.	.	.
7.	Lieut. Genl. St. Clair	.	2	9	12	7	76	70	47	38	.	2	9	233	.	1	.	.	4	13	.	4
9	Lieut. Genl. Whitmore	1	6	11	15	7	299	491	.	.	1	.	9	800					10	8	37	10
15.	Maj. Genl. Sr. Jeffery Amherst	1	4	12	20	11	93	102	20	3	55	.	1	274	.	1	.	.	3	.	12	3
22.	Maj. Genl. Gage	1	7	18	28	19	98	300	48	.	58	10	5	519	.	1	.	.	13	.	22	13
27.	Lieut. Genl. Warburton	2	3	11	13	8	102	301	.	.	77	.	5	485	.	.	.	.	9	18	33	9
28	Maj. Genl. Townshend	1	4	12	8	9	41	236	.	.	56	.	7	340	.	.	.	.	3	.	44	3
34	Maj. Gl. Ld. Fredk. Cavendish	2	7	20	36	19	258	170	165	116	8	.	.	717	.	1	1	.	38	.	66	39
35	Lieut. Genl. Otway	2	6	18	24	16	198	129	13	16	53	.	8	417	.	.	.	.	4	8	.	4
40	Maj. Genl. Amiger	2	4	14	23	15	74	199	.	.	27	12	11	328	.	1	1	.	2	.	6	2
43.	Maj. Genl. Talbott	2	4	14	27	13	78	133	28	20	29	.	.	288	.	.	.	.	5	.	.	5
46.	Lieut. Genl. Murray	1	6	9	14	8	303	160	.	.	3	129	.	595	.	.	2	.	2	.	139	2
48.	Maj. Genl. Webb	2	3	17	12	13	106	310	.	.	91	.	9	516	1	1	.	.	2	.	36	3
56	Maj. Genl. Keppel	3	7	25	36	20	296	179	60	183	.	.	3	721	.	.	–	.	22	–	6	22
58th	Maj. Genl. Anstruther	2	1	5	7	5	154	7	.	.	8	5	356	530	.	.	.	.	.	.	.	.
60.	3d Battn. Colonel Haviland	3	6	20	29	19	166	210	70	9	61	.	10	526	1	.	1	.	.	.	15	1
72.	Maj. Genl. Duke of Richmond	2	7	19	36	17	153	358	177	.	.	.	8	696	1	1	.	.	30	.	22	31
90	Colonel Grant	2	2	10	19	15	37	40	213	38	2	.	1	331	1	2	.	.	23	26	.	24
95	Colonel Burton	1	4	13	19	9	188	133	23	53	47	89	.	333	.	.	.	.	8	6	.	8
	Detachment of Royal Artillery	1	6	17	31	8	93	91	.	31	.	7	.	222	2	1	.	.	12	.	8	14
	Independents	.	1	6	10	8	241	43	3	2	.	1	.	290	.	.	.	.	1	.	35	1
	Maj. Goreham	1	1	7	8	3	201	23	.	.	2	.	.	226	.	.	.	.	.	.	.	.
	Capt. Goreham	originally			70.	Fr.	Regimt.	—		Relieved												
	Provincials	5	13	34	74	14	948	171	.	.	.	181	2	1222	.	.	.	2	.	.	114	.
	Total	37	104	321	521	263	4203	3856	867	509	570	354	437	10804	6	10	5	2	191	79	565	198

N: B: the Light Infantry and Grenadiers are Included in their Corps

Dud: Ackland
Dep. Adjt. Genl.

193

Figure 3.1. Return, "Weekly State of the Army under the Command of Lieut. Earl of Albemarle on the Island of Cuba Aug 16th 1762," TNA, WO 34/55, fols. 192–93.

while on command in Germany in 1761, Lieutenant General Howard not only noticed the irregularity, but followed up on it, writing to Townshend: "This affair is indeed of infinite consequence. . . . It certainly is impossible any Officer can knowingly be guilty of a false return, but such a thing does sometimes happen *inadvertently* and from some mistake which is easily set to rights."[94] Returns were thus reliable, regular, and usually frequent sources of quantitative knowledge about British manpower. It is not surprising that they informed Secretary at War Barrington's decisions regarding recruitment and strategy.

It is significant that by the time of the Seven Years' War, these reports on manpower were regularly recorded and sent, even from overseas. Military officers regularly made reference to returns accompanying their correspondence, and existing returns for British forces in the American colonies, the West Indies, Europe, and India demonstrate that garrisons and campaigns in all locations recorded and sent back regular returns during the Seven Years' War. Unfortunately for historians, few of these overseas returns survive: only scattered returns regarding individual campaigns or regiments have been identified in the archives, far less than the 50 percent survival of returns traced by Tabitha Marshall for British forces in North America during the American War of Independence.[95] As a result, no accurate estimate can be made about overall rates of health or illness based on these returns, although isolated runs of surviving returns can provide a snapshot of individual campaigns, such as in the case of Quebec in 1759–60 and Havana in 1762.

Among European colonial powers, Britain appears to be unique in its use of returns.[96] French military and colonial records include regular monthly lists of troops (muster rolls) and detailed hospital admission records, but these do not provide accessible quantitative information on manpower. Instead, troops are listed by name, often including individual details such as a soldier's hometown or his year of enlistment. As a result, French historians have been able to track detailed biographical information regarding French soldiers serving overseas during the Seven Years' War.[97] But this also means that general quantitative knowledge, such as how many French troops were sick at one time, is difficult to ascertain.[98] This would also have been the case for contemporary French officials. As a result, British officials, whether deciding on tactics during campaigns or, like Barrington, formulating policy and strategy, were exceptionally well-informed about rates of British manpower. Thus, when Newcastle demanded a reckoning of the state of the army, an officer responded that "Lord Ligonier can best do it from his returns."[99]

Secretary at War Barrington, as already noted, used returns not only to establish the current quantitative state of British manpower in Germany, but also to predict sickness and recovery rates and thus to determine future recruitment. Likewise, military officials used returns to identify trends in sickness and justify logistical decisions to their superiors, such as moving camp or modifying supplies. As commander in chief of forces in North

America, Amherst regularly mentions and comments on the monthly returns in his correspondence with Barrington, remarking in 1760, for example, "Your Lordship will have known by the Returns, the great number of men wanted to compleat this Army'[100] Lower down in the military hierarchy, Albemarle reported to Amherst from Havana, "You will see by comparing the enclosed returns that I have fully complied with His Majestys Instructions."[101] At the local level, commanders used returns during campaigns; during the 1759 Martinique and Guadeloupe campaign, both Hopson and Major General Barrington used returns during councils of war and in deciding on tactics.[102] Contemporaries, like historians, appear to have been unaware that returns were not used by the French, and so did not offer reflections on their unparalleled usefulness. Yet it is clear that they provided a form of quantitative expertise regarding manpower rates that was particularly useful when coordinating campaigns conducted in multiple overseas theaters.

Although returns mostly likely originated as a method to assess and control military expenditure and were further developed under the direction of the Crown, it is not surprising that their use and application were extended in eighteenth-century Britain. As historians have noted, the nature of the eighteenth-century British Parliament and the growth of the fiscal-military state encouraged the development of arithmetical techniques for governance.[103] John Brewer, for example, points out that eighteenth-century British statesmen increasingly required the expertise of skill in numbers and calculation.[104] Building on earlier practices such as bookkeeping, political arithmetic provided both the tools and rationale for what the seventeenth-century government official Charles Davenant described as "the art of reasoning by figures, upon things relating to government."[105] The writings of William Petty, Gregory King, and Joseph Massie were all indicative of this view that the workings of the state could and should be enumerated, and that quantitative information ought to serve as a guide to policy.

Given that the settlements and procedures of the 1680s and 1690s increased parliamentary control over and interest in military figures, it makes sense that returns—as detailed and accurate reports on the actual number of British forces—became both more regular and a form of public information in this period. Public information, as eighteenth-century contemporaries understood it, was not defined through widespread accessibility, but was rather more akin to universal knowledge: information that was unconcealed and impartial. Numerical data on the "real" state (unlike muster rolls) of the armed forces fit perfectly within this understanding.

Parliament not only demanded detailed numerical information regarding the armed forces out of financial interest, but also scrutinized figures through the use of returns during times of debate. For example, returns were requested in 1757 in response to Admiral John Byng's failure and subsequent court-martial.[106] Returns were also requested and discussed during the American War of Independence, the Duke of Richmond asking for them more than once, noting that "in times like these, the nation has a right to be informed of the true state of its affairs, and Parliament being the regular and authentic channel of such information, it is the duty of Parliament to give it."[107]

In his requests, Richmond explained that returns would provide "the exact number deficient or lost, by death, wounds, captivity, sickness, or desertion" among the armed forces.[108] Given that sickness was the major cause of noneffectiveness among forces, returns thereby provided exceptionally detailed quantitative knowledge on rates of health and illness in the army and navy. Not surprisingly, medical practitioners increasingly made use of returns to assess and reform medicine within the armed forces over the course of the eighteenth century. For example, the naval physician Gilbert Blane noted, in his 1785 *Observations on the Diseases Incident to Seamen*, that both he and the commander in chief used monthly returns not only for detailed knowledge on rates and types of sickness, but also "to recommend such articles of diet, or other means, as might tend to cure them, or to check their progress."[109] Returns, although initially and predominantly about military figures, were thus increasingly used as medical and health resources.[110]

Moreover, the structure of this knowledge—as numerical data—shaped the nature of medical investigations. Although historians of medicine recognize that the context of the armed forces encouraged the development of modern scientific methods of clinical medicine, including quantitative approaches, Ulrich Tröhler has convincingly demonstrated that such methods first developed in Britain. Given that returns were a uniquely Anglo-German approach to military manpower during this period, this structure of British military reporting helps to explain the development of new methodological approaches within eighteenth-century British medicine.[111]

Military returns thus fit comfortably within the eighteenth-century notion of "useful knowledge." Shaped by Baconian ideals and the Royal Society, it was tied to ideas of improvement, whether of human welfare or the wealth of nations, and thereby also frequently contrasted with mere speculation, abstract theory, or other forms of fruitless investigation. Grounded in empirical approaches to understanding the world, useful knowledge was touted as both practical and polite: "a category of knowledge, not necessarily of immediate value to those who acquired it, but having the potential to be deployed usefully."[112] Indeed, historians such as Margaret Jacob and Joel Mokyr have seen eighteenth-century Britain's adeptness at useful knowledge as pivotal for Britain's Industrial Revolution.[113] In other words, although collecting returns did not produce immediately tangible advances, they were demonstrably practical in the short term and significantly useful in the long term. By both fostering and being a product of numerical expertise in the realm of politics and medicine, army returns were part of what Joanna Innes has called the state's statistics of power.[114]

PUBLIC OPINION, PARTISAN POLITICS, AND DISEASE

As a quantitative form of manpower knowledge, returns were akin to vital statistics and other forms of political arithmetic concerned with counting and increasing population. Moreover, the vigor (or lack thereof) of the general population and the methods with which this should be evaluated were discussed and debated at length in Britain's growing public sphere. The health of the nation, and especially its laboring classes, was enumerated through Bills of Mortality in major urban centers during this period, while new medical practices, such as inoculation, were also numerically evaluated. Contemporaries considered population as the base for the wealth of nations, and eighteenth-century commentators constantly feared that populations were declining, rather than increasing. A growing population would augment trade, manufacture, and thereby commerce and progress in general, while also supplying more men for military service and greater tax revenues. Historians have demonstrated that such views persisted throughout the eighteenth century and, not surprisingly, were related to the development of medical statistics and concerns about the health of the nation, as well as broader concerns regarding the moral state of the nation.[115] In times of war, such concerns over population were especially marked, and particularly when Britain confronted France, which had nearly three times Britain's population by the 1750s.[116]

John Brown's widely read treatise, *An Estimate of the Manners and Principles of the Times*, relied on the maxim that a strong and large population was the basis for a strong and powerful nation. First published in 1757, Brown's work ran through seven printings within one year. Brown's chastisement of British commercially induced luxury and effeminacy was timely, as many struggled to find reasons for the loss of Minorca and defeats in North America, as well as the reliance on foreign troops to repel a feared French invasion. According to Brown's analysis, it was Britain's "exorbitant degree of trade and wealth" that had weakened the entire society, through its bad effect on manners, which "seems to have fitted us for a Prey to the Insults and Invasions of our most powerful Enemy."[117] Brown charged that Britain was demonstrably weaker as a result of trade and commerce, not only because the nation's population had allegedly declined over the previous fifty years (as evinced by parish records), but also because the population was physically weaker due to intemperance and diseases common in commercial urban centers. As a result, Britain's military and naval strength necessarily suffered, especially in comparison with that of France. Yet all was not lost, as Brown concluded that the political and physical strength of a nation could be reformed under proper leadership that not only checked and controlled commerce and trade, but would also coerce the nation into a more correct mode of living.[118]

Like Brown, political theorists such as Montesquieu, Rousseau, and Hume argued that it was the nature of government that determined population size and strength: good government resulted in population growth, while "depopulation became an accepted sign of despotism."[119] The vigorous debates on how exactly the strength of the nation should be enumerated and evaluated, as well as whether such quantitative data evinced a declining or increasing population, were thus discussed within the assumption that the state was responsible for the strength of its population and expected to intervene in such matters.[120] For example, John Bellers's *An Essay towards the Improvement of Physick* argued for parliamentary intervention in British medicine on the basis of financial calculations on the life of each laborer (and his offspring) thereby saved.[121] The lower orders, whether laborers, sailors, or soldiers, were thus widely recognized as integral to Britain's power as a great commercial and maritime empire, and good officials were those who would encourage their physical and moral growth. In this context, the health and welfare of troops were of direct political significance to the British nation. Donald Munro recognized the importance of this concern, noting in the preface to his work on military medicine:

> In a commercial country like our own, where numbers of hands are constantly wanted for the carrying on our Manufactories, we have a strong political Argument to add to that drawn from the Dictates of Humanity why the life of every individual should be most carefully attended to.[122]

Such concerns were at the heart of eighteenth-century philanthropic endeavors. Voluntary hospitals and charitable societies for foundlings such as Jonas Hanway's Marine Society combined Christian morality with a patriotic desire to improve the health and welfare of the lower orders, thereby safeguarding and increasing the British nation's key resource. War was an effective impetus for the foundation of these societies, and the Seven Years' War particularly so. In 1756, Hanway commented, "The nation is upon a trial of experiments, and it is a noble and useful, not a wanton trial; and the more necessary, as war consumes our people."[123] Hanway's Marine Society, established in 1756, is a salient example of how concerns over the strength of the nation in times of war coincided with charitable considerations regarding the health and welfare of the lower classes and troops. The Marine Society took responsibility for young boys who otherwise, it was feared, would waste away or become criminals on the streets of London, turning them instead into responsible Christian sailors, productive members of the nation's struggle against France.[124] Such charity, and the moral and religious example it set, would ensure the continued success of British troops, the British Empire, and British manufacturing and commerce. Hanway described God as "the *sovereign disposer of empires, and the great arbiter of the fate of nations*," warning his readers in 1760, "If we expect a continuance of success, and hope to reap any *national advantages* by our victories, we *must* show our virtue as a *nation*."[125] Moral, religious, and humanitarian motives were thus fused with practical and patriotic concerns.

As Hanway demonstrated in his praise of two military leaders in Germany, Prince Ferdinand and the Marquis of Granby, these men were admired not only because of their military prowess, but also by reason of their humanitarian virtues. Both were known for considering the well-being of their troops, Granby giving his men £1,200 out of his private accounts. According to Hanway, what made these men great in the eyes of their troops and of the British people was not only valor, but also the attention they paid to the welfare of their men.[126] Conversely, troops suffering from disease, especially if alleged to have been caused by improper management and provisioning, were a sign of irresponsible political and military leadership, faults that could lead to battlefield reverses for a commander.

Thus, in Britain's public sphere, whether traced through published texts or charitable associations, the strength of the population—particularly of thc lower orders—was considered a key political concern. Political and military leaders were held responsible for the strength of the nation, especially through due attention to health and welfare. During national periods of crisis, such as war, these concerns were sharpened and more frequently articulated. For these reasons, the loss of manpower during campaigns, and particularly through disease, was a vital political issue.

Discussions of the loss of manpower were also part of a broader debate on the merits of British involvement in Continental affairs. Opposition politicians, or those that can be loosely called "Tory" or "patriot," advocated what historians such as Daniel A. Baugh have termed a "blue-water" policy. Tories held that Britain's defense depended on naval command of European waters and that Britain's wealth and power resided in colonial and maritime commerce, rather than in an empire of territorial dominion.[127] Thus, they called for a foreign policy that was "essentially defensive in Europe (and European waters) and aggressive overseas. Overseas aggressiveness was aimed at enlarging the maritime and commercial base of England's naval power while at the same time reducing that of actual or potential enemies."[128]

Skepticism regarding Continental involvement was necessarily part of such a strategy. Not only did the Whig commitment to maintaining a balance of power in Europe require deficits and taxes on the consumer goods that the poor and middling classes relied on, but also opposition politicians such as Pitt made involvement in colonial affairs instead of European campaigns a matter of principle and patriotism. As Shebbeare had characterized it in his pamphlet against a Continental campaign, the American colonies were considered the natural progeny of Britain, while Hanover and the German provinces were foreign and unnatural burdens, a position that easily buttressed popular nationalistic and xenophobic sentiments. Trade with the American colonies, especially the West Indies, was seen to—and indeed did—provide much of Britain's commercial wealth, whereas the German dominions appeared to cost the nation much.[129]

Critics charged that Continental warfare was costly, not only in terms of subsidies, but also in terms of lives of men who otherwise could be contributing to the wealth and strength of the nation, either by protecting its overseas colonies or by laboring at home. In a best-selling and influential pamphlet, Israel Mauduit claimed:

> The resources of our enemies are infinite. France exceeds Great Britain in the number of its people, and by the nature of its government, is able to send out as many of its subjects to its military services, as their King shall be pleased to order: and besides its own superior resources, France has Switzerland, Italy, Germany, and Flanders to recruit out

> of. What has England to oppose to all these? Nothing but the bodies of its own subjects, which can very ill be spared from its agriculture and manufactures, and the levies from the districts of Hanover and Hesse. . . . Can England then, by its money alone, be a match for all Europe? Money may, in a qualified sense, be allowed to be the sinews of war; but it must find men to make up the flesh and substance of our armies, which, in the present state of Europe is impossible.[130]

Other critics of the Continental campaign concurred, repeatedly emphasizing the loss of manpower in Germany occasioned by both the climate and lack of provisions. Since these affected French as well as British soldiers, one anonymous critic counseled that pulling out from Germany would save the lives of many British soldiers while leading to the death of many French soldiers forced to garrison Hanover, concluding "upon the whole, the wisest thing we could do, would be to save our own people by transporting them back to England, and leaving our enemies to rot in this rotten country."[131]

It was common to remark that in Germany more lives were lost because of the harsh climate and conditions there, and especially because of the mismanagement of provisions, than were lost in battle.[132] Mauduit demonstrated how disease and mismanagement in Germany were directly linked to the loss of national strength at home. He polemically compared British and French policy, noting that more populous France easily raised an army of 200,000 even in peacetime, allied with "Saxon, Wirtemberg, and other corps, *natives of Germany, and inured to the food and climate of that country.*" Britain, with its smaller population and its demand for agricultural and manufacturing laborers, could not do the same. Comparing Britain with France, Manduit rhetorically asked, "Which country can best afford to send its subjects to cut each others throats, or rot in the hospitals of Germany?'[133] As critics repeatedly stated, Germany was a sickly environment for British troops, with its foreign climate and foreign food, and alongside problems with provisioning, it was an especially expensive campaign in terms of finances and manpower. In the sphere of public opinion, disease was used to bolster the unpopularity of the Continental campaign and articulate its problems, particularly its cost to national manpower. The *Annual Register* summarized affairs in Germany during 1760, and remarked that British troops and horses were ill-supplied, concluding:

> Whatever were the causes of this scarcity; it was bitterly felt by the troops, and was accompanied by diseases which thinned them ex-

> tremely. This raised a general discontent in the army, which was speedily communicated to England, where the people . . . did not confine their complaints to the conduct of the war, but began to fall into an almost general dislike of the very system upon which it was pursued. Much of the old dispute between the naval and continental schemes was renewed; and enforced with many additional topics.[134]

Complaints regarding official ill-management of German campaigns became especially prominent in 1761, when British officers home on furlough spread reports of disease and poor supplies. Newcastle impatiently inquired of military officials stationed in Germany whether the complaints were true, and requested that they be silenced. He wrote to Granby, "It is incredible what mischief [British officers on furlough] have done by their Imprudent Discourse. . . . The Distress of the Army is universally talk'd of, & their want almost of every thing, and the decrease of their numbers is likewise much observed upon."[135]

Newcastle's concern was not only over public disapproval; he and other British officials were worried that such reports made them politically vulnerable and strained relations with Prince Ferdinand. In January 1761, Newcastle thanked Colonel Yorke for publishing a report in the main Dutch newspaper that assured readers that British troops were well provisioned and happy under the leadership of the prince. In February 1761, Newcastle included, under the heading "Measures to be taken for war, or peace," efforts to put a stop to the negative reports about Prince Ferdinand and the Commissariat.[136] By April, Newcastle faced a Parliamentary Enquiry into the Commissariat and the Treasury, alongside the demands of John Stuart, Third Earl of Bute, to end the war on the Continent. Newcastle directed Barrington to write a narrative on the Commissariat and the Treasury for the Enquiry, showing that the Treasury had judiciously managed the public funds and the army's supplies.[137]

In Barrington's narrative, the complaints were organized under eight headings, including the ill management of hospitals. While Barrington rebutted this complaint by asserting that the hospitals were not under the direct supervision of the Commissariat or the Treasury, the other points were not so easily refuted. Barrington and British officials stationed in Germany did not deny that troops wanted provisions and forage and, thereby, suffered from disease while on campaign. Rather, they denied that the improvement of these conditions was within their power. Barrington and Newcastle noted that the Treasury had granted regular monthly sums of over £150,000 for army supplies and that reports of peculation could not be substantiated.[138] They concluded that the physical and logistical difficulties of campaigning in Germany were to blame, specifically a lack of navigable waterways by which to provide supplies and forage. Moreover, the countryside was regarded as agriculturally poor, and was soon entirely destroyed by years of continual warfare and unusually long campaigning seasons.[139]

Modern historians give credence to Newcastle's conclusion. They point out that no firm evidence of corruption in the Commissariat exists and that the main problem was the nature of the war itself—the long duration of the campaigning season, armies stationed in small, agriculturally underdeveloped areas for six years, and the rapid marches and movements of troops while on campaign. All of these were unusual characteristics that did not plague British forces when on campaign in Germany during the wars of the 1730s and 1740s.[140] Officials provided for the welfare of troops, despite extravagant costs, but they also recognized that under the circumstances of German campaigns during the Seven Years' War, much was largely beyond their control.

That concerns over troop welfare were also partisan concerns was admitted. Devonshire, for example, believed Pitt wanted an Enquiry into the Commissariat only as a way to criticize Newcastle.[141] As secret negotiations for peace with French officials opened at this time, while Bute and others were calling for an end to the Continental alliance, any criticism of the conduct of European campaigns was also criticism of the ministry. When writing to Ferdinand after the Enquiry was completed, Newcastle fully acknowledged this precarious situation, explaining that he had not written until Commissariat affairs were more settled, as "the war in Germany is not approved or supported by many among us, & the strongest & most affecting reason they give against the continuance of it, arises from the enormity & daily increase of its expence."[142]

Political concern with troop welfare was also indirectly demonstrated by the censorship that officials enforced of the reporting on campaigns. While the exact mechanisms of this censorship and the degree of control over reporting are difficult to ascertain, it is clear that censorship of letters and reports was common.[143] When Admiral Byng was court-martialed in 1756 and 1757, and subsequently executed, one of the many issues discussed in the public sphere was the modification of Byng's dispatch. The censorship of key words and phrases in the published version of Byng's dispatch, including sickness among his crew, served to disparage his actions and advantage the ministry, demonstrating that the ministry commonly practiced censorship of military relations.[144] An anonymous pamphlet arguing for the removal of British troops from Europe not only described those troops as "rotting by peacemeal [*sic*] in the wilds of Germany," but also asked:

> Are we to imagine, because we do not hear the groans, perhaps the reproaches, of our starving, slaughtered, expiring countrymen, in Westphalia, that none such are vented? Because, perhaps by the rigid rules of war and politics, the complaints of the survivors do not come to our ears; because the military law does not even admit of such complaints being either published in the camp, or transpiring into the public, can we imagine they do not exist?[145]

Correspondence from military and naval officials was frequently censored, allowing political officials a degree of control over what reports of campaigns reached the public. Captain George Rodney at Portsmouth wrote to George Grenville in 1757, "As I find the Post Office has thought proper to detain the letters that were sent from the officers of the Fleet employed on the late expedition, I fear those I did myself the honour to write to you have met with the same fate."[146] Military officer Sir John Irwine complained of these same censorship measures in a letter to George Sackville, after the second British attempt on the coast of France. He castigated the military leadership of the campaign for trying to procure "for us a more flattering and favourable paragraph . . . in the Gazzette," rather than planning an attack with a sensible strategy. Irwine noted not only that the report published in the *London Gazette* (the official government paper, and that from which other London papers received foreign and military news) reduced the actual number of killed and wounded, but that he was unable to write to Sackville any earlier as all communication from the army had been disallowed by officials for fear of what it might have said concerning the failed attack. Irwine explained:

> If I had wrote, my letter never would have reached you. We have for some time past been treated like people guilty of high treason, we have not only been confined, but in effect debarred the use of pen, ink, and paper; for the two last expresses that left the fleet carried only the General's and Commodore's letters, notwithstanding people gave assurances that their letters contained no news, only accounts of their health, yet these assurances had no weight.[147]

Such control over correspondence demonstrates that officials were well aware of and concerned about the role of public opinion, especially with respect to the condition of troops. The health and welfare of the troops was an integral part of debates concerning the conduct of the Seven Years' War. As political theory and national debates held officials responsible for troop health, and also directly linked the welfare of troops to the strength of the nation, disease among troops was politically explosive. This was especially true for the campaigns in Germany, which were generally unpopular and vulnerable to criticism from opposition politicians, and in which disease among troops was linked to poor provisioning and irresponsible governance. Indeed, because the health of British troops became a topic of political debates and a cause of public disaffection, reports about it were decreed worthy of official censorship.

The campaigns in Germany during the war demonstrate the workings of early modern medical military practice in its traditional forms. Typhus and dysentery, the common crowd diseases of the eighteenth century, had more to do with proper provisioning and management than with any specific medical treatment. The concern with supplies, camp order, and military discipline were directly related to sanitation and health concerns more generally. Once ill, soldiers were immediately sent to hospitals, which also required careful management. Military hospitals were criticized by both medical and political officials during the war, while the secretary at war was responsive to such criticism and was willing to follow the advice proffered by medical army men. Yet executive and legislative reforms of hospitals and other institutions long recognized as sites of crowd diseases were not effected until the later 1770s, when they were encouraged by individuals such as John Howard, alongside broader changes in the role of these institutions. Despite Barrington's efforts, British troops did suffer from disease while in Germany, and even the medical men attached to the hospitals recognized that these institutions bred and spread disease. They understood what needed to change in order to make hospitals more salubrious, and orders given by military administrators demonstrate that medical advice on hospital administration was taken into account. By the same token, orders and instructions relating to the regulation of army camps also demonstrate that officers strove to improve sanitation and that, when these orders were followed, the health of the troops improved. By June 1761, a British official reported to Grenville that, according to returns of the army in Germany, the number of sick had decreased to 12,000—or 13 percent—with a prospective sick rate a third of that.[148]

The rates of sickness during the early 1760s do not necessarily demonstrate that officials had not learned from previous experience in Germany. When responding to reports of sickness among troops in Germany during the early 1760s, officials explained that this campaign was more difficult than previous ones in German countries and, hence, more prone to disruption due to disease and disorder. Pringle's famous work on military hospitals, full of suggestions on how to improve the salubriousness of these institutions, was written as a result of his experience of campaigns in Germany during the War of Austrian Succession. Cumberland's Military Papers from the 1740s and the 1750s include Pringle's detailed and handwritten recommendations for improving military hospitals. As it was under Cumberland and Barrington that a hospital board of military medical officials was first established in 1756, it is clear that Cumberland took Pringle's advice seriously and applied it to his second campaign in Germany, that of the Seven Years' War. The measures taken by officials in this war to try to reduce rates of sickness among British troops were not novel, although the experience of disease during campaigns and the nature of military medicine contributed to new developments in British medicine over the course of the eighteenth century. In other words, although administrative change was effected and lessons learned from previous wars were applied, there were no particular novel medical techniques or tangible innovations as a result of the German campaigns. Rather than looking for decisive changes in medicine during this period, it is more useful—and accurate—to see a gradual transformation in the development of eighteenth-century medicine through the frequent experience of warfare.

Moreover, this approach shows how the medical expertise developed in military contexts helped to encourage innovations in domestic, civilian medicine. Military medicine was an integral part of British civilian medicine, as demonstrated in the careers of individual military medical practitioners. Eighteenth-century medicine was shaped by the experience of campaign diseases and military hospital medicine: an increasing focus on the health of the general population, particularly through preventative techniques and institutional approaches to crowd diseases such as typhus and dysentery; increasing use of quantitative methods to frame disease categories and medical practice; and the increasing use of empirical methodology were all eighteenth-century medical developments that can be traced, in part, to the nature of military medicine in Europe during the Seven Years' War.

By the same token, European military medicine demonstrates striking similarities to colonial medicine in this period. Particularly as Germany was described as a foreign climate with a foreign diet, causing sickliness among newly arrived British troops, campaigns in Germany sound remarkably analogous to colonial campaigns during the war. In Prussia, for example, besides combat casualties, the war caused a shortage of laborers, harvest failures, and epidemics, resulting in the loss of 10 percent of its total population.[149] The descriptions of British military officers and medical personnel stationed in Germany during the war, commenting on the spread of disease and the famine brought in its wake, lends credence to such estimates. Warfare in Europe was therefore similar in many respects to colonial warfare: it too was beset with logistical difficulties and high rates of sickness and mortality. Indeed, as this chapter demonstrates, European and colonial warfare were similarly described and experienced by British contemporaries: conducted in sickly and foreign environments, both exhausted finances and military forces, and posed both physical and political dangers.

The nature of British politics and of the British press in the eighteenth century meant that manpower was carefully scrutinized by both the public and political officials. Given the debates over foreign policy concerning the Continent and the broader context of political arithmetic, reports of sickness among troops became ammunition in political arguments. Barrington's actions to remedy problems in the military hospital, Newcastle's concern regarding the Enquiry into the Commissariat, and official censorship of campaign reports demonstrate that politicians concerned themselves both with the welfare of troops and with reports about it. By the same token, the British public and officials—both military and political—were remarkably well-informed about rates of disease and health among the armed forces. Regular quantitative returns are a salient example of this distinctive form of British expertise, relevant to political, military, and medical knowledge. Although British officials were able to restrict what was published concerning mismanagement or mistreatment of troops during campaigns, and certainly more so than in the colonies, as chapter 2 demonstrated, rumors and accusations circulated nonetheless.

During the Seven Years' War, Britain escaped many of the worst consequences of warfare. Yet the British public was concerned with the state of British troops abroad, as it was of both political and moral importance. War was cause for political scrutiny, criticism, and national self-reflection. Sickness among soldiers was evidence of physical, political, and moral disorder, because it showed ill discipline in the ranks, ill administration and corruption among officials, and the declining strength of the British nation.

CHAPTER FOUR

The Royal Navy's Western Squadron: Trials, Innovation, and Medical Efficacy

The Royal Navy was the key to British victories during the Seven Years' War. Naval blockades of enemy ports caused financial and logistical crises for enemy governments and logistical, strategic, and diplomatic crises for enemy military administrators from India to the American West. In this respect, the navy dictated the terms of engagement for all warring factions in the war. Moreover, triumphs such as Quebec in 1759 and 1760, Havana in 1762, and Fort William and Pondicherry in India are best described as amphibious operations. In colonial warfare, the navy was essential for more than just the transportation of troops and supplies; marines and seamen were expected to take part in the hard work of preparing for siege warfare, while naval artillery was integral to weakening enemy fortifications and batteries.[1]

Closer to home, the strategy of the Western Squadron is credited with the collapse of French naval power, protection of colonial trade and operations, and prevention of the invasion of the British and Irish coasts. Stationed at sea for long periods, the Western Squadron could operate continuously and successfully only by maintaining the health of its men. Historians have, therefore, credited the Admiralty's procedure of sending out fresh provisions with the success of British imperial forces during the Seven Years' War. Unlike in studies of the army, naval historians have long been aware of the role of disease during warfare and, therefore, the importance of medical care. Studies of disease and medicine in the Royal Navy credit naval administration, and not contemporary medicine, with efficacious medical care and disease prevention. Indeed, naval historians such as N. A. M. Rodger argue that naval administration maintained the health of the fleet *despite* contemporary naval medicine.[2]

A detailed examination of the Western Squadron and the naval medical board during the Seven Years' War demonstrates that there was no such disjunction between administrative demands and medical concerns. Instead, naval medical officials combined contemporary medical theory with what was administratively possible, and thereby developed sophisticated methods of scientific research and medical expertise. This chapter begins with a discussion of the health of seamen and the obstacles to maintaining it during the Seven Years' War. It then focuses on the development of the Western Squadron and especially on the effect that fresh victuals during the war had on rates of sickness. As the Sick and Hurt Board and the Admiralty recognized, sending fresh provisions to the Western Squadron was provisional and precarious, rather than a long-term solution to the problem of maintaining the health of seamen when at sea for extended periods of time. The chapter concludes with an examination of the correspondence of the Sick and Hurt Board during the years of the Seven Years' War, establishing that its medical research into cures and preventatives for scurvy *other* than fresh vegetables was not evidence of ignorance or negligence, but instead reflected what was achievable within the constraints imposed by ships at sea and the practical demands of naval administration.

The discussion below helps to solve the conundrum that has long puzzled naval and medical historians: why scurvy continued to plague the Royal Navy after the mid-eighteenth century if James Lind had demonstrated the efficacy of lemon juice in the 1750s and the Victualling Board had solved the problem of scurvy through the regular transport of fresh provisions in 1759–60. Rather than supposing that the fault lies with eighteenth-century medicine and an uninformed naval medical board, this detailed examination of naval medicine establishes the scientific nature of eighteenth-century medicine, especially in response to the challenges of war. It also demonstrates the complexity of evaluating medical efficacy in historical perspective, as short-term stasis can cause historians to overlook long-term innovation. This is clearly shown in comparison with the French navy, as contrasting the two warring navies highlights the institutional strength of British naval medicine as a forum for research and innovation. The nature of British naval medicine during the Seven Years' War thus provides a clear demonstration of the fundamental role of the British state in eighteenth-century medicine, adding to what has been shown for medicine in the British Army.

NAVAL OPERATIONS, DISEASE, AND HEALTH

The opening years of war proved particularly difficult for the Royal Navy. As naval historians recognize, one of the constant problems plaguing navies in the eighteenth century, and a factor that distinguishes eighteenth-century naval operations from today, is that significant demobilization occurred upon the end of each war. As a result, navies not only had to find and train a large number of men upon the first rumor of hostilities, but also to build, repair, and outfit ships within a short space of time. As Rodger explains, this problem of mobilization was more pressing for Britain during the eighteenth century than for other European powers, as Britain relied on its navy more than other nations and also used the threat of its naval power as diplomatic pressure before declarations of war.[3] Difficulties with mobilization explain why it was not until 1759 and 1760 that the Royal Navy won any spectacular victories, as it took four years before Britain achieved its full naval capability of 300 ships and just over 80,000 trained seamen.[4]

It was not simply a problem of finding a sufficient number of men, let alone men with sea experience. The search for seamen led to the impressment of land men, many of whom introduced disease into the fleet, and especially the infectious and fatal typhus fever.[5] The early stages of war thus corresponded with high rates of disease within the fleets.[6] In the first naval operation of the Seven Years' War, that under Edward Boscawen in North America (1755), typhus raged among the ships and was introduced into the rest of the fleet upon its return to Britain in 1756. In their explanation as to why John Byng was sent with so few ships to Minorca in March 1756—and ships badly manned and delayed at that—Admiralty officials cited sickness in the fleet as one of their central defenses. As noted in chapter 3, in the official published version of Byng's dispatch regarding his failure to protect Minorca from the French, political officials censored his reference to sickness in the fleet. To counteract this, Byng questioned his court-martial witnesses to establish high rates of sickness and undermanning among the ships of his squadron.[7]

Similarly, in the early cruises of the Western Squadron, sickness in the fleet forced Admiral Edward Hawke to return to port, much to the dissatisfaction of Admiralty officials.[8] Sent out to cruise in the spring of 1755, almost a year before war was formally declared between Britain and France, Hawke was forced to return in September with sick rates averaging 19 percent.[9] Over the next week, Hawke wrote at least three letters to the Admiralty, explaining and defending his decision to return, repeatedly emphasizing that it was ill health that caused him to end his cruise and not his unwillingness to remain on station.[10] Although both military and naval officials were concerned with manpower, crews weakened by disease were of pressing significance to naval officials, as ships below strength were unable to sail, let alone return home. The health of seamen was thus a central concern for eighteenth-century naval officials.

As well as peaking in the early years of a war, disease increased in proportion to the duration of a ship's voyage. Scurvy, the scourge of long-distance sailing, was one of the main ship diseases associated with the global wars of the mid-eighteenth century.[11] As discussed in chapter 1 with regard to North American campaigns, contemporaries understood that scurvy was the product of a lack of fresh provisions, although the disease was explained as resulting not from a lack of a specific vitamin, but rather from the onset of putrefaction.[12] Along with John Pringle, the naval physician James Lind argued, on the basis of various experiments and years of observations and experience (including Lind's two years as a naval surgeon on Channel service), that scurvy was a disease of putrefaction caused by a number of factors. Most important among these was a damp environment, and especially the moist and often unventilated and cold air in which seamen worked and slept, and a diet based on salted meats and unleavened bread. His much-cited trial with lemons on the HMS *Salisbury* notwithstanding, Lind did not argue that a lack of fresh fruits and vegetables was the main cause of scurvy.[13] Indeed, his observations as a naval surgeon and physician led him to argue explicitly against such an understanding of the disease. He explains that he had witnessed scurvy on HMS *Salisbury* while cruising in the Channel, despite the fact that the sailors had only recently consumed many vegetables while on shore. Nevertheless, Lind did recognize the benefit of fresh fruits and vegetables to the health of seamen while at sea:

> Although it is a certain and experienced truth, that the use of greens and vegetables is effectual in preventing the disease, and extremely beneficial in the cure; and thus we shall say, that abstinence from them, in certain circumstances, proves the *occasional cause* of the evil: yet there are unquestionably to be found at sea, other strong sources of it; which with respect to the former (or want of vegetables) we shall hereafter distinguish by the name of the *predisposing causes* to it.[14]

Lind thus identified the damp and cramped conditions on board ship as the *"principal and main predisposing cause"* of scurvy, along with a diet lacking in fresh provisions, especially fruits and vegetables, as well as a constitution liable to such a disease.[15] In sum, disease in general, and scurvy in particular, was best prevented through exercise and a healthy diet, especially one that included fresh provisions, and if that was not possible, one that included what were called "antiseptics" and "antiscorbutics": citrus fruits, vinegar, types of grass, ginger, wine, beer made with spruce—all items that had been shown to retard the rotting and putrefaction of meat in various trials.

Lind and other officials, including naval officials, recognized that it was thus the circumstances of ships at sea that posed the greatest challenge to crews' health. Regular stops in harbor were therefore the optimal preventative for sickness.[16] This is demonstrated in the terminology used: pit stops were called "refreshments," for both the ships themselves (being scraped and cleaned) and the men. Specifically, time on shore provided fresh air (dryer air than on board ship) and fresh provisions, both of which were widely identified as the best cures, as well as the best preventatives, for scurvy. Although the men might be granted only a few days leave once a ship arrived in port after a cruise, what was more certain was that fresh provisions would be served: when in port, on so-called flesh days, fresh meat was granted to men four days of the week.[17]

One should note the emphasis on fresh meat: eighteenth-century references to "fresh provisions" do not necessarily include fresh fruits or vegetables. As salted meats were considered part of the fundamental cause of disease, fresh meat was considered conducive, if not essential, to the men's health. While this may be frustrating to historians hoping to find dietary improvements containing vitamin C, fresh meat would definitely have been healthier than preserved salt meat. Standard victualing practice in the British Army and Royal Navy was for salt meat to be preserved in large amounts of salt and brine for months if not years; soldiers and sailors were instructed to boil the meat a number of times while scraping off the salt in order to render it softer and more easily digestible. According to the eighteenth-century theory of putrefaction, salted meat was an especially unhealthy part of a soldier's or sailor's diet. Lind maintained that "experience shews, that flesh long salted is of very difficult digestion. It requires perfect health, together with exercise, plenty of diluting liquors, vinegar, and many other correctors, to subdue it in the first passages."[18] Serving seamen fresh provisions, which always consisted of fresh meat and usually included fresh vegetables, was thus part of long-standing health practice.[19]

THE WESTERN SQUADRON AND THE HEALTH OF SEAMEN

Contemporaries were aware of the health problems posed by the operations of the Western Squadron. The squadron was not an innovation of the Seven Years' War; the term can be traced back to 1705, even though such a squadron had little practical effect until the wars of the 1740s.[20] Having a fleet of ships constantly cruising to the "westward"—west of approaches to the coast and along the Channel off Brest and Ushant—meant that incoming British merchant vessels could be protected, while French fleets and supply ships were prevented from setting out for the colonies or preparing for an invasion of Britain. The strategy of the Western Squadron was never comprehensively or clearly elucidated by either Admiral Edward Vernon or George Anson, under whom the practice first developed in the 1740s. Instead, by the mid-eighteenth century, what had begun as a practical experiment proved to be a viable strategy, albeit one requiring continuing modifications.[21]

Naval historians emphasize the problems inherent in such a stratagem. It was difficult for such a squadron to cruise for extended periods, partly because of the geography of the region near Brest, where wind, rocks, and tide combined to threaten its safety.[22] More significant still, a cruising fleet could not maintain its station for an extended period of time without losing much of its manpower to sickness.[23] The effectiveness of the Western Squadron over 1759–60, when it maintained a near-constant blockade of French shipping, should thus be seen as a tangible demonstration of British seapower: as naval historians have been keen to emphasize, the Western Squadron was the result of British naval supremacy, not simply a method for its achievement.[24] The Western Squadron during the Seven Years' War thus provides a salient opportunity to examine the problem of the health of seamen. As its success depended on the ability to keep ships constantly on cruise, it presented difficulties similar to those encountered on other naval campaigns during the war, including those in India and the West Indies. Although not burdened by tropical diseases such as yellow fever or malaria, the Western Squadron exemplifies the increasing logistical, administrative, and medical demands placed on eighteenth-century navies, especially as ships could be required to stay at sea for periods longer than ocean crossings. It simultaneously represents the new exigencies of mid-eighteenth-century global warfare and the Royal Navy's ability to cope with such demands.[25]

The problem of maintaining the health of the crews in the Western Squadron was apparent to commanders and Admiralty officials. Naval officials were also aware that there were disastrous long-term consequences to long cruises, beyond simply not having enough sailors to man the ships properly while at sea. If a cruise continued for too long and too many men fell sick, the navy, and not simply those crews, would suffer from not having enough seamen fit for duty for months to come.[26] Sickness disrupted strategy not only for a certain fleet, but for the overall strategy of the Royal Navy.

Letters from the commanders of the Western Squadron in 1757 and 1758 repeatedly describe how ships that had been at sea for periods beyond a month became sickly and were sent to port for refreshment and cleaning (removing weeds and barnacles from the bottom of the ships to ensure fast and efficient sailing). During the sailing season of 1758, even under First Lord of the Admiralty George Anson's experienced command, sickness and a lack of seamen were still a problem.[27] Correspondence during these early years of the war establishes not only that sickness did indeed reach dangerous rates when ships remained at sea for more than three months as part of the Western Squadron, but also that naval officials recognized the key treatment for such sickness was for a ship to return to port and allow the men the refreshment of land.

As significant as Hawke's feat at Quiberon Bay may have been for Britain's overall victory, his success relied on maintaining a large fleet, fully manned and healthy, so as to sustain a close and continuous blockade of Brest for eight months before the Quiberon battle and still show up in full force on the day of battle. As Rodger succinctly summarizes the triumph of 1759, "It had never been possible for a fleet at sea to remain healthy for so long."[28] Because of the regular supply of fresh provisions, accomplished through the administrative efficiency of the Victualling Board and the Admiralty, naval historians have argued, "scurvy was no longer a serious problem in British warships."[29] Yet, as Daniel Baugh has noted, if these measures were so successful in preventing scurvy, it remains to be explained why they were not implemented during the American War of Independence, as well as why lemon juice—as recommended in Lind's 1753 publication—was not instituted throughout the Royal Navy until the 1790s.[30]

In order to explain this disjuncture between innovations preventing scurvy during the mid-eighteenth century and their institutionalization years later, historians have looked to the nature of eighteenth-century medicine, characterizing it as too theoretical to be of use to the navy, or finding fault with the navy's medical board, partly composed of nonmedical men, with little insight into or authority over naval medical matters. By the same token, the accomplishments of fresh provisioning for the Western Squadron have been credited to nonmedical boards, particularly the Victualling Board and the Admiralty. For example, while recognizing that naval officials may have been aware of Lind's medical theories, historian Stephen Gradish argues that in the case of fresh victuals for the Western Squadron, inspiration came from Anson, organization came from the Victualling Board, and pressure to institute such measures came from both the Admiralty Board and naval officials such as Hawke and Boscawen.[31] Rodger not only concurs that naval administration must be credited but also concludes that "any true history of eighteenth-century naval medicine . . . must in part be a history of medical knowledge gained by demolishing, or at least circumventing the power of the medical establishment."[32]

By contrast, a detailed examination of the operations of the Western Squadron challenges these characterizations on a number of points. First, the provisioning of fresh meat and vegetables was an outgrowth of contemporary medical advice and practice, rather than running contrary to it. Second, the problem of scurvy was not solved through the actions of the Victualling Board, specifically the sending out of fresh provisions. And, third, detailed more fully in the last section of this chapter, such measures stemmed from contemporary medical understanding. Their lack of implementation in the later years of the war and during the following wars stemmed not from ignorance, medical misunderstanding, or a failure of medical authority, but from the recognition that such measures were not administratively feasible, given the operational demands placed on fleets.

As discussed previously, the supply of fresh provisions had long been advocated by medical authorities, and fresh provisions for the Western Squadron was an outgrowth of the already-established practice of providing fresh meat for ships when in port. Amounts varied; the HMS *Pallas* received 3,600 pounds of fresh beef over three weeks in July 1758, which equaled roughly six bullocks for a crew of 240.[33] Following standard procedure, the meat was cut up in order to be served to the sick, and what was left over was served to the entire ship's company.[34] This practice was gradually modified during the summer and autumn of 1759. During this period, the Lords of the Admiralty were explicit about the importance of maintaining a constant blockade of Brest, in the midst of intelligence concerning a French invasion that required supplies to assemble at Brest. Responding to Hawke's complaint of a lack of supplies, the Lords immediately sent out more provisions, assuring Hawke that this would "enable you to continue on your station where it is more necessary than ever for you to remain as long as possible at this very critical conjuncture."[35]

During the same period, officials began to supply the Squadron with vegetables, a procedure that historians consider both key and innovative.[36] Yet, the amount sent, and the regularity with which vegetables were transported, are difficult to ascertain. While regular records of fresh meat received on board exist, and such shipments were carefully noted, the arrival of vegetables does not appear to have been given the same importance. For example, the charge for vegetables was somewhat muddled, as the pursers charged the vegetables as if they were "a gift to the seamen," and hence not on their accounts, while the board appears to have charged the cost to each ship's account.[37] As well, the records concerning condemned vegetables do not state what was wrong and exactly how much was thrown overboard. This deviation from standard procedure again suggests that vegetables were not subject to the same rigorous administrative scrutiny as meat and regular provisions.[38]

As for fresh meat, by early August 1759, officials suggested that, quantities allowing, it could be given to healthy seamen as well as to the sick. Admiralty dispatches, Hawke's orders, and lieutenants' logbooks document an evolving practice of providing sick men with fresh meat as a matter of priority, while surplus provisions were occasionally distributed among healthy crew members.[39] The procuring of fresh provisions, including vegetables, was thus an extension of a common practice directed toward curing sick seamen when ships came into port, long recommended by medical authorities such as Lind. Only gradually did it develop into a measure applied to the entire squadron sailing under Hawke, just as the Western Squadron itself was initially a cruising squadron and only under dire necessity, from fear of a French invasion, became a continuous blockading force off of Brest.

The impact and success of this supply of fresh provisions, regardless of Lind's high praise and the victory of Quiberon Bay in November 1759, are not necessarily clearly established. Hawke and Admiralty officials were obviously pleased when such fresh provisions reached the fleet. Writing to the Admiralty on 28 August 1759, Hawke commented, "The little fresh meat we have had has already showed it self in very salutary effects."[40] Yet, just three days later, Hawke complained to Pett, the victualing officer at Plymouth, that Pett must ensure fresh provisions would soon again be sent as "we have been now sixteen weeks within a few days from Spithead, & the men falling down in the scurvey [*sic*]."[41] While Hawke noted that most of the seamen were healthy, he repeatedly remarked in his correspondence that the crew of HMS *Foudroyant* was very sickly.[42] As returns for the fleet under Hawke did not survive, the actual rate of sickness among the squadron cannot be clearly established. Yet comparing muster tables from ships among the squadron in 1759 with those from 1758 (that is, before the regular supply of fresh provisions was sent out) reveals no dramatic differences in sick rates for the same time of year and cruise.[43]

In many ways the blockade was a precarious operation, and maintaining it became more difficult the longer it lasted. By the middle of December 1759, Hawke reported that his ships were short of supplies and some were becoming sickly, while for him, "I have now been thirty one weeks on board, without setting my foot on shore, and cannot expect that my health will hold out much longer."[44] He wrote to the Admiralty early in January 1760, "Every plan of operation I formed after the 1st of Decem[be]r has proved abortive, through bad weather and want of provisions and necessaries."[45]

There were constant problems with the small victualing sloops, especially during the rough winter weather. After Hawke's decisive battle in Quiberon Bay, few more were sent out, and Lind reports that scurvy consequently afflicted the crews. Throughout most of his cruise in 1760, Boscawen not only reported sickness among his crew, but also found provision transports damaged by the rocks and described their supplies as "so small and uncertain that it will be of very little use."[46] Likewise, under Augustus Keppel during the latter part of 1760 and in 1761, the squadron in the Channel suffered from sickness, including scurvy. When victualers did reach Keppel, he noted that problems other than bad weather plagued the supply of fresh provisions: many of the sheep had died before reaching his fleet, while vegetables other than potatoes, onions, and cabbages "generally get here in such a condition from being rotten, that the good intent of their Lordships directing such Supplys became useless, as well as expensive."[47] Moreover, in June 1760, Boscawen reported to the Admiralty, "Captain Hughes of the Tamar that convoy'd the Transports with Bullocks and Sheep from Ireland tells me that he is afraid the Populace will not suffer more to be shipp'd at Cork."[48] Overall, such provisioning would have been very expensive and thus difficult to continue financing over a long period of time, in addition to the various practical problems that plagued supply transports.[49] As a result, provisioning at sea was never regular or dependable.

While stationed in Quiberon Bay in early 1761, Hawke requested a sufficient number of ships in order to rotate the fleet and send ships to port frequently, "to preserve their companies, be enabled to perform the duties of the station, and save the exorbitant expence of victuallers, which after all but little answer their intended purpose."[50] Even after the success and glory of the battle at Quiberon, Hawke described the sailing during the blockade as especially harsh. After his return home early in 1760, he wrote, "Indeed I have had a very long tiresome and fatiguing cruize, and as hard a piece of service to go thro with, as cou'd be put upon any Man; but thank God I waded thro it at last."[51] Hawke claimed that cruising during the blockade warranted special recognition from the Admiralty, not just because of victory over the French, but because of the difficulty encountered while at sea.[52] Like other naval commanders, he recognized that the conditions of constant blockading were exceptional and unusually harsh, notwithstanding the supply of fresh meat and vegetables.

The supply of fresh provisions, including vegetables, for the four months between July and November 1759, did facilitate a great naval victory over the French. But because of financial constraints and logistical difficulties, this operation was not continued for long after Hawke's victory, nor could it be widely or regularly instituted to ensure dependable operations of a Western Squadron for an extended period of time. While the Western Squadron's battle and blockade in 1759 were remarkable achievements, it is apparent that a permanent Western Squadron was not yet possible. The main reason for this was the health of crews. Fresh provisions, regularly provided onshore, were identified by medical officials and naval officials as the key to maintaining health at sea, yet attempts to supply active-duty ships at sea stretched naval capabilities during the 1750s and 1760s.

THE SICK AND HURT BOARD AND MEDICAL TRIALS

Alongside this short-term measure of regular supplies of fresh provisions, the naval medical board continued to research ways to prevent and cure scurvy among crews at sea. From 1756 this board, called either the Sick and Hurt or Sick and Wounded Board, was composed of four commissioners (each with an annual salary of £300) alongside a secretary (£200) and clerks, aided by officials and medical practitioners stationed in various ports.[53] Its responsibilities during the Seven Years' War entailed caring for sick and wounded seamen and managing the medical practitioners in the navy, including naval hospitals. The board was also charged with the care of prisoners of war, discussed in chapter 6. Given this remit, the board has been characterized by naval historians more as an administrative committee than as a medical authority, and criticized on this account.[54] Although by 1756 two of the four commissioners were medical men, historians have pointed out that the board did not even have enough authority to introduce medical initiatives and, overall, had "little to do with ships at sea."[55]

While the correspondence of the Sick and Hurt Board during the Seven Years' War does not suggest that the commissioners considered themselves authorities beyond the power of the Admiralty, it does demonstrate that they conceived of themselves as a medical body responsible for evaluating cures and preventatives that were practicable. In this respect, not only were they fully aware of the constraints inherent in shipboard life, but they also combined medical knowledge with bureaucratic practicality. Moreover, the Admiralty regularly requested advice from the board on medical matters, demonstrating that the Sick and Hurt Board was recognized as a source of naval medical expertise. While it is true that by today's standards most naval diseases were not curable in the eighteenth century, contemporary medical authorities were optimistic that naval diseases could be managed, both medically and bureaucratically.

Historians have overlooked the medical expertise of the Sick and Hurt Board in part because many of its initiatives do not conform to modern categories of biomedicine. Portable soup, for example, was one of the best-known and in some ways most successful medical initiative of the Sick and Hurt Board during this period. Made of beef and mutton left over from the salted naval rations, it was formed into small cakes that were easily stored on board. These were then mixed with boiling water and served to the men as soup, often with vegetables or grains. It was trialed on board ships from 1757 and was praised for preserving the lives of the sick until they reached the naval hospitals on shore.[56] Under the direction of the Sick and Hurt Board, portable soup was widely instituted throughout the navy, while its method of preparation was standardized.[57] By 1759 it was being requested by the army, and its production had expanded to Plymouth and Portsmouth.[58] Indeed, by the end of the war, portable soup had become part of the standard diet at naval hospitals and remained a naval issue throughout the eighteenth century.[59]

The medical expertise of the Sick and Hurt Board has also been overlooked because it is clear that, according to modern biomedicine, such initiatives would not have prevented or cured diseases. Yet this approach fails to recognize the long-term significance of the Sick and Hurt Board's procedure, even if the initiatives trialed would have had little success in preventing scurvy. For example, when trying out portable soup, surgeons were instructed to "make very nice and particular observations on the effects of it, on the Sick more especially those afflicted with the Scurvey and to report to them at the end of every Cruize their opinion of its efficacy and utility."[60] Such instructions are found again, when the Sick and Hurt Board reported that eight and a half bushels of dried apples had arrived from North America, "to make experiments with them on seamen ill of the scurvy."[61] Under the authority of the Sick and Hurt Board, medical suggestions were first instituted as trials or experiments, with surgeons reporting their observations to the board. If found successful, the board formally regulated the production and issue of such items. While it appears that portable broth was the only successful initiative during the Seven Years' War, the evaluation of various other suggestions reveals the medical theory and practice of the Sick and Hurt Board. Moreover, it reveals the scope of the Admiralty's investment in medical care for seamen and the priority and authority it granted to the Sick and Hurt Board in its pursuit of effective health-care solutions for the men.

While contemporary medical theory was used to explicate a proposed cure, the board repeatedly also stressed the need for trials to demonstrate the safety and efficacy of a proposed cure. In December of 1757, for example, the board rejected Mr. Leake's (first name unknown) proposal for a trial of his medicine, as Leake would neither disclose his medicine's contents nor knew anything about sea scurvy.[62] The board also turned down a proposal to use oil as a cure and preventative for scurvy on the theoretical grounds that such a treatment would produce putrid fevers in the conditions of a ship, noting that the individual who proposed the remedy had conducted no experiments that demonstrated anything to the contrary.[63] When the board refused to try Richard Dunn's medicine to cure fluxes in May 1759, they explained that it was not only because Dunn had not studied medicine, but also because he would not disclose its ingredients. The board recommended that he "find proper people who would voluntarily take his medicine and told him we would attend to the effects of it."[64] Similarly, the board was wary of the publican William Adams's "infallible cure for the flux." Although Adams claimed that the recipe was originally from India, and that he had tried it on himself and others with success in the 1740s, the board still insisted that Adams produce people or certificates that attested to its more recent success.[65]

If the safety and relative efficacy of a proposed medicine or preventative was established by medical theory and by certificates, the board then allowed the medicine to be tried on a small number of seamen at a naval hospital. When Edward Hogkin was granted permission to conduct a trial on his cure for the flux, officials at Haslar Hospital selected twelve patients on the board's direction for Hogkin's use. When the board reported Hogkin's medicine ineffective among these twelve, the Admiralty canceled the planned further trial at Plymouth Hospital.[66] Similarly, Robert Douglas was allowed to try his cure for scurvy on four patients at Haslar, under no less an authority than Lind. Upon further examination, however, the board concluded that not only was Douglas's cure not original, the main ingredient having already been published in Lind's *Treatise on the Scurvy*, but they also considered it impossible to judge the efficacy of a cure for scurvy among sailors on shore given that their diet contained fresh provisions.[67] As Douglas insisted that his cure could work at sea as well, the board recommended a sea trial. The orders that accompanied Douglas upon this experiment are especially significant. Vice Admiral Saunders, as commander in chief in the Mediterranean, was instructed

> to give the said Mr. Douglas all possible assistance for his making the proposed experiment, and that due care be taken that the persons put under his cure are such as are really afflicted with that distemper, and that while under cure they have no other assistance of diet or otherwise than such as the sick of His Majesty's Fleet at sea are generally supplied with; as this is a circumstance particularly to be attended to, to ascertain the real efficacy of the medicine; and as it did not appear upon the experiment made last year in the hospital at Haslar that the patients under his cure and enjoying the benefit of hospital diet etc received the least peculiar Advantage.[68]

The commissioners of the Sick and Hurt Board were thus fully aware that a useful cure for scurvy must be one applicable to the circumstances of a ship at sea. This distinction, and the commissioners' understanding that a valid cure for scurvy in the navy had to be effective in the absence of fresh provisions, was again made in the evaluation of wort as a cure for scurvy, as proposed by Dr. McBride. The commissioners stated that they considered wort ineffective on shore, but suggested that it might be useful at sea, where fresh meat and vegetables, "which chiefly contributes to the cure on shore, cannot be had."[69] Again, in response to a suggestion to carry fresh fruits to sea, the commissioners noted "lemons and oranges and apples would be very useful on a cruize at sea if it was practicable to carry and serve such quantities as would be necessary."[70] Although fresh provisions had been supplied to ships in the Western Squadron during the preceding years, the Sick and Hurt Board and the Admiralty thus understood that such operations could not be widely instituted in the navy. The board's continuing search for a cure for scurvy, rather than representing a denial of the advantages of fresh provisions, simply represented a search for a practical cure that could be applied throughout the navy in its far-flung operations.

As they had remarked during their evaluation of Douglas's cure for scurvy, the commissioners were well acquainted with Lind's suggestions in his *Treatise on the Scurvy.* The problem was the logistics and cost of supplying such items to ships during naval operations, a concern that was characteristic of an administrative, as well as a medical, body. The commissioners, however, did not consider a cure beyond their grasp, especially if one applied contemporary medical theory and demonstrated the efficacy of cures through experiments. According to Lind, contemporary medical theory, and empirical observations, the remedial qualities of oranges and lemons could be found in other so-called antiseptics too, such as wort, vinegar, and apples. The medical challenge for the commissioners of the Sick and Hurt Board was to find a cure that was affordable and available in sufficient quantities to supply around 70,000 seamen and that could be stored for months at a time in damp and cramped conditions.

This procedure developed piecemeal in response to the Admiralty's requests for medical guidance in evaluating suggested medicines. From the outset, medical efficacy was framed within administrative and financial demands. The earliest extant correspondence of the Sick and Hurt Board includes a request to examine a medicine in more detail, "his Royal Highnesse being not willing to put the Government to the charge thereof, till such time as hee can be satisfyed of the reall vertue of the sayd Medicine."[71] Although providers would clearly benefit should their medicine be adopted by the navy, suggested remedies were expected to be supplied initially without compensation: the Admiralty directed "that the surgeons of his Majesty's ships should not be obliged to pay for this Medicine for the present, or 'till a farther tryal is made of the efficacy thereof."[72] By the 1740s, procedures had evolved to allow the testing of medicines in foreign, or hot climates, as well as domestic ones.[73] By the Seven Years' War, a standard procedure emerged that allowed assessment of a medicine within different naval contexts: first a trial in one hospital ashore, then a second trial at another hospital, then on board a limited number of ships, and finally a widely administered trial on ships while at sea, relying on surgeons' reports to evaluate the efficacy of a medicine at sea.

Rather than focusing on individual initiatives through the lens of modern biomedicine, studying the Sick and Hurt Board through its procedures demonstrates its role as a center of medical expertise. It functioned as the hub through which Admiralty requests for medical research passed, providing onshore naval officials with informed opinions and reports gathered from squadrons and naval hospitals based at home and throughout the colonies. It is clear that the board did not consider itself as the fount of all medical knowledge, but was instead recognized as the authority on obtaining such practical advice. When the Admiralty received Lind's suggestions for maintaining the health of seamen, they requested the board's opinion. The board, as modern administrative bodies do, asked trusted physicians to give their opinion, and then forwarded what they selected as relevant to the Admiralty. Notably, these physicians concluded that Lind's suggestions "are not quite practicable tho' they seem very rational."[74] Repeatedly, then, contemporaries—whether university-trained physicians, experienced naval surgeons, or the commissioners of the Sick and Hurt Board—recognized that Lind's proposals to prevent scurvy and maintain the health of seamen were efficacious. What inhibited their widespread implementation was the impracticality of instituting such measures throughout the navy, as was the case for the supply of fresh provisions to the Western Squadron. This fact was easily grasped by the Sick and Hurt Board, ideally placed to oversee both medical research and administrative possibilities, providing medical and bureaucratic naval expertise. Under the board, medical trials were standardized, following procedures that were themselves effective and scientific, even if these did not produce effective and practical medicines during the Seven Years' War.

FRENCH AND BRITISH STRUCTURES OF MEDICAL KNOWLEDGE

Although the type of medical trial practiced by the Sick and Hurt Board was not widespread in the mid-eighteenth century, there is nothing to suggest that the commissioners of the board thought they were inventing a new scientific method. Trials, experiments, and an emphasis on systematic observation can be traced back to the sixteenth and seventeenth centuries, to the so-called new science. Yet, these earlier trials were limited in scope; indeed, often they merely involved the medical practitioner testing on himself.[75] What was different in the case of the Sick and Hurt Board was its ability to institute systematic trials on a large number of individuals. Having men under their command and large numbers under their care in hospitals and on board ships, naval medicine was perfectly suited to clinical trials and observations, providing an institutional framework ripe for such an innovation.

While historians of science have identified an "experimental enthusiasm" in eighteenth-century public spaces and the marketplace, what is suggested here is that such practices also emerged in state institutions, within the context of naval medicine.[76] As a result, the history of medicine in the navy not only provides a fruitful arena in which to research medical developments, but in this case also refines our understanding of the history of British scientific medicine. Whereas historians of eighteenth-century medicine have characterized this period as one in which consumers and a vibrant public sphere shaped medical transformations, the history of naval medicine is a reminder that the British state played a significant role in eighteenth-century scientific innovations.

The Sick and Hurt Board did not seem aware that its medical practices involved a theoretical challenge to standard medicine. As had been the case in the development of the Western Squadron, it instead appears that the board believed it was simply instituting practical solutions using available resources. With hindsight, such small practices did indeed change the nature of medical inquiry and theory, especially reinforced by the development of hospital medicine during the later eighteenth century.[77] By instituting standardized clinical trials on groups of anonymous men in the navy, asking for specific observations in order to make judgments regarding the efficacy of the substance on trial, and assuming that these trials could be replicated throughout the navy in a variety of climates by low-level practitioners, the board was challenging the usual case-by-case or individual approach to evaluating therapeutic efficacy. Although the medical trials conducted by the Sick and Hurt Board were in many ways simply an extension of an already-established practice, this extension had wide-ranging repercussions for the nature of medical practice and indeed for the relationship between sailors and the Admiralty and, more broadly, the British state. By the end of the eighteenth century, such standardized views of the bodies of sailors meant that medical practitioners could statistically evaluate the health and medical care of sailors.[78]

In their use of experience and practical skills through experimentation and trials, and in their position as trusted advisers to Admiralty officials, the commissioners of the Sick and Hurt Board served as medical experts, searching for practicable and useful knowledge that would support the imperial projects of the British state. Through this process, the Sick and Hurt Board also developed its own method of expertise. Its expertise emerged within a specific institutional context; moreover, this context appears to have been distinctively British. Although naval medicine was shared across the Channel, with the writings of leading physicians such as James Lind translated into French, there were important structural differences between scientific medicine in these warring European nations.[79] In many ways, the French Navy had a more extensive structure of naval medicine than did the Royal Navy, with numerous naval hospitals containing specialized schools established in the seventeenth and early eighteenth centuries.[80] However, the French Navy lacked any central board that dealt exclusively with health matters.

Although the Académie de Marine was founded in 1752, this society hardly touched on medical matters, and it is not clear that its suggestions could or would be implemented. While bureaucratically impressive, the French Navy had no central administrative hub that evaluated the health of French sailors, or a centralized mechanism to implement health-related reforms. Compared with British naval medicine, French naval medicine was decentralized and fragmented.[81]

As historian of the French Navy James Pritchard remarked some years ago, what is most useful in naval contexts is not so much histories of science and medicine per se, but an examination of how scientific advancement was furthered and retarded by structural organizations. The French Royal Academy of Science was certainly a leading center for scientific research and the understanding of nature. And yet, such research did not necessarily translate into solving political, commercial, or military problems of the day. In the case of nautical science, which Pritchard examines in depth, it was the institutional strength of French science that appears to have hindered navigational expertise, with problems conceived in theoretical terms, rather than as practical obstacles.[82] As both Pritchard and Rodger have observed regarding the complexity of assessing eighteenth-century naval technology, any improvement needs to be measured within the practical constraints of the time. Rodger rightly points to the difficulty in comparing French and British design, suggesting that instead of asking how scientific such technology was, or how it compared with that of other nations, the question should be "how well they corresponded to each country's strategic priorities, and how wisely those priorities had been chosen."[83] For the Royal Navy, the Sick and Hurt Board was a long-term investment whose benefits were not fully reaped until the wars of the later eighteenth century. It provided an efficient and systematic method of solving medical problems, even if those solutions remained out of reach during the Seven Years' War.

When compared with France, in the long term the Royal Navy benefited from an institutional advantage when it came to health, yet it is not clear that it suffered from a short-term disadvantage. Instead, what becomes apparent is the complexity of making health comparisons between the two navies. Statistical comparisons are not enlightening: records are unreliable and confusing, often grouping desertions and deaths from all noncombat causes together, and rates of death do not accurately represent health problems. For ship crews in particular, sickness could be just as debilitating as death among seamen, and different diseases had markedly different results in terms of deaths and long-term debility. Moreover, as noted, rates fluctuated throughout the course of a war. On the French side, major epidemics of typhus, such as at Brest in 1757–58, proved more problematic than diseases such as scurvy.[84] High rates of disease and death due to disease among French seamen were also the result of high rates of imprisonment in British prisoner-of-war institutions (examined in chapter 6), providing yet another difficulty in compilations of disease numbers. Historians of the French Navy have noted that France faced grave manpower problems during the Seven Years' War, with disease a serious factor. Pritchard demonstrates that the main cause of the manpower shortage was the "crown's state of financial malnutrition which left the navy unable to pay its crews and drove seamen to resist the levies, desert in large numbers, and flee the country."[85] The extent of the French Navy's financial problems may thus obscure the significance of disease during the Seven Years' War. The Royal Navy's Sick and Hurt Board may have been a luxury that the French Navy could not afford, but then again, the Western Squadron was exorbitantly expensive, while also effective.

The care and money invested in maintaining the health of sailors during the war, whether through fresh provisions or through the search for a practical cure for scurvy, demonstrate that the Royal Navy, like the British Army, considered the welfare of these men integral to its mission and relied on contemporary medical knowledge to preserve it. Naval medical care and medical trials during this period indicate the resources and authority available to the British state in the context of naval operations. The administrative resources, manpower, and finances expended on providing fresh provisions to the Western Squadron during 1759, and more sporadically in the years after, were remarkable, as were the efforts of the Sick and Hurt Board in trials evaluating medical suggestions and implementing successful innovations, such as portable soup.

In many ways, the supply of fresh provisions to the seamen of the Western Squadron parallels the development of the Western Squadron itself. A fleet stationed in the westward approaches had long been recognized as an excellent strategy, but the logistical problems of having such a fleet stationed along those coasts for an extended period of time proved almost impossible to solve. Gradually, cruises were attempted for longer periods, until in 1759 a fleet sustained a blockade of Brest for eight months. This blockade was recognized not only as unusual, but also as draining the strength of the Royal Navy as a whole. While in the short term such long cruises could certainly ensure the security of British coasts and colonies, in the long term such cruises could wear out the British fleet and its men for years to come, rendering the Royal Navy vulnerable in future campaigns, as was the case in the 1770s and 1780s. Likewise, medical officials had long recognized that fresh provisions would benefit the health of seamen, and when sick seamen were landed on shore, or when ships came into harbor, fresh provisions were supplied. Practical constraints, however, made such provisioning impractical in the long run for ships at sea.

More broadly, this detailed examination of the Sick and Hurt Board's activities demonstrates that naval history and medical history should not be studied as challenges to each other, or indeed in isolation from each other and from wider historical developments. The Sick and Hurt Board in the eighteenth century cannot be accurately characterized as simply a naval administrative body, but neither can it be defined as a body concerned only with medical research and care. This is clearly demonstrated when medical theories and methods are studied within their contemporary administrative context.

Comparing the navy with the army, it appears at first glance that the navy was able to maintain a better standard of health among crews, especially because naval officials were able to institute stricter controls to maintain the health of sailors, owing to the practice of impressment and the tighter control over men on board ships. Yet this assumption can be challenged on a number of fronts. First, as Rodger's detailed examination of the "disordered cohesion" of life on board ships demonstrates, naval officials commanded not through threats and strict discipline, but rather through persuasion and the recognition of seamen's traditional rights and privileges.[86] Second, there was significant overlap between medical services in the army and navy, especially since almost all operations were amphibious. As noted, during the expeditions to the coast of France, provisions for both sailors and soldiers were provided by the navy. James Maxwell, one of the commissioners of the Sick and Hurt Board during the war, had previously served as a medical official with the British Army and corresponded with Viscount Barrington (the secretary at war) regarding the medical services of the army.[87] The Western Squadron was thus in many ways an unusual operation, in that it involved the navy in isolation. Third, the nature of a ship on cruise, with its damp and crowded environment, and the lack of fresh provisions, was in itself the greatest challenge to the health of sailors during this period. Fourth, there was no significant difference between the sick rates of military and naval troops. Whether on campaign for four months, or at sea for four months, both the army and navy during the Seven Years' War experienced average morbidity rates of 20 percent, and when campaigns or cruises continued for longer, rates dramatically increased. With archival material physically separated, historians of warfare tend to separate their studies of the army and navy, giving the illusion that during times of war, operations and conditions were also disparate.

Yet there were important differences between the army and the navy during this period. Most significant, naval operations were clearly centralized around Admiralty offices, which was reflected in the structure of naval medical care. The establishment of permanent and large naval hospitals during the Seven Years' War meant that many sick sailors were sent back to Britain for care, while sick soldiers were more often treated in field hospitals, and army veterans often settled in various colonial outposts upon the end of war. As a result, the medical care for sailors and disabled sea veterans was more centralized and regulated than that of the army. The structure of medical care in the navy, and the power of the fiscal-military state that supported it, were thus more clearly discernible by the public, not least because of the imposing naval hospital buildings.[88]

The British state was also visible in the practice of medical trials and experiments. As historians of science have pointed out, the development of experimental science depends not only on obtaining bodies on which to try methods, but also on the judgment and authority of the individual who conducts the experiment.[89] Robert Douglas and other applicants whose trials were deemed failures by the commissioners protested that this was because they had not been able to conduct the trial entirely as they had wished to. In this context, it was the British state that gave naval officers and ships' surgeons the authority to oversee such trials, and this suggests the nascent development of later practices regarding state regulation and standardization, overseen by experts acting as intermediaries between the state and theoretical knowledge.

The Western Squadron's achievements in 1759 were impressive. As Hardwicke recorded in his notes for Byng's Enquiry during the late 1750s, when the Western Squadron was in place, "the French Fleet was kept in, our coasts and colonies are unmolested, the French Trade, and the Succours intended for America have been in part intercepted, and our own Trade in the midst of War enjoyed all the Security of Peace."[90] Yet it was widely recognized that the cost and dangers of its implementation were considerable:

> These Benefits are not cheaply gained, a Fleet superior to what the Enemy can send out must be always employed . . . , cruizers in all weather, and often with Tempestuous and contrary winds wears out the ships, the masts and rigging and it ruins the Health and costs the lives of the Seamen, it often disables a ship in a week which has been three months in preparing and it demands a great part of our naval Force.[91]

Hardwicke's notes were compiled to defend the decision not to send out a greater force with Byng, a decision that officials recognized had resulted in the loss of Minorca to the French. Working with impressive, if still limited, resources, naval officials appreciated that keeping the Western Squadron constantly on cruise was of the utmost strategic significance in 1759. They accordingly directed resources to ensure the squadron's success, and specifically, the maintenance of sailors' health. Yet officials also recognized that such health provisions could be supplied only for short periods, that it was not a reliable or practical medium-term solution, and that it posed a great risk to Britain's naval capabilities in the long term by undermining the availability of naval resources for years to come. Under these circumstances, the Sick and Hurt Board searched for a reliable and practical solution to ill health among seamen; in the process, it also developed a thoughtful, methodical, and skillful method of medical research.

CHAPTER FIVE

Adaptation and Hot Climates: Fighting in India

In the early 1750s, the surgeon William Wills published an entertaining account of his time with the British East India Company. Leaving behind his life as a young surgeon in Bristol, Wills sought "a much speedier Fortune by going Abroad" and was appointed surgeon's mate on a British East India Company ship.[1] Adventure and wealth with the East India Company called Wills, as it did other young men who traveled to India as "writers" (lowest-level company staff). These men hoped to move up through the company hierarchy, maintained by strict seniority, and to amass increasing fortunes along the way. Perhaps the most successful East India Company surgeon in this period was John Zephaniah Holwell, who became governor of Bengal in 1760 and who was reputed to have amassed £96,000 during his career in India. Like Wills, Holwell had served an apprenticeship as surgeon before he sailed to India as a surgeon's mate. He successively held the posts of surgeon to a company factory (trading post) and assistant surgeon to the company hospital at Calcutta before becoming principal physician and surgeon to the presidency in 1746. Holwell not only learned about Hindu theology and become fluent in Arabic while practicing medicine in India, but also became involved in broader company affairs, especially revenue management, and was on the council of Fort William when Siraj ud-Daula attacked Calcutta in June 1756, later publishing and publicizing his account of the attack and his imprisonment in the infamous Black Hole.[2] By contrast, although Wills was promoted to full surgeon, his frequent and private surgical appointments with the sole white woman on board his second East India Company voyage led him to be imprisoned and court-martialed before returning to England.

While Wills and Holwell represent the extremes of East India Company careers, their paths demonstrate the fluidity and diversity of medical practice within the company, and the motivations common to medical practitioners who traveled out to India around midcentury. Surgeons appointed to company ships easily became surgeons to company factories or troops, or were appointed to settlement hospitals, which served soldiers and merchants of the company. In the East India Company, just as individuals held both civilian and military posts, and military officers engaged in private trade, so medical men serving in India were simultaneously military men, company servants, and private traders, having chosen medicine as one route among many to achieve wealth and status.

This chapter examines how the Seven Years' War changed the nature of British involvement in India, as demonstrated in the nature of medical practice and theories of disease. As a consequence of campaigns during the Seven Years' War, the company was regarded as a territorial, if not imperial, power by 1765 (the date of the *diwani* grant), and its responsibilities could no longer be described as simply trade and business. This resulted in reforms that standardized the medical practice, just as later reforms increased parliamentary scrutiny of the company's activities and curtailed private trade. At the same time, the scale of the Seven Years' War drew more British troops to India than ever before, which afforded British medical practitioners and military authorities the opportunity to make observations on an unprecedented scale about the effect of India's climate on the health of European troops. One immediate consequence was that British medical theory became more pessimistic about European ability to adapt to India's climate, suggesting instead that India's native population was intrinsically, biologically, different. This, in turn, was to influence the nature of British rule, warfare, and lifestyle in India during the later eighteenth and nineteenth centuries.

This chapter first examines the nature of medical practice in the East India Company before discussing medical care provided to troops, and British medical theory concerning India. It then details how medical theory informed campaigns in Bengal and the Carnatic during the Seven Years' War and the role of disease in siege warfare in particular. As in other theaters of war, the consideration of disease influenced campaign strategy. In India, this was compounded by the difficulties in recruiting men (especially when competing with Royal recruiting) and in transporting them from Europe. The campaigns of the Seven Years' War were larger in scale than any previous ones. They altered not only the nature of British involvement in India, but in the context of medical theory and observations, also

British conceptions of health and disease. Consequently, Britons changed their conceptions of themselves and their relationship to the Indian environment and population.

As in other colonial locations, particularly the American colonies, British forces did not fight only against French troops, but were embroiled in Indian conflicts. The British relied on Indian allies in these contests, making use of preexisting rivalries. Such alliances overlapped during the war, and contemporaries stationed in India were often unclear as to where one war started and another ended.[3] As a shortage of manpower was a perennial problem in India, British military administrators considered campaigns against Indian forces and the French alike, as they presented the same drain on manpower and resources. For these reasons, this chapter surveys battles that involved British forces during the 1750s and 1760s, not only those fought against French forces as part of the Seven Years' War.

The parameters of British military activity in India during this period are complicated also by the nature of the British East India Company: although a private corporation, it relied on British state authority and resources, particularly during the Seven Years' War, when regular forces were essential to its campaigns. It coordinated its demands for manpower with those of the British state and relied on its expertise by, for example, having the Royal Navy examine surgeons for use on East India Company ships. As P. J. Marshall points out, "In retrospect, the Seven Years War can be seen as a significant stage in the incorporation of the East India Company into the British state."[4] This chapter thus provides an overview of the British experience of war and disease in India during the era of the Seven Years' War.

Historians have examined the fundamental role of medicine in British India. As David Arnold points out, Western medicine has been seen as "one of the most powerful and penetrative parts of the entire colonizing process, [and] one of the most enduring."[5] Such studies focus on the later period of British rule; by contrast, this chapter discusses medicine and disease in the genesis and formative period of British imperialism. Examining the role of medicine and disease in 1755–64, when British commercial interests became territorial and imperial powers, confirms the importance of medicine in Britain's imperial rule of India. Whereas studies of the late eighteenth and nineteenth centuries establish how the British used medicine to dominate indigenous populations, environments, and cultures, this chapter's focus on the early period of British colonial development demonstrates that medicine was initially a tool for survival, rather than control. It was the experience of the Seven Years' War that transformed European medicine into a tool of empire, and thus a form of expertise. The physical experience of thousands of British soldiers—more than had ever served in India previously—consolidated changing conceptions of European bodies and convinced officials that European authority could be maintained only through European-style discipline, both bodily and military, rather than through adaptation. This chapter thus identifies the Seven Years' War, and particularly the physical experience of the war, as crucial to the development of tropical medicine and, consequently, to British imperialism.

EAST INDIA COMPANY MEDICINE

The practices of medical personnel in company service around midcentury were varied and flexible. Company surgeons did not live by their salaries alone. Like other company servants, they participated, within limits, in private trade and moneylending to amass personal wealth.[6] They were also granted what Surgeon General Daniel Campbell called "Indulgencies," or financial subsidies from company trade revenues.[7] Indeed, the salaries of company surgeons during the 1750s and 1760s implied that medical practitioners depended on such supplementary income. In 1759, when a senior merchant at Fort St. George was granted an annual allowance of £81, a military lieutenant £92, and the chaplain £178, the surgeon's mate was granted £73, while a surgeon at Bombay was granted only £81, and the head surgeon at Fort St. George £114.[8] Campbell, who had come to India in 1759, asked for an increase in his allowance in part because he claimed that he did not engage in private trade.[9] The company recognized the financial implications of curtailing private trade, for in response to the surgeon general's petition, the Board of Inspection increased his stipend by three and a half times its original amount.

In his petition, Campbell outlined his present and past responsibilities as surgeon in the settlement, noting that he traveled great distances to treat patients and had also served the army and the company factory. Such a variety of responsibilities was not unusual among company medical practitioners. For example, James Ellis had gone to India in 1758 as an assistant surgeon, arriving in Calcutta in 1759. He served at various company posts, briefly serving with the army, before being appointed as full surgeon in 1760. He then served as a surgeon to the army, becoming senior surgeon in 1764, and then first surgeon in the Bengal Establishment in July 1765.[10] Not only did company surgeons serve the civil servants and the army interchangeably while rising rapidly through the ranks; they could also be promoted to the rank of physician. One such case was that of

Andrew Munro, who in December 1756 was promoted from hospital surgeon to the company physician at Fort St. George.[11]

As in North America and the West Indies, colonial military medicine encouraged fluidity between the traditional professional categories of surgeon and physician. In contrast to metropolitan medicine, it provided unusual opportunities for advancement because expertise in a foreign environment could be considered sufficient to support the promotion from surgeon to physician. Yet conditions in India encouraged even greater fluidity than in other colonial locations during the war. Indeed, professional distinctions in India were so interchangeable that the terms "physician" and "surgeon" were very loosely applied to medical practitioners with the company. During the 1750s and 1760s, the surgeons to the settlements were sometimes simply grouped together as "doctors." Medical practitioners regarded themselves as equivalent to both physicians and surgeons, and company officials concurred. Company officials stated that many surgeons already practicing held the degree of physic and yet called themselves surgeons. Moreover, since surgeons stationed in India had "the Advantage of long practical Knowledge of their Profession in this particular Climate," company officials claimed they were physicians in all but name.[12] As was the case in the West Indies, and as Lind remarked in his treatise on diseases of hot climates (including India), it was the direct experience of foreign climates that made a medical practitioner fit to advise on the health of Europeans stationed there.[13]

Medical practitioners with the company certainly gained a variety of experiences through their service in India. Before the reforms of the late 1760s and 1770s, surgeons moved easily within the company's precincts, and particularly between military and civilian posts.[14] Since the sick and wounded company troops were sent to the company's settlement hospitals, the division between military and civilian medical practice was not strict either, especially in times of war.[15] Surgeons also did more than practice physic. Many were merchants, some served as soldiers, and others as company administrators.[16] William Fullerton, for example, was one of the seven doctors who fought at Calcutta in 1756, and was better known for his military leadership, great wealth, and adoption of native culture than for his surgical practice (fig. 5.1).[17]

Medical practitioners experienced fluidity not only within the company, but also beyond its ranks, as company surgeons were frequently used by Indian rulers.[18] For example, Dr. William Forth served as physician to Alivardi Khan, nawab of Bengal, in April 1756.[19] In times of war, this trust in medical practitioners could be exploited for military and political ends.

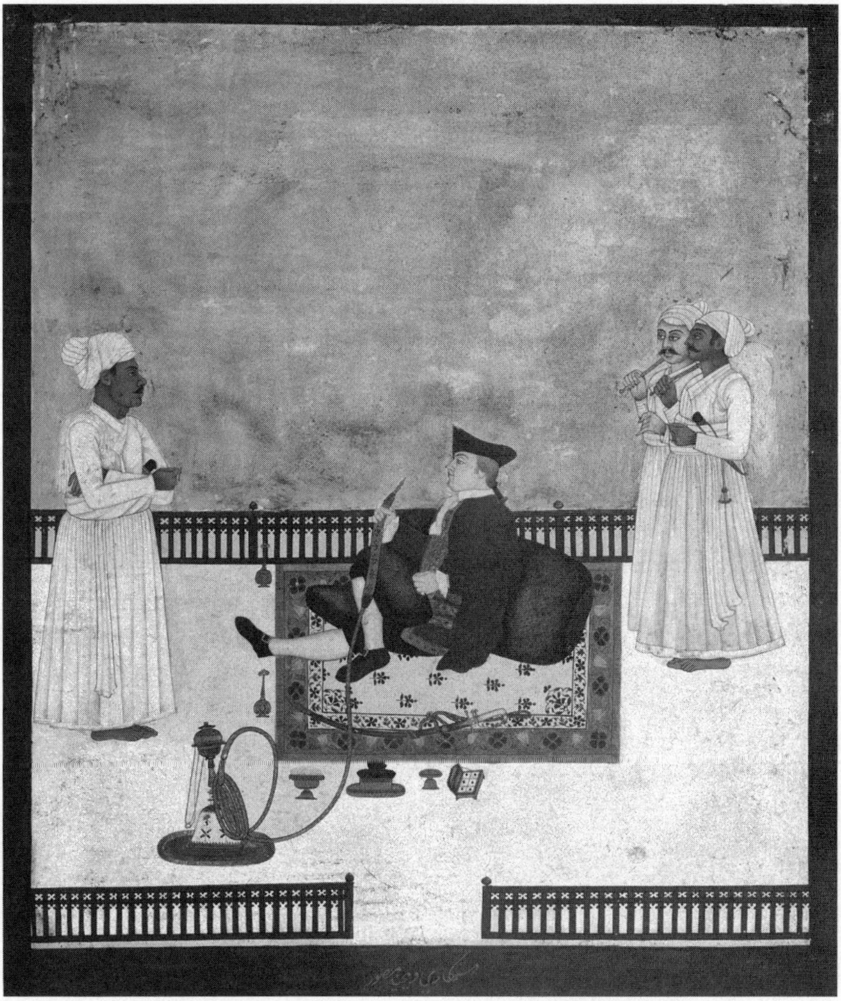

Figure 5.1. *Officer of the East India Company, Probably the Surgeon William Fullerton, on a Terrace, Smoking a Huqqa Directing a Servant*, by Dip Chand, Company School. Watercolor. Murshidabad or Patna, India, ca. 1760–63. © Victoria and Albert Museum, London.

In December 1756, the Select Committee at Fort William engaged Doctor Forth to stay on at Chinsura, and from there "to transmit us from time to time such intelligence as he may judge to be of any consequence to the Company's affairs." Forth was enthusiastic in his task, regularly reporting to company officials on his conversations with the nawab and others at the court, as well as the movements of the nawab's troops.[20] Medicine was thus an integral part of company affairs, and surgeons were active participants in company and private commerce.

Compared with both metropolitan medical practice and that in the British Army and Royal Navy, medical service in India was more flexible, and boundaries between medical positions and between medical and nonmedical practice were more porous, allowing medical practitioners to gain a variety of medical experiences, as well as private wealth, while also rising quickly through the ranks. This suggests that ambitious and intelligent men seeking adventure and profit, but not always possessing rigorous medical training, were drawn to the medical service in India. Given the scarcity of sources, few details are known about the background of these men, but it is clear that before the reforms of the later 1760s, and particularly during wartime, medical candidates were not rigorously examined.[21] Company officials and medical men believed that knowledge of disease was best acquired through firsthand experience in India, especially as medical publications concerning the climate of India were not common until the later 1760s and 1770s. Consequently, the British medical service was comparable to the company's civil service: both required on-the-ground training, and provided opportunities for swift advancement. The men who enlisted in the civil and medical departments were similar, too, insofar as they regarded medical practice and a clerical career in India as a respectable, learned, and professional path with which to gain experience and wealth, and not necessarily as an end in itself.[22]

INDIGENOUS AND EUROPEAN MEDICINE

During this period there are scattered references suggesting that company medical practitioners made use of native medicines and methods. In general, medicines were shipped to surgeons from Britain, with the East India Company Board in London allowing surgeons to try out medicines furnished by different suppliers before choosing one with which to contract.[23] In practice, it appears that many medicines were bought locally, partly because many medicines were damaged or lost on their voyage from Europe. By the early 1770s, the board was repeatedly admonishing hospital apothecaries in India for buying medicines at local "Bazars" (unless such medicines were perishable, as the board could not control or check this type of drug expenditure). These repeated injunctions indicate that apothecaries nevertheless continued to supply themselves with local drugs.[24] Even Edward Ives, a company surgeon critical of indigenous medicine, recounted visiting a local Indian physician when he first arrived in India, recording the variety and prices of drugs available.[25]

The most comprehensive investigation into native medical practices during the 1750s and 1760s is John Zephaniah Holwell's *Account of the Manner of Inoculating for the Small Pox in the East Indies* (1767). Holwell, described as "the first European official who made a study of Indian antiquities," extensively researched the religions and languages he encountered while in India.[26] He became a fellow of the Royal Society in 1767, although his tract on inoculation was the sole medical treatise he had published. In this work, Holwell describes how he watched the Brahmins inoculate "multitudes" in India over the course of several years.[27] It was not only the success of the Brahmins' technique that convinced Holwell to reject his initial prejudice against their procedure, but also the method's explanation according to what he called "rational principles and experiment."[28] Not only did Holwell find the actual method of inoculation similar to the one usually employed in Britain, but he also praised Indian practices as they conformed to European medical theory, noting that they were demonstrably successful in the many cases he had treated accordingly, "making a necessary distinction and allowance between the constitutions of the Natives and Europeans."[29]

Holwell's adoption of Indian medical practices and his explanation of these practices according to European medical theory were not unusual. Early European settlers in India found little difference between their medical theories and those of indigenous medical practitioners. Each was based on a humoral conception of health, albeit with some minor variations. Thus, European medical practitioners in India were eager to investigate and adopt indigenous medical practices, as the few medical treatises on such practices published during the seventeenth and eighteenth centuries demonstrate.[30]

Although indigenous medicine and British experience in India continued to influence settlers' medical theories, British medical practitioners stationed in India did not maintain their enthusiasm for indigenous practices. Historians have identified a trend toward the disparagement of indigenous methods during the eighteenth and nineteenth centuries, culminating in the rejection of not only indigenous medicine, but also indigenous methods of sanitation and hygiene, and even locating the origin of disease in native populations themselves.[31] While the rise of bacteriology and its displacement of the humoral conception of health in the nineteenth century certainly encouraged such a shift, the transformation can also be traced to imperial political developments in the later eighteenth and nineteenth centuries. Specifically, this shift corresponds with attempts at permanent and larger-scale British settlement and political involvement in India, stemming from the territorial and political acquisitions of the Seven Years' War.

This transformation in British medical thinking was not confined to medical practice, but shaped broader conceptions of disease and the human constitution as well. When Europeans had first arrived in India in the sixteenth and seventeenth centuries, they had observed differences between themselves and indigenous populations, but assumed that such differences could be overcome. Not only did Europeans consider the human constitution malleable, but they also did not find India necessarily disease-ridden. With monogenesis claiming that all humans had descended from one set of parents (Adam and Eve), differences in skin color and appearance were explained by reference to changes acquired in different climates. Europeans were thus able to adapt to different climates, and therefore to the diseases associated with those climates. For these reasons Lind described Europeans moving to a hot climate as transplanted flora (as discussed in chapter 2 on the West Indian campaigns). Although European medical practitioners identified some diseases as specific to warm climates, early European settlers in India did not necessarily encounter a disease environment drastically different or more lethal than that of Europe. With malaria (albeit the nonlethal and nontropical *Plasmodium vivax* type) and plague still rife in Europe, and Asiatic cholera not yet epidemic in India, Europeans even considered parts of India more salubrious than home. Not until more rigid and essentialist biological conceptions of the human constitution developed, alongside the decline of plague, *P. vivax* malaria, and other epidemic diseases in Europe on the one hand, and the rise of cholera and other feared diseases in India on the other, did the British come to consider India an alien and dangerous climate. Theories of climatic adaptation were replaced by racial pessimism. Such a transformation fed into, and was nourished by, the shift from "a largely commercial relationship with Indian states, to one of territorial dominance" during the later eighteenth and nineteenth centuries.[32]

Holwell's treatise and other medical works dating from the 1750s and 1760s thus indicate a period of transition. During the Seven Years' War, successful British campaigns resulted in substantial gains by the company, as well as increased "penetration" of Indian state structures and new observations on British and native bodies, all of which had repercussions for British conceptualizations of health and disease in India.[33]

COMPANY TROOPS AND THEIR CARE

The Indian climate and its diseases were important considerations for the armed services. The British East India Company was perennially short of troops, especially compared with the vast armies that Indian rulers could command. The company encountered two main obstacles with regard to troops. First, the voyage to India required upwards of six months on a ship, and often more if unfavorable winds or bad weather intervened. Second, the company competed with His Majesty's Army for recruits.[34] In times of war, when regular regiments in Britain were also aggressively recruiting, the company encountered great difficulties in raising troops. The company thus relied on His Majesty's troops during war time. Royal troops were first sent to India, at the request of the Board of Directors, to fight against the French during the campaigns of the 1740s.[35] A British battalion of 1,000 men was again sent in June 1759. By 1760, four regular British regiments were serving in India with substantial support from the Royal Navy against both French and Indian forces.[36] As well, close to 3,000 European company troops were serving the board in India, a notable increase from the 500 rank-and-file soldiers commanded by some ten to twenty officers in 1750.[37]

The difference between British regular troops and company troops is difficult to delineate. Although exact figures are not known, company troops were mainly composed of European and Eurasian Christian mercenaries (often called Topasses, who were frequently part Portuguese), one-quarter of whom were of British descent.[38] It was widely acknowledged that the troops sent to serve the company in India during the early eighteenth century were of low quality, and their officers were ridiculed for their low social rank.[39] The council at Calcutta under Robert Clive complained to the Board of Directors in London about the poor quality of men sent out to India as troops, blaming the practice of recruitment by contract, whereby the company sold contracts to individuals who then provided recruits.[40] The board defended its methods by comparing them with those of the regular army. Not only did it follow the same procedure, the board also insisted that the amount it paid per man was "always considerably more than what the Government allow," adding, "We are often necessitated to take undersized soldiers, but if they are not always strong able men, we have been deceived."[41]

Disparaging generalizations about soldiers by both contemporaries and historians are common for the eighteenth century, and in-depth research often demonstrates that these generalizations are more caricatures than just portrayals.[42] By the 1770s and 1780s, the profitable acquisitions from the Seven Years' War and the publicity surrounding the spectacular victories of Clive and other officers attracted men of high status to India, with gentlemen frequently serving as military officers.[43]

Writing during the Seven Years' War, the sailor William Spavens claimed that company troops were recruited in England by being "kidnapped and kept in certain offices till the ships are at Gravesend, whither they are sent, and kept under a guard until they sail," a description contemporaries might also have used concerning the navy's seamen.[44] By contrast, a British regular soldier complained about company recruitment during the war that enticed would-be regular soldiers into the company's service through its "extraordinary proportion of pay" and promise of large rewards.[45] Stories of the kind well known for the West Indies, about soldiers and sailors doing anything to avoid being sent for service in India or deserting when their destination was announced, do not appear to have been common.

There were obvious drawbacks to serving in India, notably its distance from Britain and that company troops did not enjoy the same care and benefits as British regular troops did. Although all company servants, including soldiers, received medical care from company surgeons while on service, soldiers did not receive any benefits if they were disabled. Disabled soldiers in the regular army, by contrast, were granted a small allowance as out-pensioners or lived in Chelsea hospital as full pensioners.[46] The navy's provision for disabled veterans was slightly more generous, with the larger Greenwich hospital for live-in naval pensioners and more substantial allowances granted to out-pensioners.[47] Similarly, the Poplar Fund for seamen maimed or killed in the company's service was established in 1619 (although the mechanisms of this fund are not well understood).[48] Yet such provisions were not forthcoming for invalided company soldiers; as the directors in London made clear, "we have no fund for such a purpose, nor can we raise one."[49]

The company recognized the value of such rewards, using promises of land or pensions for veterans to attract sepoys to its service in the 1760s and 1770s.[50] Sailors on board company ships appear to have been better provided for by having closer links with existing Royal Naval medical care; company ship logs record regular deductions from all seamen's pay for the navy's Greenwich hospital, and East India Company ship medical forms were sent to the Sick and Hurt Board of the Royal Navy.[51] However, the Sick and Hurt Commissioners noted that the navy's requested East Indian medical care "has not been heretofore practised, and may be attended with some inconvenience," while also remarking on its exorbitant cost.[52] While health provision for disabled company troops would have been a welcome reward, the free medical care provided by the company to all servants and troops while on service (with the exception of care for venereal disease) was thus an expensive and effective gesture toward recruits and employees.[53]

The East India Company also invested in the men's health during the long voyage from Europe. Not surprisingly, scurvy constantly wrought havoc among troops on their way to and from India. Theories concerning its rise and prevention, as discussed at length in chapters 1 and 4, identified it with a lack of fresh provisions and the cramped unwholesome quarters common on board ships during long voyages. Even with improved sailing routes, the average distance of a voyage from England to India or China during the later eighteenth century was over 13,000 miles, and the average duration close to four months (often longer when returning to England), including frequent stops in ports.[54]

The logs of British East India Company ships regularly document the ravages of scurvy. According to Edward Ives, the surgeon onboard the *Kent*, scurvy appeared among Admiral Charles Watson's squadron sent from Britain in 1754. On arriving at Madagascar, the *Kent* had 150 sick:

> The greater part were now afflicted with the scurvy, and to so great a degree, that they had not strength enough to crawl upon the deck, and scarcely to breathe; we were obliged therefore to carry them out of the ship in their hammocks: but so salutary was the land, and the refreshments it produced, that in less than three weeks after they were put ashore, almost all of them happily recovered their former health and vigour.[55]

It was on the longer voyage back to England that higher rates of scurvy prevailed. After the *Marlborough*, for example, set sail for England from Culpee (near Calcutta) on 21 January 1758, the first sick sailors were sent ashore on 15 April 1758. By mid-October, 25 of the 170 men (15 percent) were sick and deaths were recorded. With provisions running out, the sickly and undermanned crew were put on half rations, having to throw the ship's heavy guns overboard in order to finally anchor in Kinsale road on 26 October 1757.[56]

While this is an extreme example of a hard voyage from India to England, the journey between these countries did regularly occasion disease.[57] Oranges, lemons, lime juice, and "fruit" in the form of dried currants and raisins were provisioned on board to reduce rates of scurvy, but their usefulness in preventing the disease was limited. Fresh fruit and fruit juice would have rotted or lost its vitamin content by the time it was required to prevent scurvy, and currants and raisins contain very little vitamin C, which decreased further the longer they were stored on board.[58] With India at such a distance from Britain—much farther away than colonies in North America or the West Indies—the disease was more common during these trips. As Lind had stated in his treatise on scurvy, it was in the unnatural circumstances of long voyages and long sieges that scurvy flourished.[59] Although sufferers could recover if sent on shore, scurvy was a regular complaint that demonstrates the difficulties inherent in sending British forces to fight in India, even before they arrived in its foreign climate.

CLIMATE AND DISEASE

Disease in India was inseparably linked to its climate, as was the case for the West Indies. In his treatise on inoculation, Holwell describes the climate and seasons of Bengal and their accompanying maladies. He divides the year into three seasons: the rainy, the cold, and the hot and dry. While Holwell describes the cold season as the most "desirable or delightful climate" to be found in the world, and the hot season as relatively healthy, the rainy season, lasting from the middle of October to June, often caused disease, especially if settlers were immoderate in their behavior. More specifically, the end of September was the opening of what he called "the dangerous season," during which fevers were common, and of which

> the Natives frequently recover, but the Europeans seldom, especially if they in the preceding May and June indulged too freely in those two *bewitching delicacies, Mangos* and *Mango Fish*, indiscriminately with the free use of *flesh* and *wine*; for these (*all together*) load the whole habit with impurities, and never fail of yielding Death a plentiful harvest, in the three last months of this putrid season.[60]

Such an account agrees with Lind's characterization of the relationship between disease and climate in general, and of the diseases found in India in particular. In *An Essay on Diseases Incidental to Europeans in Hot Climates*, Lind dedicated a section to the diseases of the East Indies, and specifically to those suffered by company servants in India. Like Holwell, Lind defined Bengal's rainy season as beginning in October and ending in June, noting, "The remainder of the year is healthy and pleasant."[61]

Lind characterized indigenous diseases as "malignant and remitting fevers, which rage during the wet season, and some time after it, in the unhealthy parts of the East Indies."[62] Like Holwell, he noted that these fevers attacked most readily those living intemperately.

Other medical authors observed the disease of the liver that plagued Europeans in India. According to a 1763 medical tract, inflammation of the liver was "very common in the East Indies: the soldiers suffer most from it; probably, either from the excessive heats they are often unavoidably exposed to, or from an intemperate life, though indeed the most sober do not always escape."[63] Relying on observations gleaned from the course of the disease and from dissections on dead soldiers, the author concluded that medical treatment (in the form of mercury and bleeding) was successful, even though it disagreed with metropolitan medical theories.[64] As in other colonial locations, empirical methods and other forms of firsthand experience strongly informed medical theories about disease in India.

The most constant complaint of the British in India during this period, the putrid and intermittent fevers, also produced jaundice and an inflamed liver.[65] These fevers were certainly malaria, characterized by its periodic bouts of chills and fever. Caused by a parasite infection (*Plasmodium*), malaria is transmitted by the *Anopheles* genus of mosquito in much the same manner as yellow fever. Carried in the blood system, the parasites attack the liver, producing the violent paroxysms of chills and fever; hence its appellation "intermittent" fever. The milder form, *Plasmodium vivax*, is debilitating and has episodic recurrences throughout a sufferer's lifetime, but is not usually lethal unless complications intervene. *Plasmodium falciparum*, on the other hand, is much more mortal but, if survived, will not cause relapses. Unlike the *Aedes aegypti* mosquito involved in yellow fever transmission, the *Anopheles* genus and its eggs cannot be carried long distances. Instead, the breeding habits of *Anopheles* ensure that the mosquitoes are present in warm and humid environments only, especially marshes and tropical coastlines during and after the rainy season. Consequently, the disease had long been associated with these locations, and especially with the pestilential air that seemed to arise from such conditions; the term "malaria," in fact, is Italian for "bad air."[66]

According to eighteenth-century nosology (disease classifications), fevers were defined according to their symptoms, and hence by the classical division into continual, intermittent, and remittent, with periodic fevers further subdivided into quartan or tertian, depending on the number of days between episodes.[67] British medical practitioners of the period were familiar with the form of malaria common in the marshy areas of Britain into the nineteenth century, known as "ague." However, the European form of malaria was the less lethal *P. vivax*, whereas it was the mortal variety *P. falciparum* that threatened in the tropics. In India, British medical practitioners observed the difference between the malarial fevers: not only did the practitioners classify tropical fevers as specifically putrescent and more malignant, but the British in India also suffered from a more deadly version of the disease. As in theories of typhus and scurvy, putrid air and the excessive heat and humidity were understood to encourage the natural process of putrefaction, resulting in higher rates of putrefaction in the natural environment and in an individual sufferer's body during the course of disease.[68] As the surgeon James Stevenson, stationed in India, summarized it to Pringle, "The most prevailing diseases on this Coast are intermitting and remitting Fevers, Fluxes & nervous disorders. . . . These Fevers attack with much the same symptoms as in Europe, but more violently."[69]

Lind's section on diseases in the East Indies followed much the same pattern as his section on diseases in the West Indies: he included lengthy excerpts from those who had been stationed there, demonstrating how first-hand observations underpinned his medical theories. Surgeons stationed with the East India Company and British forces during the war provided most of these accounts, such as the Royal Naval surgeon Edward Ives. As in other locations during the war, Lind relied on unpublished accounts and a network of correspondents who served with British armed forces. Ives, for example, served in India between 1754 and 1757 but did not publish his account until 1773. Lind also used these observations on diseases and the environment in India as he had done for the West Indies: to show that the diseases were all similar in their origin, tied to the nature of hot climates. The West and East Indies, along with Africa and parts of America (as well as a few locations in Europe), formed a coherently foreign disease environment, presenting similar challenges to the health of Europeans.[70]

Lind's overarching argument was thus that all hot climates, which were the same foreign environments in which British colonialism was consolidating, were medically unified. Because of this, his book is considered the foundational text for tropical medicine, a discipline that Michael Worboys has described as the "main scientific expression of Western medical and health policy for the Third World" for most of the twentieth century.[71] Lind's treatise should thus be seen as an integral part of the British imperial process—drawing on observations gleaned from the experience of British armed forces serving abroad, while also providing advice that would shape the nature of future imperial projects and policy. While pointing to the fundamental unity of hot climates, his view was not rigidly uniform or static; accounts of those actually stationed in places such as Africa and India demonstrated that some parts were perfectly safe for Europeans, and more malignant environments could be improved through drainage and agriculture. Thus, Lind argued that British settlement in hot climates was possible.

As the dry seasons in India were associated with good health, it is not surprising that medical practitioners were optimistic about preventing diseases among British troops stationed in India. Lind was adamant that disease in India followed the seasons, and that the ravages of the diseases could be avoided if settlements were established in healthy locations, away from damp areas, and low-lying marshes and coastlines that lacked healthy winds, just as in the West Indies.[72] By avoiding the seats of putrid air during the rainy seasons, Europeans would maintain their health even in a tropical climate. This medical dictum was widely known: even Robinson Crusoe moved his tent to a location farther away from the marshy shore soon after finding himself shipwrecked.[73]

As *Anopheles* mosquitoes prefer such locations, eighteenth-century medical practitioners were correct in their observations and recommendations concerning malarial fevers. The company naval surgeon John Clark rightly remarked that putrid remittent fevers were linked to "exhalations from the land," and hence, once ships were cleaned and out at sea, the disease dramatically lessened.[74] The *Anopheles* genus can fly only within a two-mile radius from shore, meaning that troops on board ships away from the coastline would indeed have avoided malarial fevers. But even for troops required to camp on shore, preventative methods were still available. Just as the draining of ditches and marshes is recommended today to destroy the breeding grounds of mosquitoes, and hence stem the incidence of malaria, Clark recommended that Europeans residing in India establish themselves in dry and drained locations:

> The improvements which are every day taking place at Bencoolen will soon render that settlement healthy. The residents there having totally relinquished the old town, which was wet and low, and residing at Fort Marlborough, on a drier and more elevated situation, are not so subject to sickness in the rainy months, and the diseases which appear are of a much milder nature. Upon the whole, the insalubrity of this island seems to be owing to want of culture [i.e., cultivation in an agricultural sense].[75]

As he had also argued in the case of the West Indies, Lind agreed with Clark that it was within the grasp of British officials both to establish settlements in healthy locations in India and to turn unhealthy locations into healthy settlements. He explained in his introduction to southern Asia, "The countries which are well improved by human industry and [agri]culture, such as China, and several other places in that part of the world, are blessed with a temperate and pure air, salutary to the European constitution."[76] This is not to suggest that Lind entirely discounted disease as a problem for Europeans in India. He strenuously argued that such a climate was potentially dangerous to a European constitution and that deaths from sickness were necessary considerations for military officers stationed in those parts of the world. This sickness, however, could be prevented, and therefore Lind was adamant about the importance of following medical advice to encourage seasoning to the new climate, as was also the case for the West Indies. These medical views comported with the popular understanding that disease outbreaks among troops were symptoms of disorder; they also complemented the optimism of the British that they could adapt to the climate of India. As Colonel Scott declared in his proposed 1754 plan to conquer Bengal, scurvy during the voyage to India was the only disease British troops should worry about, as "objections to the heat of the Climate being a set or hindrance to the enterprize, can be made only by those who are unacquainted with the country."[77]

Along with the judicious choice of settlements and disciplined management thereof, Europeans could also avoid disease in India by exercising moderation, especially with respect to alcohol and diet. As with yellow fever in the West Indies, medical practitioners linked fevers in India to excessive drinking and eating. While troops in India would have been tempted by the cheap and plentiful liquor available in the form of arrack, drinking alcohol also exacerbated diseases that afflict the liver. Holwell, Lind, and Clark all cautioned against overindulging in food and wine, Lind stating in the preface to his work on disease and hot climates that "violent exercises, excessive drinking, and every species of intemperance, dispose the constitution, more especially in hot climates, to the attack of the epidemic diseases of the country."[78] Military officials concurred, blaming indiscipline and drunkenness among troops in India for disease outbreaks.[79] As Colonel Scott neatly reminded company officials in his plan for the conquest of Bengal, "It must be remember'd, the preserving [of] our conquest, must depend on the preservation of our people, toward which the strictest discipline & temperance must likewise contribute."[80] With bark (quinine) recommended to treat fevers, along with discipline and wise decisions regarding the location of camps, it appeared to company and military administrators in the mid-eighteenth century that disease among European troops stationed in India could be successfully controlled.

DISEASE AND CAMPAIGNING SEASONS

Although medical practitioners were optimistic that high rates of disease could be prevented, it was apparent that European troops regularly suffered from disease while on campaign in India. According to the few hospital admission records that survive from this period, it was "fever" that sent most men to the hospital.[81] As contemporary regimental returns and historian Mark Harrison's analysis of hospital admissions demonstrate, disease rates varied according to the seasons, with admissions peaking during and after the rainy season, just as Lind, Clark, and Holwell observed.[82] Health concerns thus restricted the campaigning season in India to the period between May and October, a practice with a long tradition among indigenous Indian forces.

During the opening stages of the war, the few company troops stationed in India were in good health, and many were more worried about the nawab of Bengal than French attacks.[83] In response to increased British political interference and growing military preparations, Siraj ud-Daula, the nawab, laid siege to the company's Fort William at Calcutta on 16 June 1756. When most of the company servants fled, anywhere between 69 and 146 British men and women were locked in the holding cell that became infamous as the "Black Hole of Calcutta." Accounts published soon after attest to the widespread acceptance of medical theories concerning putrid air in a hot climate. The various narratives claimed that the incarcerated men and women who died suffered not only from a lack of air in the small room, but also because "the prodigious heat joined to the noisome stench of several wounded men who were put in with them."[84]

Contemporaries attributed the prisoners' deaths in the Hole to the cruelty of Siraj ud-Daula, and in response demanded that the company retake Calcutta. Historians have demonstrated that the Black Hole of Calcutta incident has more to do with British mythology about corrupt and vicious Indian rule, in contrast to British liberal governance, than with actual events.[85] However, British outrage is also understandable in terms of contemporary medical beliefs that saw outbreaks of sickness—in a camp, on a ship, or in a prison—as evidence of poor management, callousness, or outright cruelty. Such callous treatment of troops and prisoners (see chapter 6) was cause for condemnation of enemy and allied commanders alike.

Regardless of the inaccuracy of accounts, the retaking of Calcutta initiated British military actions in India that concluded, in 1764, not only with the end of French influence in India but also with the British company as de facto rulers of Bengal, an act that in the long term established the British Empire in India.

During the late 1750s and early 1760s, the company fought against both French and native rulers, who often overlapped, either through alliances or by playing one against the other. For British officials, disease also linked campaigns against French forces with those against Indian powers, as using troops in a campaign against the one often resulted in sickness that incapacitated campaigns against the other. For example, in the expedition to retake Calcutta in 1756–57, disease among British troops resulted in concern over a lack of manpower to fight the French in 1757. Sickness first began when company survivors of the nawab's siege of Fort William were stationed at Fulta, along with Major Kilpatrick and his troops, awaiting plans to retake Calcutta. A French company official described Fulta, situated some thirty miles south of Calcutta on the shore of the river Hughli, as having "unhealthy air."[86] The council of Fort William had firsthand experience of this, having lost both its secretary and subsecretary to fevers while at Fulta.[87] Kilpatrick, who had served in India since the early 1750s, recognized the dangers of Fulta's location, writing to his company superiors, "The Place and Situation we are in, renders it extreamly unhealthy, and I am sorry to hear that it will be but more so as the season advances."[88] Kilpatrick's observations were correct, as the log of the company ship *Delaware* stationed at Fulta confirms high levels of sickness by mid-August, along with the death of troops and officials, including the surgeon's mate.[89]

In their plans for the retaking of Calcutta, the council at Fort St. George took into consideration the rainy season and resulting sickness.[90] Torn between maintaining the health of British troops by delaying the expedition until the healthy season, and saving the health of those stationed at Fulta through immediate action, the council chose a compromise: a few of the navy's ships with 250 army troops would be sent toward Calcutta, "only without attempting any thing more until join'd by further Succours."[91] While waiting for the arrival of these forces, the *Delaware*'s log lists 31 deaths at Fulta between early August and January 1757, out of a total of 118 seamen and officers on board.[92] British officials reported on "the sickly state of the remaining gentlemen of Calcutta & the party under Major Kilpatrick of which only 30 men fit for duty."[93] Moreover, the troops sent by the council at Fort St. George, arriving in December 1756 and February 1757, were not all healthy.[94]

The high levels of sickness meant that when British forces attacked at the end of December 1756, there were only 700 Europeans fit for action, fighting alongside 1,200 native troops. Once troops landed, Eyre Coote called for an immediate attack so the troops would not suffer ill health by sleeping on shore during the night. The next day, the company and regular troops sailed on to Tannah fort, while the sepoys marched alongside the ships, on shore—standard procedure to prevent the exhaustion of European soldiers. In early January 1757, British and company troops continued their march on Calcutta, skirmishing with the nawab's forces throughout. Meanwhile, Clive continually complained of a shortage of troops. Writing to Admiral Watson on 20 January 1757, Clive explained that he had only 300 rank-and-file Europeans in camp, and asked for reinforcements from among Watson's Royal troops, adding, "You are very sensible, Sir, that with sickness and other accidents how far this force falls short of what was intended to act offensively against the Nabob of Bengal."[95] Although relations between Clive and Watson were acrimonious at the outset of the expedition, these appear resolved by this point: the following day Watson acceded to Clive's request, even providing extra troops from the ships under his command.[96] Returns of the troops camped at Barnagore, near Calcutta, show 181 troops sick out of a total of 733—a high, but not disastrous, sick rate of 25 percent.[97] Clive wrote to the company's committee in London early in February, claiming that he could not attack the nawab and his forces at Calcutta until reinforcements arrived.[98] Clive's grievance is substantiated by British observations that even Siraj ud-Daula's native troops had succumbed in large numbers to the season's diseases.[99]

Open battle finally commenced on 4 February 1757. With the success of European troops established, Siraj ud-Daula signed a treaty with company officials in mid-February, assuring them the right to trade and to fortify Calcutta, as well as returning possessions and reimbursing company officials for damages suffered during the siege of June 1756.[100] The expedition to retake Calcutta during the rainy season meant that European manpower was weakened on account of sickness throughout, and thus resulted in longer-term shortages of manpower for the following campaigns.

It came as no surprise when Coote read the notice of the declaration of war between France and Britain in March 1757 to his troops.[101] For some time, company officials had been worried that their forces were not strong enough to withstand attacks from the French while fighting off native rulers. Company officials were right to be anxious about fighting against two enemies in India, for both Clive and Watson were short of men throughout January and February because of sickness.[102] With Calcutta retaken, British officials turned their attention to the French Compagnie des Indes, storming the French post at Chandernagore, around twenty miles north of Calcutta, in mid-March 1757.

In his attack on French posts, Clive repeatedly took the health of his troops into consideration. He stationed only a few troops in Calcutta so that they would not fall sick from overcrowding, ordering the remainder to Chandernagore "as being the more healthy place."[103] Clive also resisted plans to send forces back to Madras, suggesting instead that they remain encamped around Calcutta until August as he felt the journey would "be long and painful to the troops."[104] His strategy proved successful, as returns of the troops under his command in April 1757 list among the European rank and file only 176 sick out of a total of 1,397—a low sick rate of only 13 percent that was maintained through to June 1757.[105] The health of the troops benefited British and company military endeavors. By the end of June 1757, forces under Clive and Coote had taken Cutwa, then marched through Calcutta and fought Siraj ud-Daula's army with spectacular success on 23 June 1757 at the battle of Plassey, helped by the Royal Navy.[106]

Yet the company's position was not secure, for French troops still threatened from various French Compagnie des Indes posts. In pursuit of the French, British forces marched upriver from Plassey and well into Bihar. Both sepoys and the European troops complained of hardships during the march, and the sepoys also about their distance from their families.[107] With the onset of the rainy season in 1757, the troops under Coote began to fall sick again. A council of war decided early in August to abandon the pursuit of the French, in part because of sick rates.[108] Following medical advice, Coote proceeded to quarter his troops at Patna in the company's factory and in a French building, ensuring that the men were not crowded and that their quarters were kept clean for the sake of maintaining their health.[109] Despite these measures, troops continued to fall sick.[110]

As for Clive, the early months of the rainy season in 1757 began optimistically. After the success of Plassey and his first battles against the French forces in Bengal, Clive wrote to the Court of Directors in London on 22 August 1757, "The sinews of war are in your own possession, and there wants nothing but supplies of men and military stores to keep up your influence, and preserve all your privileges and acquisitions."[111] Even in the midst of these victories, Clive knew well the necessity of maintaining the health of his troops. He informed the Secret Committee that he had garrisoned the troops in a healthy location, as "the lives of men are very precious at this critical juncture."[112] Notwithstanding his care, as with the troops under Coote, men soon fell sick during the rainy season.

By mid-October, Clive requested reinforcements because of sickness among his troops.[113] The troops quartered at Chandernagore under Archibald Grant similarly fell sick during the unhealthy months of September and October. According to the monthly return dated 29 October 1757, out of the total 407 troops, a remarkable 290 soldiers were listed as sick—a sick rate of 71 percent. Grant assured Clive that he was doing his utmost to rectify this situation. He blamed sickness on the lack of a proper hospital, and told Clive that a new one was being built. Grant's description of the sickness reflects the prevalence of disease theories focused on putrid air in hot climates, explaining, "Tis imagin'd that the mortality that has happen'd has been in a great measure owing to the putrid and corrupted air with which the former [hospital] must be filled, from the numbers that have been in in [*sic*] it."[114]

Even when medical advice was followed and precautions were taken, more troops from Britain were necessary for large-scale campaigns against native forces and the French, particularly as such campaigns increasingly extended beyond the healthy season. The growing sickness was reflected in the monthly returns and in commanders' urgent requests for reinforcements. Writing to the company's committee in London in January 1758, the committee at Fort William detailed their need for more men to be sent from Britain in order to maintain their holdings, especially given that the French were sure to attack.[115] The returns indicate that sepoys were affected as much as European troops, or even more so.[116] The opening years of the war clearly established that disease was a constant presence and concern during Indian campaigns. For British officials stationed in India and those directing strategy in London, decisions regarding diplomacy, strategy, and logistics (recruitment, contracting, transport, and the like) revolved constantly around the manpower challenges posed by sickness.

SIEGE WARFARE, PONDICHERRY, AND HOT CLIMATES

As was the case in North America, the West Indies, and Europe, warfare in India during this period was often characterized by long sieges, in which an attacking force besieged a fortified holding, battering its defenses with land and naval artillery and attempting to cut off supplies. Besides small skirmishes and artillery exchanges, open battles were fought rarely—usually once one side had exhausted its provisions and strength.[117] In India, warfare during the Seven Years' War was little different, although it was constrained by the unhealthy rainy season, and European troops were vastly outnumbered by native sepoys. Beginning in 1758, British forces stationed in India continually besieged, or were besieged by, French forces, until the last French post in Bengal fell to the British East India Company in 1761.

Because sieges forced troops to crowd into small holdings with limited provisions and fragmented sanitary and medical arrangements, siege warfare resulted in high rates of sickness. As at Quebec and Havana, this meant that military and naval officials worried more about their troops falling under strength because of disease than because of battle wounds—a particular concern in foreign climates. Eighteenth-century medical theories regarding putrid air, especially that produced in crowded and unventilated areas, seemed vindicated by such instances of sickness. The wars in India, like the famous example of the Black Hole of Calcutta, served as further confirmation of contemporary medical knowledge and of the significant role that disease played in campaigns. The details of siege warfare also highlight the nature of European colonial war, where cultural practices such as prisoners of war and medical provision served to reify European identity in foreign environments.

After additional French forces arrived in India in April 1758, the French besieged the British Fort St. David, situated near Cuddalore, off the Carnatic coast and approximately 100 miles south of Madras. Alexander Wynch, the British official in charge of the garrison of St. David, reported to Governor Pigot that when the French first arrived, he had 158 rank-and-file European troops fit for duty.[118] The European troops at first helped with the hard labor of improving defensive works against French artillery, but in the heat of the climate, they soon balked at such tasks.[119] By 21 May, Wynch reported only 120 Europeans fit for duty, along with 70 Topasses, 20 marines, and 200 sepoys.[120] About a week later, the besieged were reduced to salt provisions while the fort's water supply was no longer fit to drink. The combination of crushing heat, salt provisions, and limited water is a hard one, and discipline appears to have broken down. By 31 May, half of the sailors were recorded as drunk, with only the sepoys fully accounted for. With no expectation of a naval squadron appearing anytime soon, the British surrendered on 2 June 1758.[121]

The French continued their offensive in 1758, retaking positions in the Carnatic, despite tensions in the French command between Thomas, comte de Lally, and the Marquis de Bussy. In December 1758, the French began their siege of one of the central British strongholds, at Fort St. George, Madras. British garrison returns before the siege list around 1,100 Europeans and 1,800 sepoys in the fort, with a low sick rate of 8 percent.[122] As with all sieges, the besieged British troops suffered from both bombardment and a shortage of provisions. The British forces also suffered from sickness throughout the siege; records indicate rates as high as 60 percent, before naval reinforcements in February 1759 lifted the siege.

With their failure at Fort St. George early in 1759 alongside the loss of possessions in the Northern Circars, French operations began to falter, particularly because of the strength of British naval blockades and increasing French financial strains. After British forces took Conjerveram in March 1759, the British continued to chase retreating French forces, even though Colonel Draper reported increasing sick rates among the troops under his command during May and June.[123] By January 1760, British forces had successfully attacked Wandiwash under Coote's command (with the constant naval support of Pocock), capturing almost all the French stations along the Coromandel Coast, and were slowly closing in on the last main French holding, Pondicherry.

Located in southeastern India, on the Bay of Bengal, Pondicherry was the chief French settlement in India, first established as a trading center in 1673, and of vital strategic importance to the French. British troops first arrived at Pondicherry in May 1760, and were reinforced late in the summer. Along with crucial support from the Royal Navy under Admiral Charles Stevens, Coote commanded the siege of Pondicherry and its surroundings. By August, Coote had already intercepted letters from Lally, the French commander at Pondicherry, that detailed the scarcity of provisions among the French.[124] The British besiegers were also suffering under the conditions of the siege, Coote reporting in late September that he had almost 600 sick men, and 115 killed and wounded, of a total of 2,000 Europeans and 6,000 sepoys.[125] A few days later, Coote requested more men from the fleet, as otherwise he would "be obliged to raise the blockade of Pondicherry, for want of men to occupy the different posts."[126]

Lally's position was more tenuous than Coote's. As the British forces were unable to destroy the fortifications, they were content to starve the besieged into submission.[127] Early in November, Coote intercepted more letters from Lally, in which the French commander stated that without provisions and aid from the French fleet, he would soon be forced to surrender. On 28 November, Coote recorded in his journal, "[French] Deserters dropping in daily who all agree in the distressed situation of the garrison, each man being allowed no more than half a measure of Rice per diem."[128] By 11 January, deserters stated that the French could not hold out a week longer, and indeed, the French surrendered the fort on 15 January 1761.[129]

Reports about the terrible conditions within the French garrison during the nearly eight-month siege circulated freely outside the fort. When British prisoners were taken during a skirmish early in January, Lally released them, lacking the provisions with which to feed them.[130] Upon the French surrender, a British official wrote from Fort St. George: "I believe they [the French] would have given us some trouble before they would have given up, had they not been obliged to it for want of provisions. They actually lived some days on camels and dogs flesh & were miserable objects to look at when they surrendered."[131] Although French-controlled factories—including Pondicherry—were eventually returned at the 1763 Peace of Paris, the successful siege of Pondicherry meant the end of French political and military power in India in the short term, with Lally executed in 1766 for his role in the surrender.

Yet for British forces in India, the taking of Pondicherry did not mean an end to military campaigns. British forces were still required to secure, and then expand, their holdings against native powers. French commanders were an enemy that British military and naval officials knew and understood, and one that appeared to act according to established conventions of war.[132] This understanding was only enhanced by a shared European awareness that they were acting in an alien and hostile environment. Correspondence between Coote and Lally during the siege of Pondicherry demonstrates that they respected one another and agreed on proper military codes of conduct. Medical provisions, for example, were allowed to pass into enemy territory so that the sick and wounded could be treated. Lally wrote that Indian and company men "know no right but that of force." By contrast, he, "as a European and a King's man I fulfilled my duty towards you and Mr. Cornish, and sent each his Surgeons, and assure you your scorbuticks will be taken as much care of here, as if they were with you."[133] Even in the midst of warfare, gentlemanly and polite behavior, detached professionalism, and similar social backgrounds united officers. When taken prisoner, for example, officers dined with their captor officers, and were expected to live in relative ease and comfort.[134]

As concerns disease and health, such gentlemanly codes of conduct meant that the officer class of a besieged force could escape much of the worst of warfare. But officer status was no defense against the climate, as fevers such as malaria would have struck individuals regardless of social rank. What did differ, however, was the medical treatment available to sufferers. While doses of quinine and other medicines would most likely have been similar for the rank-and-file troops as for officers, the remedy that surgeons in India increasingly recommended was a change of air. This was a logical application of contemporary theories of fevers, and would have removed troops from malarial and the hotter locations, just as hill stations did for the British during later imperial rule.[135] What distinguished officers from the rank and file in this period is that officers had the option to be sent back to Britain for a change of air, while this was too difficult and expensive to apply to the rank and file, who could at most be moved to another settlement in India. Both Coote and Clive received leave to return to Britain for the sake of their health during the war, Clive going to Bath to take the waters, perhaps as much for his nervous complaint as for any ailment resulting from his service in India.[136]

Letters written by officials during the war contain requests, almost always granted, for military and naval officers to take leave to return to Britain for the sake of their health, but none for the rank and file to do the same. Admiral Charles Watson refused leave granted him to return to England for his health, a decision that cost him his life, as he died in 1757 from sickness in Calcutta. This refusal contemporaries declared as worthy of a British hero, Edward Ives extolling that "so predominant in his breast was the spirit of patriotism, and the love of glory," that the admiral stayed in India and "resolved still to expose himself to the hazards of a climate, peculiarly fraught with danger and disease."[137]

Returning to the moderate, healthy climate of Britain was believed by contemporary medical practitioners to be crucial to recovery. The case of the naval officer Thomas Latham, commanding captain of the *Tyger*, illustrates this. Letters by company surgeons describe his long-standing bilious complaint of four years: a liver disorder (most likely malaria along with other afflictions), the disease most common to Europeans fighting in India. The surgeons emphatically declared that Latham could be cured only by returning to Britain, and accordingly Pocock granted Latham leave to return on 15 February 1759. As Latham was reluctant to ask for leave, his advising surgeons canvassed the surgeons attached to the naval squadron, as well as those stationed at the company's settlements, for medical advice. Surgeon George Johnson conveyed the general consensus:

> Your whole frame is so extremely relax'd from your tedious long illness, its almost impossible your health should be re-established in a warm climate, which probably may be effected in a cold one, therefore

> [I] advise you as I have done before at Bengal, and Madras to return to England as soon as possible, for the longer you continue in India the more dangerous will be your Disorder.[138]

This medical advice is significant not only in that it so closely resembles that offered by physicians such as James Johnson and Thomas Trotter, who had experience with British troops in India during the later eighteenth and early nineteenth centuries, but also in how much it begins to differ from Lind's view of tropical climates and disease.[139] Whereas Lind argued that Europeans could adapt to a hot climate, albeit by following a strict regimen and choosing and managing their settlements with care, surgeons serving the British troops in India advised Latham that nothing could help him but a return to his native country.

Changes in British attitudes toward the climate and diseases of India can be traced to the Seven Years' War. Throughout the war, disease rates fluctuated widely from levels as low as 10 percent during the healthy season to debilitating rates of 60 or 70 percent during the rainy season and during sieges. Whereas Colonel Scott could write in the early 1750s that the conquest of Bengal presented no serious obstacle in terms of health to European troops, save scurvy on the voyage over, surgeons serving during the war were not so optimistic by the time Bengal had been firmly secured under British control in 1764. The timing of this shift is hardly surprising, as it is only in the period of the Seven Years' War that large numbers of British troops served in India.[140] Before the war, central stations such as Bombay had only a few hundred European troops in their garrisons (supported by many more native soldiers). But with the coming of war, thousands of company and British Army and Royal Navy forces were sent to fight in India. These roughly 4,000 European troops were not overwhelming numbers, compared to the tens of thousands fighting in North America and the West Indies. Yet the impact of the experiences of these men in India on medical theories was momentous.

The campaigns won by British and company forces during the Seven Years' War had revolutionary consequences, establishing a territorial empire and ending French influence. Much of the period's historiography focuses on this shift, tracing continuities and pinpointing fundamental changes.[141] In explaining the overwhelming British victories during the war, military historians have noted that the British approach in the later 1750s, including tactics and technology, was no different from that of earlier periods. The only change was an increase in resources: the arrival of Clive and Watson with their troops, as a full-fledged amphibious campaign. The British campaigns in India were thus remarkably similar to campaigns elsewhere during the war, such as at Havana. Additional resources, carefully implemented by taking into consideration local conditions such as disease and climate, resulted in victories that were unachievable during the 1740s.

These victories fundamentally changed the nature of British involvement in India. By the close of the Seven Years' War, the British East India Company could rightly be regarded as an imperial power—a political and territorial power, no longer just a commercial organization. Such a shift had broad repercussions beyond the scope of administration. Company officials came to adjust their political and cultural approaches to life, trade, and diplomacy in India. They no longer felt constrained to accept native practices, instead introducing their own cultural mores.[142] This shift included the introduction of new European medical practices and theories, instead of adopting indigenous ones.

British attitudes toward India's climate and its associated diseases were changing, especially once larger settlements were established after the successful conclusion of the war. These changes had obvious repercussions for British troops in India. Although use of sepoys had started in the 1740s, the practice expanded after their success in the Seven Years' War, with at least 25,000 sepoys stationed in Bengal by the late 1760s, until British forces in India came to consist almost entirely of native troops under the command of British officers. Indeed, the one marked difference for India, compared to other theaters of the war, was the number of native troops enlisted into military service: there were at least twice as many sepoys as European troops, although during this period they were used similarly to American provincials and black troops in the West Indies, as auxiliaries.[143]

When first employed, sepoys had not been regarded as more physically robust substitutes for Europeans, but rather as laboring troops who filled the constant shortage of European troops. Indeed, initially, their habituation to the Indian climate was viewed as a liability, as British officials theorized that such men were enervated and lacking in discipline.[144] While sepoys were expected to perform harder duties than European troops during the Seven Years' War—for example, marching on shore while European troops sailed alongside in ships, or doing the hard labor on fortifications—this was because they were considered inferior in terms of military experience, not because of health considerations. Similar considerations—difference in military status and combat worthiness—explains why American provincials were utilized for noncombatant labor in the American and West Indian campaigns. There is no mention in correspondence during the war of sepoys being recruited because their constitutions were stronger or better suited to the Indian environment, and the few returns that include sepoys during this period do not demonstrate a marked difference in sick rates. A return from June 1757 has British regiments with a sick rate of 13 percent and sepoys at 8 percent, a discrepancy that would not have struck military officials as significant, while a return of 16 December 1757 shows the sepoys in garrison having a significantly higher sick rate than the European troops.[145] Similarly, the four other returns that include sepoys never indicate a difference of more than 13 percent in sick rates between Europeans and sepoys, and not once did this difference occasion remarks by British officials.[146] However, given that a proportion of native troops may have carried genetic resistance to *falciparum* malaria, rates of death may well have been lower for native troops, and differential resistance to disease between European and native troops would have become apparent in the long term.[147]

The constant sickness of European troops and the problems encountered in transporting more men to India did influence the recruitment of sepoys, as this shortage of European troops impelled British officials to exploit native sources of manpower. Still, British officials relied heavily on their European troops and strove to prevent sickness among them. Clive, Watson, and other officials repeatedly expressed concern about the location of troop settlements and about the timing of operations during healthy and unhealthy seasons. The attention that commanding officers paid to the health of their troops was remarkable, especially when compared with late nineteenth and early twentieth-century campaigns: surgeons during the Seven Years' War took part in councils of war and influenced military strategy to a degree that would strike more modern commanders as inappropriate. To quote Clive himself, in a report to the British East India Company's board in London, the lives of men were deemed "very precious."[148] As established in previous chapters, maintaining troop welfare in the wars of the Age of Reason was seen as a strategic, diplomatic, political, professional, and moral imperative.

Discipline, as British officers and medical practitioners all agreed, would maintain health as well as lead to military success in the midst of a dangerous environment. For these reasons, British officials distinguished sepoys from European troops on the basis of discipline, encouraging the regimentation of sepoy battalions and training under British officers.[149] After all, according to British interpretations, it was Europeans' superior discipline that had won so many battles between small numbers of European troops and large numbers of native forces. Native troops were believed to be cowardly and weak, in part because of the effects of a hotter climate on their bodies and character; this weakness demanded that they be officered by Europeans, who would lead by example and instill regular discipline and courage.[150] As Major Caillaud explained, reflecting on the situation of the British in India during the Seven Years' War, "To a greater degree of natural courage, to more skill in the art of war, and to discipline, and order opposed to confusion and irregularity we owe our superiority over the Asiatick."[151] Discipline over British bodies and control over the foreign environment and its diseases were proving out of reach for the British in India. Yet discipline could be introduced among native troops to maintain control over the company's recently extended holdings, and it could account for remarkable military success in India. The shift from commercial influence to direct rule was accompanied by a shift from the use of sepoys as auxiliaries to their use as frontline troops. These shifts were accompanied by a shift in medical knowledge, from earlier notions of adaptability to a belief in biological fixity and theories of race. India, a hot climate like the West Indies, was a distinct and foreign environment for Europeans, where European intervention could possibly transform an unhealthy location into one salubrious for British settlement. Both British dominance in India and the role of sepoy armies there were explained by this new medical knowledge. The role of the British was to manage, since they were best suited for it; the role of Indians was to work and fight.

CHAPTER SIX

Imperial War at Home: The Welfare of French Prisoners of War

Few Britons would have been exposed to the nature of warfare in India. As Adam Smith wrote, just after the end of the Seven Years' War, in "great empires the people who live in the capital, and in the provinces remote from the scene of action, feel, many of them scarce any inconveniency from the war; but enjoy, at their ease, the amusement of reading in the newspapers the exploits of their own fleets and armies."[1] Unlike in the colonies or on the Continent, hardly any fighting took place on British soil, most of it limited to coastal raids and invasion attempts. Historians recognize that warfare, especially imperial warfare, entered the lives of British civilians through sermons, religious fasts, extraparliamentary displays of patriotism and ministerial criticism, and by means of an impressive national and international network of newspapers.[2] However, many on the home front also experienced the physical presence of war firsthand. Those living near ports and centers of supply, for example, were certainly aware of the demands and ravages of warfare. These towns were vital links between the center of the metropole and the imperial periphery, and although not witnessing warfare itself, they were part of its preparations and its effects. More generally, Britons experienced the course of the war through exposure to the unprecedented number of prisoners of war held on British soil, many of them in port towns.

According to British records, a total of nearly 65,000 French prisoners were captured and brought back to Britain during the Seven Years' War, with well over 25,000 held on British soil by 1762.[3] Yet the significance of these enemy prisoners is not simply that there were more than ever before. In addition to their unprecedented large numbers, the predominantly French prisoners became the focus of published writings and philanthropic campaigns as their imprisonment dragged on and as French financial support for them waned. The treatment of these prisoners and public discussions of the nature of their care thus articulate the close relationship that eighteenth-century Britons saw between military victory and the welfare of soldiers and sailors. As one correspondent to the *Public Ledger* explained, British care for French prisoners "adds lustre to the character of this our nation, [which] must not less celebrate its name to the world, than its many glorious triumphs, whereby they have become our captives."[4] The direct result of imperial victory, the prisoners were a tangible manifestation of British success in imperial warfare, and their increasing numbers throughout the war demonstrated the inability of the French to capture an equal number of British forces for prisoner exchanges. Moreover, their deteriorating health was a manifestation of the decline of French power. In response to the 1758 withdrawal of the French king's bounty (a fund for the sustenance of French war prisoners abroad), the British public raised thousands of pounds to buy prisoners clothing and shoes, explicitly linking British superiority to the financial, military, and moral weakness of the French state. Caring for the welfare of French sailors and soldiers was thus represented as a patriotic, and distinctively British, act. Whereas the French were portrayed as impotent in their inability to fund their own forces or callous in not caring for their own men, the British public saw themselves as powerful and cosmopolitan philanthropists, able to rise above the petty distinctions of national enmity.

Understanding the fundamental linkages between welfare, military victory, and public opinion is vital to accurately understanding the history of prisoners of war during the eighteenth century. If the role of public opinion is overlooked, then accusations of mistreatment—as in the case of the Black Hole of Calcutta—may be mistaken for factual and objective reports. In contrast to most histories of eighteenth-century prisoners of war, this chapter examines not the experience of being a prisoner, but the regular administration of prisoners of war in Britain, showing that reports of ill treatment need to be recognized as accusations and rhetorical claims, a part of wartime diplomatic negotiations, and a central plank of attempts to influence public opinion and morale.[5] Few studies examine the administration of prisoners during the early and mid-eighteenth century, resulting in a preponderance of studies that recount prisoner treatment in the American War of Independence, the Napoleonic Wars, and the American Civil War without considering the precedents and early modern conventions that shaped prisoner-of-war administration in the later eighteenth and nineteenth centuries.[6] By the same token, historians have tended to focus on extraordinary or problematic cases of prisoners, whether during rebellions or wars with non-European powers.[7] In this study, prisoner welfare is contextualized within eighteenth-century warfare and social conditions more broadly, illustrating how an appreciation for administration, strategy, and public opinion can yield a clearer understanding of the history of the welfare of prisoners of war.

Building on the analyses of chapters 2 and 3, this chapter delineates the central role of public opinion in the welfare of the armed forces. Because public opinion played a significant role in British wartime policy, the administration of prisoners was part of debates in the public sphere. Just as military victory was seen as linked to and earned through the maintenance of troop welfare, they were similarly linked to the British state's responsiveness to public attitudes regarding care for French prisoners. Prisoner welfare not only bolstered public support for the government, but also aimed to intensify public, financial, and manpower pressure on the French king by prolonging the incarceration of French troops in Britain. This chapter opens with an overview of the presence of prisoners in Britain during the war, before detailing the administration of their care. Public discussions of their treatment are then analyzed to demonstrate how Britons understood the relationship between troop welfare and state power. The chapter concludes with a discussion of humanitarianism, public opinion, and the British state, illustrating how expertise in manpower was essential to convincing an increasingly powerful public sphere that British administration of the war was militarily effective and morally sound.

PRISONERS OF WAR AND STATE ADMINISTRATION

Although prisoners of war were not evenly scattered throughout Britain, many Britons, particularly those residing in urban centers and port towns, would have encountered them during the Seven Years' War. With tens of thousands of these enemy prisoners held in local institutions and with thousands of officers on parole, contemporaries remarked on their presence. Horace Walpole, constant diarist, recorded during the invasion scares of 1759: "We were defenceless at home, and could not assemble above twelve thousand men. Our towns were crowded with French prisoners. They were removed up into the country and committed to the guard of the militia."[8] Others described a more peaceable coexistence with the French prisoners. Hannah More, for example, hosted French officer prisoners with her parents, serving as their translator.[9] In total, Britain and Ireland received 64,373 (rank-and-file) prisoners during the war, with near 15,000 held in the British kingdom in 1757, and numbers peaking at 26,157 in 1762.[10] Key centers for rank-and-file prisoners included Bristol, Exeter, Bideford, Portsmouth, Plymouth, Sissinghurst, Winchester, Kinsale in Ireland, and even as far north as Edinburgh. Numbers varied: by 1761, some towns (such as Liverpool) held fewer than 80, while others (such as Plymouth) held more than 5,000.[11] Newspapers also spread information about the prisoners to British communities farther afield; in 1761, they claimed, "the Number of French prisoners now in England is said to amount to little less than 35,000."[12]

These numbers represented a marked increase over previous wars. During the War of Austrian Succession, Britain brought back less than half the number of prisoners that it would during the Seven Years' War, and the most it held on British soil at one time was 7,754 prisoners, in 1747.[13] Figures for the War of Spanish Succession are less detailed: by 1707, British authorities had captured just over 18,000 prisoners in total, and exchanged between 2,000 and 4,000 annually thereafter.[14] The increase in the number of prisoners demonstrates both the growing size of armed forces over the course of the eighteenth century, and European warfare's expanding global scope, as prisoners captured at sea and overseas were brought back to be held in Britain.[15]

During the Seven Years' War, the presence of prisoners was felt not only because of their number, but also because of the duration of their confinement and the consequent deterioration of their health and welfare. Standard conventions during this period usually had prisoners exchanged or ransomed within fifteen days of their capture, particularly when taken after battle on the Continent.[16] However, French prisoners held in Britain during the Seven Years' War were mostly captured at sea, and no exchanges were agreed on between the French and the British after January 1758.[17] Because the British regularly captured far more French sailors than the French did British sailors, and because of the lack of a cartel (an agreement for exchange), these captured French seamen remained in British prisons for years, if not for most of the war—a lengthy incarceration that was unprecedented. Moreover, the plight of these French prisoners was further worsened when the French bounty was stopped in December 1758.[18] Britons were aware of the financial strain caused by these enemy prisoners. Horace Walpole complained, "The prisoners now brought from Louisbourg raised the numbers of that nation captive here to twenty-four thousand; and the King of France, to increase the burthen of our expence, withdrew his allowance to them."[19] As will be examined in more detail, the British public responded by organizing subscriptions and other philanthropic endeavors on behalf of the starving and sickly French prisoners.

Prisoners of war were administered by the medical board of the Admiralty, the Sick and Hurt Board, discussed at length in chapter 4. The board oversaw prisoners through a network of prisoner agents, stationed at each locale where prisoners were held. Perhaps unsurprisingly, a number of these agents were medical men, serving the prisoners and the Admiralty as both surgeon and agent.[20] Their medical background may explain why they were known and trusted by the board, and it would also have been useful in their duty of assessing the welfare of prisoners. However, much of an agent's activities were financial and administrative. The account books of Matthew Limbrey, agent at Exeter during the Seven Years' War, document total costs near £14,000 and list more than twenty contractors and workers whom he employed.[21] As a result, many agents—particularly in centers holding a substantial number of prisoners—were merchants or men of local standing, as the position required capital, financial expertise, and mercantile networks.[22]

Traditionally, prisoners were maintained by the host country, which was to accommodate and feed them in quantity and quality comparable to what its soldiers and sailors received when on campaign. During the Seven Years' War, rules and regulations, which included the weekly allowance of victuals, were to be posted in the language of the prisoners in each prison.[23] Upon the end of a war, or as part of negotiations for cartels for exchange during a war, each side would present accounts for these costs and demand reimbursement, subtracting what the other side had paid for hosting enemy prisoners. It was thus a system maintained through the principle of reciprocity, with each side using prisoners as bargaining chips. During the 1740s, for example, the Sick and Hurt Board investigated what the French were giving to British prisoners in France so that they could supply the same in Britain, assuring French authorities "that the Treatment our People find in France, will be the measure of the Treatment of their People here, in England."[24]

Although the cost of maintaining prisoners was thus paid under the assumption that it would be reimbursed, the financial and administrative burden of prisoners was immense, and particularly as a result of the notable increase in numbers and duration of confinement of French prisoners during the Seven Years' War. The Sick and Hurt Board struggled to find sufficient accommodation for upwards of 26,000 men, often modifying older institutions such as prisons, hospitals, or a disused royal residence, in the case of Winchester.[25] Victuals and other necessaries were provided through the usual military system of contractors. Contemporaries remarked on the demands that these prisoners made on national consumption patterns, with a committee against the new duty on cider calculating the "extraordinary" charge resulting from having supplied thousands of prisoners with drink throughout the war.[26] Moreover, the prisoners had to be carefully guarded by militias, which further encumbered local populations through the demands of quartering. At Winchester, where over 3,000 prisoners were stationed within a local population of around 5,000, the publicans at one point threatened to shut their businesses in revolt against the burden of quartering the prisoners' guards.[27] It was also not lost on authorities that these were enemy forces: beyond the fear of prisoners taking part in invasion attempts, agents and related officials were at times suspected of treason.[28] Smugglers took advantage of prisoner exchanges for their own purposes, providing another reason for officials' uneasiness with prisoners.[29] Local populations also resented the influx of hundreds to thousands of foreign men, often because sailors and soldiers carried infectious diseases.[30] It was not unusual for the Sick and Hurt Board to receive requests for additional funds to ease the problem of "the fears of the Inhabitants, the Generality of whom will not receive sick [prisoners] themselves or suffer others who are included to Quarter them to do it, lest an infectious Disorder should thereby be introduced."[31] By the close of the war, the Sick and Wounded Commissioners explained the unprecedented size of their debt by reason of the "Number of Prisoners of War subsisted in the latter of those years, *more* than in the former," calculating that prisoners were costing them near £15,000 a month.[32]

Prisoners were not usually maintained solely through the host's provision of food and accommodation. They were also traditionally given regular amounts of money remitted directly by their home country, enabling them to buy clothing and fresh food from nearby markets, as was also the case on campaign. Such payments, called the king's or queen's bounty, allowed the home country a degree of control over the provisioning of their men. During the 1740s, for example, a British consul stationed in Spain encouraged Newcastle to continue the bounty to British prisoners held in Spain. Regardless of regulations under which Spanish authorities were to provision the British prisoners, the consul claimed "a great difference between being subsisted by His Majesty's Bounty, and being maintained by [the Spanish] Court, since it is with great backwardness its officers have complied even with the payment of the small allowance they have hitherto granted the Prisoners."[33] Given that this was a payment made without promise of reimbursement, and that it was paid to men who were providing no active service to a home country during war, such regular disbursements were yet another heavy financial burden in wartime.

Both sides thus recognized that the confinement of prisoners of war was expensive and problematic, and the release of prisoners, through an exchange or wholesale cartel, was always the desired solution. Exchanges could be ad hoc arrangements, agreed and negotiated informally, in which prisoners were usually exchanged man for man and rank for rank, with much discussion of which ranks were equivalent. A formal cartel, or agreement of exchange, could regulate the details of regular, man-for-man exchanges or the payment of ransoms, and it could also be a formal legal contract in which all prisoners on both sides would be returned to their home country. In 1712, for example, the Sick and Hurt Board explained that the War of Spanish Succession never saw "a cartel settled between us and France for the exchange of prisoners," although regular exchanges on the basis of a verbal agreement had been practiced from 1703, until "there arose difficulties as to lieutenants and ensigns of men-of-war."[34]

Precedent was one of the most common arguments made during exchange negotiations. Authorities frequently referenced what had been applied in previous wars in order to make their case, reminiscent of legal arguments. For contemporaries, negotiations and arguments about exchanges were a mixture of appeals to law, custom, and humanitarianism or morality, buttressed by practical strategic motivations. Indeed, this is what gave the laws of nations—what today would be called international law—their potency: that they answered arguments and claims made on the basis of humanity. Abiding by the laws of nations meant that one was a civilized and humane nation, while it was also through the application of laws during wartime that humanitarian conditions would be achieved. As a 1758 pamphlet arguing for the exchange of seamen claimed, "An Exchange of Prisoners is one of the *capital Laws* of *War* among *civiliz'd Nations*," also noting that such exchanges would encourage other seamen to enlist, ensuring naval strength.[35] With war accepted as a natural, if not necessary, part of international relations, early modern laws of war governed the conduct of war (*jus in bello*), more so than the justness of war itself (*jus ad bellum*). And as the good treatment of noncombatants was one of the fundamental principles of humanitarianism and just war theories, the treatment of prisoners was a key issue for deliberations on how to wage war in a humane, enlightened, and pragmatic manner.[36] Emer de Vattel's influential treatise, *The Law of Nations*, translated into English in 1759, is characteristic of eighteenth-century optimism about both the rationality of laws of war and the present "humanity with which most nations in Europe carry on wars at present."[37] Vattel reiterated early modern conventions that prisoners taken during war should not be killed or made slaves, but could be fettered, if necessary. For Vattel, the increasing use of prisoner-of-war exchanges and officer parole, methods by which the natural misfortune of imprisonment could be avoided, were yet another demonstration of "the humanity of the Europeans."[38]

Alongside legal precedent and humanitarian conventions, exchanges were demanded because they were widely recognized as the most practical method for resolving the problem of imprisonment. Although poor conditions were often complained of, authorities and prisoners used these to petition for an exchange, rather than to focus on reforming conditions. In 1704, for example, the Sick and Hurt Board directed the authorities to agree on exchanges, as this would "best conduce to the Relief of Her [Majesty's] Subjects."[39] The French prisoner Du Donjon complained of his "malheur" in being held prisoner, explicitly specifying that his misfortune lay in not being released through an exchange.[40] The acceptance of poor conditions during imprisonment was implicit in how prisoners were chosen for exchanges: the aged, wounded, and ill were first exchanged, since these were men "least able to endure the Hardships of Imprisonment."[41] This mirrors views of civil imprisonment during the first half of the eighteenth century, in which incarceration was most commonly applied to those awaiting trial, rather than as punishment in and of itself, and in which provisions and improved conditions were obtained by paying the jailor.[42] As the 1758 pamphlet on exchanges stated, imprisonment was one of those "unavoidable Evils of War," its misfortune lessened only through exchanges.[43] Similarly, the threat of ending exchanges demonstrates both their import and the widespread acceptance of poor conditions when confined. In response to reports of poor treatment of English prisoners in France in 1705, the Sick and Hurt Board wrote to the French Commissary at Calais, warning that if this occurred again, "the exchange of prisoners will certainly be put a stop to."[44]

What this also demonstrates is the diplomatic and strategic uses to which reports and petitions of poor conditions were put. Authorities were aware of this: in 1704, the Sick and Hurt Board forwarded reports of ill treatment of English prisoners in France to the Earl of Nottingham (the secretary of state), noting that they supposed "the French may use the English thus out of Designe to move her Maj[esty] the sooner to consent to a Cartell."[45] In this case, officials warned against being pushed into an agreement that would disadvantage the English in the long term, and instead pursued a policy of retaliation as a form of negotiation for improving prisoner conditions. English correspondence mixed moral outrage—describing French practice as "contrary to the usage of all Christian and

Civilized Nations"—with threats and negotiations. Authorities reduced the allowance and amount of straw given to French prisoners, and directed agents "to read this order publickely to the Prisoners" and encourage them to write about it to the French court, making it clear that these retrenchments would remain in place until the French king improved his treatment of English prisoners held in France. The Sick and Hurt Board even suggested that particularly literate French prisoners be given a copy of the new order to include in their letters.[46]

Similar action and rhetoric were applied in the 1740s, when British authorities threatened that Spanish prisoners would be treated "in the same rigorous manner" as they heard that British prisoners were being treated in Spain, unless the Spanish approved a cartel and improved their treatment of British captives.[47] British officials explained, "This would not be from any motive of Cruelty or Barbarity, for that the English were incapable of, but only to try whether a little less good nature on our part might not procure a little more humanity on theirs."[48] Reports of ill treatment were thus part of wartime negotiations, particularly for cartels, which were themselves central to wartime strategy.

As demands for or refusals of cartels demonstrate, prisoners were not simply the by-products of battles or symbolic spoils of war. Even taking into account their administrative and financial demands, prisoners were valuable strategic assets, particularly within the context of eighteenth-century imperial warfare. In 1704, one English official explained how the capture of French privateers early in the war, to the number of 7,000 prisoners, meant that "French privateering was almost broke, and that, if the same success had continued, the French King would have been disabled to man his ships." On the other hand, since this success had been reversed, English ships had been taken, "interruption of trade and losses sustained, her Majesty's revenue much lessened, the nation weakened, the subject ruined, the enemy enriched, strengthened and encouraged; [and] her Majesty's sugar plantations are much exposed for want of English men-of-war and Jamaica especially in great danger."[49]

The policy of capturing French privateers and merchantmen was remarkably successful during the Seven Years' War, resulting not only in the crippling of French privateering and naval power, but also the protection of British colonies and overseas trade. As the French historian T. J. A. Le Goff explains, this detention, compared with other Franco-British wars of the eighteenth century, was, "above all, decisive during the Seven Years' War." He concludes that the British capture and detention of so many French seamen was a significant factor in the shortage of French naval manpower, exceeding even the disastrous impact of typhus.[50] Contemporaries were aware of this: Admiral Rodney wrote to George Grenville late in the war, upon having captured a privateer near Martinique, that he had "given directions (since my command in these seas) never to exchange any men belonging to the French privateers, but to send them prisoners to England, which I hope in time will entirely clear these seas of such vermin."[51] Capturing French seamen, and, importantly, holding them captive throughout the war, were a significant and successful part of British imperial strategy of colonial defense and commerce protection during the Seven Years' War.

On the part of the British authorities, refusing to agree to exchanges required both a military and a moral advantage.[52] Militarily, the French had far fewer prisoners than did the British throughout the war, meaning that the French desired an exchange, while the British could afford to refuse. In 1758, French officials noted that it would be difficult to convince British authorities to agree to a cartel, given that the British held over 20,000 French sailors, privateers, and merchantmen crews, whereas they held only around 3,000.[53] This imbalance increased throughout the war, leaving French officials with little power in their negotiations. In terms of moral leverage, the French also confessed that, apart from problems early in the war, they could not complain of poor treatment. In 1758 French officials noted that negotiations for a cartel were frequently complicated by complaints of ill treatment by both sides, but admitted that "it is certain that the treatment given to English prisoners is in some respects inferior to that which the French enjoy in England," explaining that British officials provided more straw and blankets.[54] Moreover, British officials made it clear that French prisoners were cared for, even after the discontinuation of the French king's bounty. In 1759 the Sick and Hurt Board wrote to French officials, observing the lack of clothing among French prisoners, and diplomatically explaining that they were sharing these reflections "so that you could take whatever measures appear most proper to you, in order to guard them from the inconveniences of the approaching winter."[55] They concluded their letter by noting that in Liverpool, the agent and the local population had donated clothing to succor the French prisoners stationed there.

THE WELFARE OF FRENCH PRISONERS AND PUBLIC OPINION

It was not only in Liverpool that Britons provided for the French prisoners. When the French royal bounty ended in December 1758, many were made aware of the poor conditions that resulted. When French prisoners were marched from Dundee to Edinburgh Castle as a result of the 1759 invasion scare, a letter to the Edinburgh paper recorded that locals witnessing the "almost naked [prisoners], conducted along the high street of Edinburgh to the castle," were immediately moved to offer clothing for them. Civic pride, as well as compassion, was at stake: the letter noted that similar charity had already been implemented at Sissinghurst Castle in Kent.[56] Based in London and serving as a national organization, the Committee on French Prisoners was the largest organization focused on this philanthropy. It first met in December 1759 at the Crown and Anchor Tavern in the Strand, and collected more than £4,000, spent on thousands of hats, shoes, shirts, coats, and other clothes sent to prisoners stationed throughout Britain.[57] In addition to this committee, various similar groups raised and distributed charity locally—for example, in Penzance, Exeter, Bristol, Winchester, Portsmouth, and Plymouth.[58]

The structure of these charities mirrored that of commercial joint-stock enterprises, and was typical of philanthropic groups in Britain during the eighteenth century, many of which also linked wartime national concerns with improvements in welfare for the lower orders.[59] Merchants and officials of local standing often chaired these organizations, while funds were collected through public subscriptions. Locations at which individuals could donate were usually advertised in newspapers, while all subscribers could examine accounts and other administrative details. In the case of the Committee on French Prisoners, which published a full account of its administrative and financial proceedings in 1760, a minimum number of subscribers needed to be present for decisions to be made, and information regarding what was required throughout Britain was gathered through notices "in the public-papers" as well as through a network of private correspondence.[60] Local agents and the heads of the local guarding militia were the hubs through which specific requests and charitable items were conveyed.

Similar to other voluntary charitable organizations of the time, the various working groups for the welfare of French prisoners were keen to provide public and exact accounts, thereby avoiding accusations of corruption and further encouraging subscriptions. Indeed, charities on occasion offered themselves as a solution to officials' corruption. When reports of poor treatment circulated in Belfast, and when militia and civic officials concluded that this was due to abuses committed by the agent, a committee was formed to raise funds and remit money directly to the prisoners, thereby bypassing the agent and effectively putting him out of a job.[61]

In Edinburgh, where disagreement over the extent of the prisoners' needs prevailed, the trustees of the charity (men "of considerable fortunes," and therefore men of credit) conducted an inquiry into the state of the French prisoners and published their findings.[62] They also noted that they would keep an exact record of all sums given and expended, "and every person who contributes to the value of a shilling, shall have free access to inspect this book."[63] Likewise, the London-based Committee on French Prisoners published its full proceedings "for the satisfaction of the public," explaining that these "exact accounts" would allow donors to "judge how properly their benefactions have been applied."[64] Expert and transparent administration, similar to that demanded through military returns (examined in chapter 3), would ensure that the welfare of prisoners was properly conducted.

These charities were not without their detractors. Indeed, the number of publications on the charities' internal procedures, and their public accounting methods, were either a response to criticism or an effort to stave off speculation of malfeasance, just as accessible manpower reports on the army and navy were a means to answer or avoid parliamentary inquiries. In Belfast and Edinburgh, the publication of letters and other papers relative to charity for the prisoners was a response to local controversy over the motivations and methods of the charities. For example, the 1761 pamphlet on events at Belfast explained, "To free the charitable conduct of these gentlemen from reproach, and to prevent it from losing its proper influence by any misrepresentation, is truly a charitable office, and one reason why a candid state of Facts is here submitted to the decision and impartiality of the Publick."[65] Moreover, the nature of care given to the French prisoners was also publicly debated. An anonymous letter published in the *London Chronicle* early in 1760 railed against charitable organizations for French prisoners, complaining that it was "*Charity without knowledge*, and sister to blind Zeal." These donors did not realize that they were causing worsening conditions for British sailors held in France, as the charities propagated "false representations of the miserable conditions" of French prisoners held in Britain, which would surely result in reprisals on British prisoners in France.[66] Jacobites were mentioned as behind the scheme; likewise, in other contexts, Quakers and other "particular religious" groups were denigrated as the instigators behind such unpatriotic activities.[67]

The most common criticism raised, and defended against, was that such charity either infringed on the responsibilities of the British state, or demonstrated its weakness. The anonymous letter in the *London Chronicle* observed how poorly such charities reflected on the government, adding darkly, "I am sure such a proceeding must naturally tend to throw an odium on the present Administration, if it were not designed to do so."[68] Defenders of the charity explained that the government was responsible only for subsistence: food, medical care, and accommodation. As "there is no precedent for cloathing, the French may possibly demur to this circumstance; for which reason the [British] Ministry may be better pleased, that the liberality of individuals should be shewn on this occasion."[69] Likewise, Samuel Johnson's introduction to the proceedings of the Committee on French Prisoners pointed out that the charity provided only for those items that "we know that for the prisoners of war there is no legal provision."[70] This was why charity was strictly confined to buying shoes and clothes for the prisoners: these were the items that would otherwise have been obtained through the French bounty, and that were not the responsibility of the British state. Charities made it clear that they never gave French prisoners ready money, nor did they give items that overlapped with official provisions. The charities were careful to work with the British state, rather than critiquing its methods or power.

Charities for French prisoners were therefore similar to eighteenth-century British charities more generally. Eighteenth-century charities were part of what historians have termed the mixed economy of welfare, in which private charity, the state, and the church worked together to alleviate problems associated with poverty, conditions in prisons, and illness.[71] The Committee on French Prisoners, for example, relied on the state's network of militia officers and agents in its activities, working alongside them to improve conditions for French prisoners. Rather than seeing private charity to the poor as filling a gap or identifying problems, contemporaries did not focus on the differences between actors, but instead worked in tandem toward a common goal. As discussed in chapter 3, this goal was to maintain, if not boost, the population of the nation, particularly by ensuring the health and vigor of the lower classes. In times of war, this translated into a focus on manpower, specifically in competition with the enemy's manpower. As a result, depriving the enemy of manpower was of vital national significance, and voluntary charities enthusiastically worked alongside government officials to achieve this.

Charitable trustees and subscribers were explicit that their activities buttressed the power and glory of the British state. As the trustee of a charity at Cornwall explained, "That as our victorious troops have proved an overmatch for our enemies at the fatal decision of the sword, so will our numberless subscriptions to cloath them convince the whole world, that we are as much their superiors in the gentler passions of mercy and benevolence."[72] Contemporaries grouped the charities for French prisoners together, alongside the Marine Society and groups raising funds to clothe British troops overseas, as military charities: "calculated either to preserve, or to encourage, the sailor and the soldier engaged in our service."[73] According to merchant and philanthropist Jonas Hanway, these organizations demonstrated how British commercial genius was reconciled with its martial virtue, as giving money to such activities was likened to the sacrifices that troops made on the field of battle. As Hanway and other commentators often remarked, British generosity to French prisoners demonstrated not only British military power, but also Britain's wealth as a flourishing commercial nation, and its leadership as a Christian and humanitarian country.[74] Charity and attention to welfare combined practical, humanitarian, and religious motives. Charity to the enemy was thus a patriotic act.

This charity was also portrayed as distinctively British, not only a result of Britain's unique commercial wealth, but also a form of national, if not Protestant, philanthropy. Published writings often contrasted British generosity with French pretense. As one contributor to *Owen's Weekly Chronicle* claimed, after having returned from captivity in Bayonne, "The Bayonners have not that humanity which many in England have, to raise contributions for the relief of the poor naked soldiers. The French pride themselves much on being the politest of nations: and certainly they are so, if politeness consists in fine compliments, and external gestures of the body, without any intention to perform what is said."[75] Likewise, Oliver Goldsmith not only boasted that the English were more generous than any other nation (suggesting that this may derive from their greater wealth), but also cited the example of charities for French prisoners to demonstrate the unusual rationality and magnanimity with which the English distinguished themselves. He explained that "the men who were brave enough to conquer, were generous enough to forgive."[76] Goldsmith surmised that such donors, rising above divisions of party, religion, and nation, were truly citizens of the world. Hanway also asserted that charity for French prisoners demonstrated a distinctively British trait, claiming that it was well known that "many of those [French prisoners] who were relieved, expressed a due sense of *british generosity*."[77]

Although the British state provided the overwhelming majority of financial and administrative support for French prisoners of war, it also required the support of the British public, and it is certain that officials helped to shape opinions and practices through the traditional outlets of pamphlets and newspapers. Given the discussions and appeals to the public through published accounts, public opinion played a key role in the management of prisoners during the Seven Years' War, even though it, and the methods for managing it, may not have been as sophisticated as in the later eighteenth century.[78]

In recognizing the role of public opinion historians must acknowledge that writings on the welfare of prisoners were rhetorical attempts to persuade, most often aimed at the public, either in order to pressure officials to negotiate or concede strategic gains, or to empower officials to continue allegedly successful policies. In the Seven Years' War, the British public was successfully convinced not only that French prisoners were well cared for, but also that such attention to their welfare was part of British moral and military strength. What adds credence to the central role of public opinion is that the French, perhaps unsurprisingly, interpreted British treatment and the welfare of French prisoners differently. Le Goff details a mortality rate of 12.5 percent for French prisoners detained in Britain during the war, demonstrating that this was one of the reasons why the Seven Years' War was the most deadly war of the entire eighteenth century for French seamen.[79] On the one hand, this is only a slight increase over the 10 percent mortality recorded during the War of Austrian Succession, and is comparable to mortality rates during long campaigns and detention in civil institutions at the time. On the other hand, the deaths of over 10,000 French seamen while under British care would have been problematic, regardless of what percentage this represented. British authorities recognized this, for, as Le Goff points out, they were reluctant to release comprehensive death accounts after either the War of Austrian Succession or the Seven Years' War, as they feared that these figures would be misused as anti-British propaganda at home and abroad.[80] Moreover, French publications from the time of the war paint a markedly different portrait of British treatment of prisoners of war than that circulating in British publications. Robert Martin Lesuire's *Les sauvages de l'Europe*, first published in 1760 and reprinted twice during the war, repeatedly describes British mistreatment of French prisoners within its narrative of a French couple's visit to a violent and dysfunctional England. It is just after disembarking that the travelers are first horrified to see French naval prisoners violently stripped of their belongings and thrown into miserable English prisons run by cruel English jailors. In the 1764 English translation, the translator explained that such misinformation was the result of "infamous falshoods [*sic*] which were published in every political pamphlet in France and Flanders, during the last war, on this very subject."[81]

Lesuire's account makes clear the significance of the welfare of prisoners. As the French travelers' wise Chinese guide explains, they should not be surprised to see such displays of English barbarism. The mistreatment of prisoners, whether by putting them in irons or by stealing their personal possessions, "is the practice of all savage nations."[82] Vattel expressed the same sentiment in his treatise on the laws of nations. Accusing one's enemies of neglecting the welfare of prisoners of war was a common rhetorical strategy that powerfully appealed to both morality and legal conventions. Ill treatment of prisoners and accusations of ill treatment were part of military strategy, aiming to pressure enemy officials through public opinion. By the same token, humane treatment of the enemy and reports thereof were also part of patriotic war efforts. The British treatment of French prisoners combined utilitarian motives—particularly strategic ones—and moral ones. Indeed, eighteenth-century Britons were explicit that charities needed to be practical and administered efficiently in order to accomplish their Christian and humanitarian goals, as well as the nation's military goals. Thus, sound and expert administration and humanitarianism were fundamentally linked, not only in providing for the welfare of forces, but also in the attainment of victory.

VICTORY AND THE END OF WAR

British victory was portrayed not only as the result of campaigns won through the exertions of its vigorous armed forces, but also through the extension of Christian charity and provision for the welfare of people—soldiers and civilians, friends and enemies—living under British dominion. As a contributor to the *London Chronicle* newspaper remarked, praising British generosity in the treatment of French prisoners, "The glorious successes of his Majesty's arms has so distressed the French in general, that they cannot assist their friends and relations in England."[83] Caring for the welfare of French prisoners was an act of patriotism, and simultaneously showed the superiority of Britons in their ability to rise above the petty distinctions of nations. As Hanway, among others, made clear, it was both cause and effect of British imperial prowess: the prisoners and Britain's wealth were the consequence of victory, but it was Britain's undoubted moral leadership that allowed such victories, for it was precisely such acts of benevolence and humanity that enlisted divine favor.

Moreover, the welfare of French prisoners demonstrates the working relationship between the British public and the British state. The unprecedented length of detention of French prisoners was a key part of British strategy to protect overseas trade and colonial campaigns by depriving the

French of much-needed skilled manpower. As the treatment of prisoners played a significant role in wartime negotiations for or against exchanges, the welfare of these prisoners was a practical strategic concern. The British public enthusiastically took up this cause, following the administrative model of other charities concerned with the welfare of the lower orders in Britain. Indeed, charities for French prisoners were so ubiquitous during the Seven Years' War that a 1760 satire on charity, "the mad extravagance of the present age," used charities for French prisoners as its target.[84]

For the British state, the issue of French prisoners did not end with its victorious conclusion to the war. Instead, as was often the case, negotiations over the reimbursement of prisoners' maintenance dragged on for years. The British bill for their care of French prisoners amounted to 26.5 million livres, while the French claimed an outstanding bill of 2.5 million livres. From the middle of 1763 and throughout 1764, British officials repeatedly presented their claim of 24 million livres (roughly £1.2 million) to French officials at the French court. This amount was not even the full British claim: British officials noted that this did not include expenses incurred after 11 January 1762 or those of the British East India Company. However, as they soon learned, "considering the present involved state of the French Finances," full payment could not be expected in a timely manner.[85]

Each side debated various details of repayment, demonstrating that the legal definition of prisoners (when and where troops were taken prisoner, for example) had serious financial implications. This subject, along with the Canada bills and Dunkirk, threatened the Franco-British peace settlement. As treasurer, George Grenville was painfully aware of Britain's overall debt of £133 million, noting that the French debts were not only a financial concern. He explained to the Earl of Hertford that "however welcome that sum of money may be to us," the reimbursement of the prisoners' maintenance was more important as a sign of France's intentions in complying with the Treaty of Peace: "If [France] breaks them in the first instances that comes before the public, there is scarce a man in this country who will rely upon their good faith in those which still remain unperformed."[86] Indeed, the problems securing repayment were known to the public: they were not only discussed in the newspapers, but also used as part of partisan attacks on the ministry.[87] With French officials offering nothing more than a repayment of 15 million livres, at one point even suggesting that it be paid over the course of fifteen years, and with constant reminders of the terrible state of French finances, British officials despaired of coming to a settlement.[88] In January 1765, it was finally agreed that the French would pay the British £670,000 (roughly 15 million livres) in thirteen installments over two years "for the Discharge, and total Extinction of all the Pretensions and Demands, on the part of Great Britain, for the Maintenance and Subsistence, and all other Expences whatever, incurred on account of French Prisoners."[89] Parliament approved the proposal, as presented by the king, although it was no secret that the settlement disadvantaged the British.[90]

In Britain's next war, conventional exchange and repayment structures were absent within the context of what was a British civil war, while the role of public opinion and its relationship to the welfare of prisoners were sharply demonstrated. During the American War of Independence, the welfare of prisoners played a significant role in the shaping of public disapproval of British imperial authority, and, indeed, continues to do so. As one analyst of the history of prisoners of war explains, "The treatment of prisoners of war in the American Revolution has, in many ways, become part of the mythos of the Revolution itself. During the American Revolution and afterwards it was cited as proof of British injustice, and it would be invoked by lawyers nearly 150 years later as an example of abusive treatment."[91] The nature of historical accounts of captivity during the American War of Independence itself demonstrates the potency of accusations and rhetorical strategies, for instead of examining administrative details and legal precedents to establish responsibility for prisoner welfare, these accounts focus on the experience of imprisonment. Histories of prisoners during the American War of Independence often take narratives of British inhumane treatment at face value, with little historical analysis devoted to establishing which officials were financially responsible for provisions and accommodations, how this was negotiated, or why exchanges—long considered the only real solution to poor conditions—were stopped.[92] Rather than considering prisoner welfare as an administrative issue, one that had traditionally been negotiated by governments alongside strategic accusations and counteraccusations of ill treatment, the history of prisoners of war became centered on personal experience, sentiment, and the rhetoric of inhumanity.

The difference in accounts of British treatment of prisoners between the two wars also reflects the differing outcome of these wars: when Britain was victorious, its treatment of prisoners was understood as contributing to its victory. During the American War of Independence, however, military reverses made Britain increasingly susceptible to accusations of mistreatment of prisoners. Reports on ill treatment reflected the ebbing of Britain's support in both Britain and America, while also demonstrating that it deserved to lose. Much of the power of laws of war and reports on the welfare of troops thus derived not only from legal formalities and administrative realities, but also from the sway of public opinion. Just as the taking of prisoners was important for the war effort and for morale, how prisoners were treated was of concern to the public. During the Seven Years' War, Britons were adamant that French failure to abide by its responsibilities demonstrated French weakness, something they were keen to emphasize through a display of their own superior, Protestant, and distinctively British practices. Authorities could lose credibility and political legitimacy if they did not appear to fulfill their responsibilities, including answering to the demands of a vibrant public sphere. As the care for French prisoners during the Seven Years' War shows, accusations and reports on the welfare of armed forces were a powerful part of the conduct of eighteenth-century war, integral to strategy and public support.

EPILOGUE

During the American War of Independence, public disapproval of prisoner-of-war conditions was not simply a result of wartime propaganda. More broadly, public expectations about the welfare of prisoners and prison conditions in civilian life were shifting. Historians of hygiene have noted that by the 1770s, cleanliness was tied to notions of humanity and fundamentally linked to moral concerns such as civility. As the American colonial historian Kathleen Brown demonstrates, the American War of Independence "contributed to a new sensibility about basic expectations for humane conditions, one that realigned eighteenth-century meanings of gentility."[1] At the same time, encouraged by John Howard's *The State of the Prisons in England and Wales* (1777), prison conditions became a focus of campaigns for reform. As historians have recognized, Howard's "writings on prisons were powerfully driven by a concern for public health, especially the danger that dirty prisons posed not just to the prisoners themselves, but to wider society."[2] In other words, rather than identifying evidence of worsening conditions, in the second half of the eighteenth century, historians trace a widening public interest in prisoner welfare, often sparked by concern over disease, alongside increasing public expectations for state intervention in these matters.[3] As a result, reports of terrible conditions at the hands of despotic British imperial authorities, circulated through memoirs and poems, found receptive civilian audiences in Britain and North America during and after the American War of Independence.[4] These movements had their roots in the experiences of the 1750s and 1760s. Indeed, John Howard reputedly had his eyes opened to the problem of prison conditions during the Seven Years' War, when he was captured by French privateers and imprisoned at Brest.[5] As chapter 6 demonstrates, by the time of the Seven Years' War, the welfare of prisoners was not solely a medical concern, but also a political and moral issue, discussed and acted on in Britain's public sphere.

The physical experience of the Seven Years' War shaped eighteenth-century British views and practices. In part, this was a result of the war's unprecedented scale. Drawing in more men than ever before, the British armed forces recruited 321,000 troops (army and navy) throughout the war, representing one in nine of all military-aged able-bodied men: a marked increase over the previous war's rate of one in fifteen.[6] More generally, war encourages a focus on bodies, whether through the state's enumeration of manpower, officials' focus on discipline and drill, or the public's appreciation of the spectacle and gore of battle. Michel Foucault cites naval and military hospitals as spaces in which the formation of modern disciplined bodies can most clearly be traced.[7] The account here sheds light on the physical realities behind these practices and indicates that their origins preceded the hegemonic state: military medicine was not uniformly enforced from above, but was part of a negotiated process, in which local conditions and demands could not be ignored.

The role of physical realities and local conditions was most sharply articulated in the war's colonial environments. As Frederick Cooper and Ann Laura Stoler have pointed out, a key issue underlying imperialist endeavors is defining and maintaining colonized people as "others."[8] In military terms, both colonial Americans and native sepoys were clearly of lower military rank than British armed forces, assigned to laboring duties rather than complex military maneuvers. This difference was explained by a lack of experience, not by innate incapability. Yet through the course of the Seven Years' War, Britons observed differences that seemed to indicate a fundamental distinction between their bodies and those of colonial natives, made manifest by disease. As eighteenth-century medicine interpreted disease as a symptom of disjuncture between a body and its environment, the experience of the Seven Years' War suggested to many that bodies were not as responsive to different conditions and climates as had been initially assumed. Bodies, in other words, were not always fluid, malleable entities. Instead, medical men, officers, and soldiers observed fundamental differences between the bodies of American colonists and British troops. With large numbers of British bodies send to the East and West Indies, the experience of the Seven Years' War sparked interest in confirming whether bodies from a temperate climate could, indeed, modify themselves to labor efficiently in warm, foreign environments. This was tangibly demonstrated in James Lind's *Diseases Incidental to Europeans in Hot Climates*, a text that drew extensively and explicitly on the experiences of

British troops during the Seven Years' War and the struggle to maintain European health in colonial environments. Lind's text would shape the nature of British imperial governance for years to come.

The experience of the Seven Years' War thus contributed to the eighteenth-century development of the concept of the modern body, which itself shaped the nature of modern governance and imperialism. Whereas the early modern body was conceptualized as achieving health in its balance of fluids, and was easily permeated and disrupted through activities such as bathing, and by emotional or climatic change, the modern body is conceptualized as a fixed entity, self-regulated according to its biological makeup. Early modern bodies were described as constantly undergoing a natural process of putrefaction; it was the activity of consuming (food, drink, and air) and corresponding evacuations (through bodily excretions, including perspiration) that maintained health. Health was a process, an activity—and a precarious one at that, requiring careful attention to environment and diet. Likewise, diseases were unstable entities, one easily morphing into another. This conceptualization of the body meant that differences were explained by different cultural practices and transplantation to different climates. Hence, people became "seasoned" to new environments, undergoing cultural, environmental, moral, and physical transformations. European travelers to new worlds noted differences between themselves and native populations, but theorized that these differences were not essential, as they would erode the longer one stayed in the new environment. Eighteenth-century medical theory suggested that this "seasoning" process required careful attention through moderation and self-control.

Yet the thousands of British bodies fighting in foreign environments during the Seven Years' War—whether in the American colonies, the West or East Indies, or Germany with its alien diet and climate—did not easily acclimatize. Instead, disease manifested and accentuated persistent differences, physical and cultural. American-born provincials appeared physically different from British rank and file, as their bodies responded differently to the same environment. Likewise, British bodies did not adapt to Indian environments and lifestyle; rather, guidelines of self-control suggested that discipline—a kind of distancing from local conditions—was required in order to maintain European health in hot climates and foreign environments. Instead of malleability, bodies—and by consequence, cultures—increasingly appeared to be essentially different. Modern categories of race and gender ascribe notions of inherent fixity to bodies, stamped on the individual and determined through the biological operations of heredity.[9] Scholars such as Dror Wahrman and Roxann Wheeler point to the late eighteenth century as the time frame for a shift from climatic and cultural understandings of bodily differences toward that of the immutability of bodies, and the focus on skin color as a marker of difference.[10] While the slave trade and debates over abolition shaped discussions of race later in the eighteenth century, the physical experience of war at midcentury also transformed how Europeans understood and defined themselves.[11] In essence, the war's many theaters served as testing grounds for medical theories.

A transformation in how European bodies were conceptualized is also relevant in domestic contexts. The Enlightenment historian Lynn Hunt has pointed out that changing notions of physical or bodily autonomy, along with the rise of sentimental first-person narratives, were central to the development of ideas about human rights and political liberty during the later eighteenth century, and she identifies the 1760s as the key period for these shifts in public opinion.[12] Disease and poor conditions among British troops in Germany and French prisoners in Britain were publicized as a political issue of national concern. As in the case of prison reform, the public attended to the welfare of French prisoners of war not only because they, too, were human, but also because poor treatment was barbarous. Allowing continued suffering among the lower orders was unenlightened and ill befitting a civilized European nation. As the comments of Lally to Coote during the siege of Pondicherry in India make clear, attention to the welfare of troops and the provision of medical care during wartime was central to European self-identity.

Widespread attention to the welfare of troops encouraged methods with which to gauge welfare, and to improve it. The collection and systematization of medical and numerical observations on the state of manpower throughout the empire shows the development of both an imperial bureaucracy and structures of medical knowledge. The trials managed through the navy's Sick and Hurt Board; the network of observation spanning the empire through regimental, hospital, and ship surgeons; and the collection of regular returns informed and guided central authorities—military, political, and medical. James Lind's position as an expert on colonial environments and disease, establishing the discipline of tropical medicine and thereby shaping the nature of British imperial governance, was itself a product of the structures of medical knowledge created by the British Army and Royal Navy during the Seven Years' War—particularly as Lind himself did not visit the sites on which his research was based. The British state consolidated its authority by making use of experts stationed throughout its empire; at the same time, it substantiated their expertise and their position as knowledgeable authorities. The structures of medical knowledge and imperial bureaucracy gathered information that was used not only to administer imperial military force, but also to justify strategy and policy, and thereby legitimate British authority. Expertise in manpower, which during the Seven Years' War was most tangibly articulated as medical expertise in foreign environments, both contributed to Britain's imperial state authority and was itself constructed through the functioning of the British imperial state.[13]

Coinciding with a crucial period in the development of the practice and profession of British medicine, the experience of war helped to shape medicine during the second part of the eighteenth century.[14] James Lind, John Pringle, Donald Munro, and Richard Brocklesby were not critics of the medical establishment, nor were they outside of it. Rather, their wartime experience contributed to the nature of eighteenth-century medical knowledge, with its emphasis on hospital training, observations, trials, and empirical and quantitative methodology. At the same time, their war experience also helped to boost their professional authority, not only by providing opportunities to observe and experiment, but also through access to political and social networks, and publishing on topics that were a vital national concern. The development of expertise is necessarily also a process of exclusion, and these medical men certainly excluded traditional and local medical practitioners, while appropriating their knowledge and insights, in both the colonies and the metropole. As in the case of most successful claims to expertise, these medical men left few records of this process of exclusion, claiming instead that their expert status developed naturally, rather than through purposeful cultivation.

In contrast to the usual outline of the development of eighteenth-century medical authority, these practitioners received their approbation not just by reputation in the public sphere, but were also invested with authority through its dialectical counterpart: the state and its various channels of power. Over the course of the eighteenth century, the health of the lower orders was not only of general humanitarian interest, but became politically and socially crucial, with medical men playing a key role as social and political reformers. Because manpower was one of the most highly valued natural resources for eighteenth-century European imperial powers, experts on conserving and exploiting manpower were integral to the consolidation of British state authority, both at home and throughout the empire.

British victory in various parts of the globe was secured through means beyond simply plentiful resources. As this examination of global warfare demonstrates, the workings of the British state relied on experts and local authorities knowledgeable about and responsive to local conditions, adapting to changing environments and demands. This is also demonstrated in the cost, and precariousness, of victory. Victory in the American colonies was achieved only when British officials took heed of colonial complaints about supplies and conditions; likewise, victory in the West Indies was achieved only when commanders such as Barrington adapted logistics and strategy to fit their immediate environment. In the West Indies and in the American colonies, the price of victory included increasing alienation among colonial populations. At sea, naval victories hampered the longer-term readiness of fleets, and in India, victory against the French led to years of fighting against Indian forces. On the Continent, British operations took a heavy political toll, though the cost of victory was most obvious in Prussia, which lost 10 percent of its population to troop fatalities and war-related agricultural failures and epidemics.[15]

Victory was not immediate, nor obvious: by learning from previous failures in the West Indies, officials asked for and implemented effective amounts and types of resources. Likewise, James Lind's admission that his theory of scurvy was flawed, as demonstrated during the siege of Quebec, underlines responsiveness to the experience of war. Experiences in India and the New World suggest that the colonies were often "laboratories of modernity"; likewise the extent to which the German campaigns and the Western Squadron were sites for testing and evaluating methods of health care is a salient reminder of the similarities between colonial and European experiences.[16]

Early modern medicine often seems pointless, if not absurd and harmful.[17] However, when placed within the context of early modern observations and understandings of the body, it emerges as thoughtful and even effective, given its aims. It was especially responsive to the demands of campaigning in foreign environments, as were the officials who instituted policy and strategy. The establishment of the British Empire relied on this adaptability, building on domestic practices of negotiation and local autonomy. As the case of French prisoners points out, one can trace imperial methods of reliance on, and negotiations with, local authorities to the nature of eighteenth-century Britain, itself a patchwork of regions where central authority could not be taken for granted. The experience of global large-scale war would transform British state formations, both at home and abroad. Upon the end of the Seven Years' War, with victory achieved, these methods would be redirected to the problems of demobilization and colonial reform, but with less flexibility and less success.

The remit of this study does not allow firm conclusions to be drawn as to whether the attention to the welfare of forces was novel or distinctively British. In-depth examinations of attention to the welfare of British forces in previous periods or welfare among other European forces have not been conducted along similar premises. Indeed, comparative studies demonstrate the complexity of evaluating disease and troop welfare, given that European powers used and deployed their troops differently.[18] In colonial locations, Spanish and French authorities relied more on militia and other local or seasoned troops than did the British. As a result, British authorities sent a higher proportion of regular forces, who were more effective militarily, but who also suffered from higher rates of disease. The problem of disease during the war was thus not felt evenly across European nations, underscoring why a quantitative approach to evaluating troop welfare is not necessarily historically insightful.

Moreover, European authorities themselves paid attention to different types of quantitative information on manpower. Whereas British authorities tracked disease rates through returns, French authorities relied on hospital admission records. As a result, historians know that of the 7,450 French soldiers sent to New France between 1755 and 1760 and identified by historians, 1,731 died (from various causes), while there were 1,744 admissions into the hospitals of New France. This can roughly be translated to a mortality rate of 22 percent, but a morbidity rate of 23 percent does not accurately portray the nature of hospital admissions, which were appropriate only for severe illnesses and injuries and which could include multiple admissions of one individual.[19] Moreover, unlike British returns, French records do not provide a statistical measure of troop strength at any point of a campaign, instead providing more detail on individual soldiers and hospitals. As the nature of modern statistical evidence was itself being developed during this period, it is not surprising that French and British records are not comparable. Instead, the records demonstrate differing priorities and structures of knowledge, showing how modern methods of quantitative evaluation are themselves historically contingent.[20]

However, there are substantive reasons to suggest that Britain in the mid-eighteenth century was a crucial place and time for the development of colonial military medicine and, more broadly, heightened concern for the welfare of armed forces. Given the central role of public opinion on the welfare of troops, along with the increasing cost of soldiers and sailors as trained professionals in the early modern period, eighteenth-century European states had growing practical and political reasons to concern themselves with the welfare of their troops. The British state was under particular public and parliamentary pressure to do so—or to appear to do so—from the late seventeenth century. Since Britain was aware that it had a much smaller population than France and was also committed to waging war across multiple continents, it appears that the development of methodologies to manage manpower, such as returns, were a result of Britain's unique pressures of manpower and parliamentary scrutiny. At the same time, British popular politics were decidedly vigorous during the mid-eighteenth century and, combined with a marked increase in the number of armed forces—particularly in the number of British regular soldiers and sailors sent overseas—likely resulted in considerable and conspicuous intensification of official and public interest in the welfare of British troops.

Representations of the war crafted for the British public demonstrate this interest. As discussed in the introduction, Penny's and Hayman's images of the war were displayed in public and bought as reproductions, attesting not only to public involvement, but also to concern over the nature and responsibility of British authority.[21] Penny's portrayal of the Marquis of Granby makes use of Granby's public image: the commander was popular among British troops and the public because of his well-known generosity and genuine care for his troops. Indeed, as the story goes, it was this generosity that accounts for the many pubs named after Granby, the result of gifts to disabled noncommissioned officers upon the end of the war. Alongside a successful military command, his generous gifts to the men under his care established Granby as a beloved British patriot and a model officer. These practices could not be maintained in the long term: Granby died in 1770 with debts of over £30,000.[22] Upon his death, Horace Walpole described Granby as "the idol of the army and the populace," adding: "Of money he seemed to conceive no use but in giving it away: but that profusion was so indiscriminate, that compassion or solicitation, and consequently imposture, were equally the master of his purse. Thus his benevolence checked itself, and wasted on unworthy objects the sums he often wanted to bestow on real distress."[23]

Penny's popular representation of Granby remained just that: a popular representation. In fact, as has been demonstrated, the welfare of British armed forces was essentially maintained by the British state. This resourcing required careful monitoring, unlike the indiscriminate personal charity of Granby. Regular returns of the armed forces, for example, provided the foundation on which medical practitioners, officers, and officials decided matters of logistics, strategy, and foreign policy, while medical men carefully observed, recorded, and trialed methods to preserve manpower, responding to the challenges of overseas warfare.

The care of the British state for the welfare of its armed forces was thus not only a sentimental response, but also a pragmatic effort designed to ensure victory. Just as gift giving and charity are forms of reciprocal exchange, so too did the resources spent on soldiers and sailors combine humanitarianism with military, economic, and political calculations.[24] Disease rates figured prominently in criticisms of specific officials and general policy. Such critiques can be found in both the American colonial and British press, alongside patriotic reports celebrating the care given to French prisoners. This illustrates the fundamental role of care for the welfare of armed forces in public opinion. It was this care that sustained the legitimacy of a warring British state, ensuring obligations and commitments from the public through taxation, charitable support for troops, and military and naval service.

This detailed examination of British responses to disease during the Seven Years' War provides insight into the workings of the eighteenth-century imperial British state. This was a state actively engaged in the development of scientific medicine, playing a central role in clinical trials, quantitative data collection, and empirical practices more broadly: it was not only a fiscal-military state, but a state that fostered the development of knowledge as well. Rather than a cold and distant authority, this state paid careful attention to, and invested heavily in, the welfare of its troops, even if only out of strategic and practical considerations, or in response to the pressure of public opinion. Regardless of motivations, the British imperial state during the Seven Years' War developed expertise to efficiently manage and conserve manpower during global warfare, in the form of knowledge and practices that in many cases did not come to fruition until the later eighteenth and nineteenth centuries. As the naval historian Jan Glete notes, historians of state formation should take account of two types of state efficiency. While the first, which Glete called static efficiency, focuses on using existing resources most effectively, the second, termed dynamic, is what helps to shape a state and its war effort in the long term: "the capacity for creative and innovative efforts aimed at radically improving the institution's performance in the future."[25] Although the Sick and Hurt Board's investigation into scurvy remedies did not bear fruit during the Seven Years' War, its methods and structure ensured the elimination of scurvy as a threat by the time of the Napoleonic Wars, and so were crucial to British power projection in the long term. Likewise, practices and methodologies for colonial medicine would be applied throughout the later eighteenth and nineteenth centuries, becoming key components of modern British imperial governance.

Building on studies that see a growth in the layering of eighteenth-century governmental force, authority, and legitimacy, rather than a sudden shift, this examination of the British state in the Seven Years' War shows a long-term process of innovation and transformation, formed through responses to the physical demands of global warfare.[26] The Seven Years' War was a meaningful stage in this process of state formation, featuring a gradual buildup in the scale of war, the authority of the state, colonial tensions, and the role of public opinion in public life. At the same time, examining the role of disease in war demonstrates the crucial role of warfare, the British state, and the colonies in the construction of modern medical expertise. By focusing on the physical features of early modern warfare, this study provides a view of the war from imperial authorities' vantage point: one trained on the endless and laborious task of managing manpower in the face of virulent disease in the field, political opposition at home, and the clamor of public opinion in both the colonies and the metropole.

NOTES

INTRODUCTION

1. Solkin, *Painting for Money*, 204.

2. Solkin, "Portraiture in Motion," 3.

3. Solkin, *Painting for Money*, 190–99. See also Fordham, *British Art and the Seven Years' War*; and more broadly, Hoock, *Empires of the Imagination*.

4. On conserving manpower by preventing disease, see Gradish, *Manning of the British Navy*; and more generally, Riley, *Eighteenth-Century Campaign*; Mathias, "Swords into Ploughshares."

5. [Mauduit], *Considerations on the Present German War*, 68

6. Tilly, *Coercion, Capital and European States*.

7. Rogers, *Military Revolution Debate*; Downing, *Military Revolution and Political Change*; Gunn, Grummitt, and Cools, "War and the State in Early Modern Europe." The role of navies has not been entirely neglected: Glete, *Navies and Nations*. For a recent and nuanced overview of historians' approaches to the relationship between war and the growth of the European state, see Parrott, *Business of War*, 8–18.

8. Brewer, *Sinews of Power*; O'Brien, "Political Economy of British Taxation, 1660–1815; Mathias and O'Brien, "Taxation in Great Britain and France"; Dickson, *Financial Revolution in England*.

9. Storrs, *Fiscal-Military State*; Stone, *Imperial State at War*; Scott, "Seven Years' War"; Bowen and González Enciso, *Mobilising Resources for War*.

10. Eastwood, *Government and Community*; Cookson, *British Armed Nation*; Innes, *Inferior Politics*; Langford, *Public Life and the Propertied Englishman*; Braddick, *State Formation*; Harling, *Modern British State*.

11. Blanning, *Culture of Power and the Power of Culture*, 5. See also Scott and Simms, *Cultures of Power in Europe*.

12. Black, *Debating Foreign Policy*, 2. The seminal history of the public sphere is Habermas, *Structural Transformation of the Public Sphere*, chap. 3, under the heading "The Model Case of Britain." On "the public," "public opinion," and politics "out of doors" (beyond Parliament) during this period, see Peters, *Pitt and Popularity*; Danley, "British Political Press and Military Thought"; Wilson, *Sense of the People*; Brewer,

Party Ideology and Popular Politics; Rogers and Jordan, "Admirals as Heroes"; Rogers, *Whigs and Cities*; Harris, *Politics and the Nation*; Cardwell, *Arts and Arms*; Lincoln, *Representing the Royal Navy*; Barker, *Newspapers, Politics and English Society*; Barker and Burrows, *Press, Politics and the Public Sphere*, esp. the introduction and chap. 4.

13. Rodger, *Wooden World*; Lincoln, *Representing the Royal Navy*; Conway, *War, State, and Society*, esp. chap. 3; Anderson, *People's Army*; Steppler, "Common Soldier"; Brumwell, *Redcoats*; Houlding, *Fit for Service*; Guy, *Oeconomy and Discipline.*

14. Rabier, "Introduction," 2. See also Ash, *Expertise*; Selinger and Crease, *Philosophy of Expertise*; Damien, *L'expertise.*

15. Ash, "Expertise," 12; see also Ash, *Power, Knowledge and Expertise.*

16. Porter and Brewer, *Consumption and the World of Goods*; Porter, *Enlightenment*; Porter, *Health for Sale*; Porter, *Disease, Medicine and Society*, chap. 4; Porter, *Doctor of Society*; Porter and Granshaw, *Hospital in History*, including Porter, "Gift Relation." Even historians who disagree with Porter's findings have tended to focus on similar subjects, given the fruitfulness of his cultural and social approaches to the history of medicine.

17. Porter, *Cambridge History of Science*, vol. 4; see, e.g., Fox, "Science and Government": "modest" on 124, structures "few and weak" on 113.

18. See, e.g., Stewart and Jacob, *Practical Matter*; Stewart, *Rise of Public Science*; Jacob, *Scientific Culture and the Making of the Industrial West*; Mokyr, *Gifts of Athena*; Berg, "Joel Mokyr's *The Gifts of Athena*." For a nuanced overview of eighteenth-century scientific activity that refines assumptions of British state noninvolvement, see Hilaire-Pérez, *L'invention technique.*

19. See, e.g., Drayton, "Knowledge and Empire"; Drayton, *Nature's Government*; Grove, *Green Imperialism*; Gascoigne, *Science in the Service of Empire*; Chakrabarti, *Materials and Medicine*; Harrison, *Medicine in an Age of Commerce and Empire*; Cook, "Practical Medicine and the British Armed Forces"; Hudson, *British Military and Naval Medicine*; Haycock and Archer, *Health & Medicine at Sea.*

20. Although the overlap between the armed forces and the state may not be as obvious as in other European nations, such as Prussia or France, regardless of eighteenth-century Britons' hesitancy to articulate the role of the armed forces, bureaucratic evidence demonstrates the centrality of war to British state activities. Philip Harling, for example, notes that between 1689 and 1815 "on a per capita basis, Britons spent more on warfare than any of their continental counterparts," with more than 80 percent of state funds going toward war. Harling, *Modern British State*, 42. For Continental overviews, see Contamine, *War and Competition between States*, esp. chaps. 4, 6, 8.

21. This relies on John Brewer's definition of the state: "a territorially and jurisdictionally defined political entity in which public authority is distinguished from (though not unconnected to) private power, and which is manned by officials whose primary (though not sole) allegiance is to a set of political institutions under a single, i.e. sovereign and final, authority." Brewer, *Sinews of Power*, 252 n. 1. On the difficulties of defining and identifying the British state during this period, see Innes, "Forms of 'Government Growth'."

22. This paraphrases Michael Braddick's definition of the state: "a coordinated and

territorially bounded network of agencies exercising political power." Braddick, *State Formation*, 9.

23. Innes, *Inferior Politics*, chap. 2; Slack, *Reformation to Improvement*.

24. On the importance of logistics and military administration for war in the colonies, see Chet, *Conquering the American Wilderness*; Pargellis, *Lord Loudoun*. In India, historians have noted the fundamental role of finances for the hire of mercenaries and political alliances: Bryant, "Indigenous Mercenaries in the Service of European Imperialists"; Bryant, "Asymmetric Warfare." Black, "Military Revolution?," 103, argues for the significance of "military technique (broadly conceived to include drill, cartography, logistic and financial institutions, as well as tactics)" to explain European military ascendency overseas.

25. On the British army as imperial presence, see Shy, *Toward Lexington*; McConnell, *Army and Empire*.

26. Marshall, *Making and Unmaking of Empires*, 85.

27. The classic account of British strategy is Corbett, *England in the Seven Years' War*; Baugh's *Global Seven Years War* provides a masterful overview of Franco-British strategy, policy, and diplomacy.

28. Harkness, "Americanism and Jenkins' Ear"; see also Harding, "Growth of Anglo-American Alienation"; Leach, *Roots of Conflict*; Anderson, *People's Army*; Brumwell, *Redcoats*; Greene, "Seven Years' War and the American Revolution." For histories of the war that focus on America, see Anderson, *Crucible of War*; Hofstra, *Cultures in Conflict*; Fowler, *Empires at War*.

29. Black, *America or Europe?*; Savory, *His Britannic Majesty's Army*; Szabo, *Seven Years War in Europe*; Simms, "'Ministers of Europe'"; Simms, *Three Victories*. For a recent Atlantic history of the war, see Schumann and Schweizer, *Seven Years War*.

30. Marshall, *Problems of Empire*; Marshall, *East Indian Fortunes*; Bowen, *Revenue and Reform*; Gupta, *Sirajuddaullah and the East India Company*.

31. Influenced by Baugh, *British Naval Administration*, naval history is heavily administrative; see, e.g., Gradish, *Manning of the British Navy*; Syrett, *Shipping and Military Power*; Wilkinson, *British Navy and the State*; Buchet, *Marine, économie et société*. On military administration, see Bannerman, *Merchants and the Military*. Many excellent maritime histories of the war exist; see particularly Rodger, *Wooden World*; and Rodger, *Command of the Ocean*, chaps. 18–20.

32. Marshall, *Making and Unmaking of Empires*.

33. On the centrality of the Seven Years' War to colonial warfare, see, e.g., Christiansen, "Colonial Warfare."

34. Black, "Military Revolution?" For studies that examine the European nature of colonial warfare, see Chet, *Conquering the American Wilderness*; Pargellis, *Lord Loudoun*; Lenman, "Transition to European Military Ascendancy in India." On warfare during the eighteenth century and the notion of "limited" war, often contrasted with unbounded war in the colonies, see Bell, *First Total War*; Anderson, *War and Society in Europe*; Showalter, *Wars of Frederick the Great*; Duffy, *Military Experience in the Age of Reason*; Robson, "Armed Forces and the Art of War"; Strachan, *European Armies and the Conduct of War*, chaps. 2–3. On challenges to this view, see Black, *Warfare in the*

Eighteenth Century, chaps. 2, 3, and 6; Black, *European Warfare*, chaps. 3 and 5; Charters, Rosenhaft, and Smith, *Civilians and War in Europe*.

35. Watson to Cleveland, 31 Jan. 1757, in Hill, *Bengal*, 2:200; the decision of the Fort William Committee in APAC, MSS Eur/Orme India V, fol. 55: 7 Jan. 1757; see also Bryant, "War in Bengal," 410–11.

36. On problems defining the Seven Years' War, see Danley, "'Problem' of the Seven Years' War."

37. See, e.g., Middleton, *Bells of Victory*.

38. See note 10 above; Brewer, *Sinews of Power*; Storrs, *Fiscal-Military State*, esp. Storrs, "Fiscal-Military State in the 'Long' Eighteenth Century," Scott, "Fiscal-Military State"; Bonney, introduction; Harling and Mandler, "From 'Fiscal-Military' State to Laissez-Faire State." In colonial contexts, see Greene, *Peripheries and Center*; Marshall, *Making and Unmaking of Empires*, esp. chap. 2.

39. Mackillop, "Political Culture of the Scottish Highlands"; Conway, *War, State and Society*, chap. 2; Innes, "Central Government 'Interference'."

40. Black, *Warfare in the Eighteenth Century*, 173–74.

41. Pelling, "Contagion/Germ Theory/Specificity"; Hannaway, "Environment and Miasmata"; Kessel, *Air, the Environment and Public Health*; Riley, *Eighteenth-Century Campaign*. See also chapter 5, on disease and sieges.

42. CP, MFR 687 (reel 80), box 53/38: Cumberland to Ligonier, 24 June 1757.

43. McNeill, *Mosquito Empires*, esp. chap. 2.

44. Foucault, *Discipline and Punish*; Jones and Porter, *Reassessing Foucault*; on Foucault and colonialism, see Stoler, *Race and the Education of Desire*. On colonial medicine, see Worboys, "Emergence of Tropical Medicine"; Harrison, *Medicine in an Age of Commerce and Empire*, esp. chap. 3; Kiple and Beck, *Biological Consequences of the European Expansion*; Curtin, *Disease and Empire*; Bewell, *Romanticism and Colonial Disease*; Harrison, *Climates & Constitutions*; Arnold, *Colonizing the Body*; Drayton, *Nature's Government*. For a review of colonial medicine, see Anderson, "Where Is the Postcolonial History of Medicine?"

45. On the body and medicine, see Lupton, *Medicine as Culture*; Gallagher and Laqueur, *Making of the Modern Body*; Turner, "Rationalization of the Body." On military discipline, see Van Orden, *Music, Discipline, and Arms*; Houlding, *Fit for Service*. On war and medicine, see Harrison, "Medicine and the Management of Modern Warfare"; Harrison, "Medicalization of War—the Militarization of Medicine"; Cooter, "Discourses on War"; Cooter, "Medicine and the Goodness of War."

46. Nancy Stepan, "Race, Gender, Science and Citizenship," 49 n. 26.

47. On the relationship between scurvy and discipline, see Lawrence, "Disciplining Disease"; and chapters 1 and 4 below.

48. Vigarello, *Concepts of Cleanliness*; Brown, *Foul Bodies*; Harrison, *Climates & Constitutions*; Ernst and Harris, *Race, Science and Medicine*; Hannaford, *Race*.

CHAPTER ONE

1. For surveys of early American warfare, see Higginbotham, "Early American Way of War"; and Lee, "Early American Ways of War." Detailed examinations have demon-

strated that wilderness warfare remained European in its tactical approach, although logistical demands were great, requiring extensive administrative support: Beattie, "Adaptation of the British Army to Wilderness Warfare"; Chet, *Conquering the American Wilderness*; Pargellis, *Lord Loudoun*.

2. There is no accurate term to describe British colonists whose roots lie in the American colonies, as the often used "Anglo-American" neglects Scottish, Irish, and German immigrants, among others (see Ward, *Breaking the Backcountry*, 267 n. 2). Here, I am using "provincial" to designate British American colonists and the provincial regiments (see note 87 below) just as contemporaries used it, and also as it is the most broadly encompassing and accurate available term, as the colonies were considered "provinces" of the metropole (hence "Provincial Assemblies"). By the same token, I use "British" to designate those who came to the American colonies as part of the British Army, Royal Navy, and British government.

3. The standard military medical history of the British Army is Cantlie, *History of the Army Medical Department*; Cantlie assumes no preventative medical care was attempted (see chap. 5); others, such as Frey, similarly assume a low level of medical care due to "Britain's reliance on an anachronous administrative system to supply its troops abroad." Frey, *British Soldier in America*, 29. Standard military histories of the 1759–60 siege, such as Doughty, *Siege of Quebec*; Fortescue, *History of the British Army*, vol. 2; and Corbett, *England in the Seven Years' War*; and even recent histories such as Anderson, *Crucible of War*, mention disease either not at all or only in passing, and assume no preventative medical care was instituted. For recent studies that have rehabilitated British military medicine in the colonies, see Kopperman, "Medical Services in the British Army"; Kopperman, "British Army in North America and the West Indies"; Kopperman, introduction to *Regimental Practice*; Harrison, *Medicine in an Age of Commerce and Empire*; Marshall, "Surgeons Reconsidered"; Hudson, *British Military and Naval Medicine*. McConnell and Brumwell include details of medicine and disease in their excellent social histories of the British Army: McConnell, *Army and Empire*; Brumwell, *Redcoats*, esp. chap. 4.

4. See, e.g., Anderson, *Crucible of War*; Mapp, *Elusive West*; Anderson, *People's Army*; Anderson, *War That Made America*; Ward, *Breaking the Backcountry*; Selesky, *War and Society in Colonial Connecticut*; Richter, *Facing East from Indian Country*, chaps. 5–6; McConnell; *A Country Between*; Ward, "Understanding Native American Alliances"; McConnell, *Army and Empire*; Skaggs and Nelson, *Sixty Years' War for the Great Lakes*; Flavell and Conway, *Britain and America Go to War*, pt. 1.

5. French, "Scurvy."

6. Carpenter, *Scurvy*, 227.

7. Taylor, "Clinical Manifestations of Vitamin Deficiencies"; Carpenter, *Scurvy*, 202–3.

8. Lind, *Scurvy* (1753), v.

9. See, e.g., Harvie, *Limeys*.

10. Lind, *Scurvy* (1753), 272–73.

11. Ibid., 278.

12. Ibid., 291.

13. Ibid., 287.

14. Ibid., 307.

15. Pringle, *Observations*, appendix, lxviii.

16. As few regimental returns survive, there is little quantifiable indication of numbers of sick throughout the war; Stephen Brumwell notes morbidity rates ranging from 16 percent to 55 percent based on isolated surviving returns Brumwell, *Redcoats*, 151.

17. John Johnson, reprinted in Doughty, *Siege of Quebec*, 5:81; and examples in Knox, *Journal*.

18. HL, James Abercromby Papers, Box 4, fol. 192: Pownall to Abercromby, 24 Apr. 1758. For more on the nature of British negotiations with local contractors, see Charters, "Caring Fiscal-Military State," 928–30.

19. Knox, *Journal*, 1:17–18.

20. TNA, WO 34/4, fol. 19: Murray to Amherst, 19 May 1760.

21. TNA, WO 34/5, fol. 65: Gage to Amherst, 6 Mar. 1762.

22. LO 6218 (Interrogatories for Capt. Monypenny, 12 Feb 1760).

23. Cartier, *Voyages*, 76–80.

24. Houston, "Scurvy and Canadian Exploration," 161–67.

25. Lind, *Scurvy* (1753), 222–23.

26. Carpenter, *Scurvy*, 111–38, 230–32.

27. Chaps. 40 and 42 refer to spruce beer.

28. TNA, WO 34/19, fol. 43: Duncan to Amherst, Fort Ontario, 31 May 1761.

29. TNA, WO 34/21, fol. 32: Eyre to Amherst, Fort Niagara, 15 Apr. 1760.

30. Jenks, *Diary*, 13.

31. Knox, *Journal*, 1:71–72.

32. NAC, MG18-L4, A-1826 015, "Journals 1758–1763."

33. Carpenter, *Scurvy*, 229–30.

34. See, e.g., Parkman, *Montcalm and Wolfe*; Doughty, *Siege of Quebec*; Stacey, *Quebec, 1759*; Carroll, *Wolfe & Montcalm*; Chartrand, *Québec*. Recent contributions continue this trend, albeit through new approaches: McLynn, *1759*; Olson et al., "Perfect Tide, Ideal Moon."

35. See, e.g., Flavell and Conway, *Britain and America Go to War*; McNairn, *Behold the Hero*; LaPierre, *1759: The Battle for Canada*; Anderson, *Crucible of War*; Fowler, *Empires at War*; Ward, *Battle for Quebec*; McConnell, *Army and Empire*. Ward's focus is specifically the development of North American irregular warfare, with little reference to similar practices of irregular and unlimited warfare in Europe or in other colonial contexts, while McConnell's focus is on garrison life, and not battles per se, in the British Atlantic world. French-Canadian studies often provide a broader and longer-term focus, including the battle of Sainte-Foy in the conquest of Canada, as well as reflections on the battle's memorialization. See most recently Lacoursière and Quimper, *Québec*; Veyssière and Fonck, *La guerre de Sept Ans*; Fonck, "Une victoire inutile."

36. TNA, CO 5/64, fol. 30: Murray's Journal, 13 Nov. 1759.

37. TNA, CO 5/64, fols. 34–38: Murray's Journal, 24 Dec. 1759–9 Feb. 1760; Knox, *Journal*, 2:298–305.

38. Knox, *Journal*, 2:309.

39. TNA, CO 5/64, fol. 95: Return of 24 Dec. 1759. On returns, see chapter 3 below.

40. Knox, *Journal*, 2:318.

41. TNA, CO 5/64, fol. 97: Return of 24 Jan. 1760, with a total of 1,837 sick out of 7,223 rank and file.

42. Knox, *Journal*, 2:334: order of 5 Feb. 1760; and 2:352.

43. TNA, CO 5/64, fol. 99: Return of 24 Feb. 1760, with a total of 1,976 sick out of 7,120 rank and file.

44. TNA, CO 5/64, fol. 101: Return of 24 Mar. 1760, with a total of 2,525 sick out of 6,959 rank and file.

45. TNA, CO 5/64, fol. 44: Murray's Journal, 9 Mar. 1760.

46. TNA, CO 5/64, fol. 47: Murray's Journal, 21 Apr. 1760.

47. TNA, CO 5/64, fol. 103: Return of 24 Apr. 1760.

48. Fraser, "Capture of Quebec," 163.

49. TNA, CO 5/64, fols. 49–50: Murray's Journal, 27–28 Apr. 1760.

50. Johnson, in Doughty, *Siege*, 5:120–22.

51. Malartic to Lévis, 23 May 1760, in Lacoursière and Quimper, *Québec*, 258: "Je ne crois pas M. Murray en état de faire d'entreprises; il n'a pas plus de quinze à seize cents hommes en état de servir; encore plusieurs ont-ils le scorbut. Il me disoit hier, me témoignant de la confiance, qu'il lui tardoit que tout cela finît; qu'il n'aimoit pas ce pays-ci; que presque tout son monde étoit malade et n'etoit pas reconnoissable."

52. SHD, A1 3624, fol. 21, Vaudreuil, Montréal, 3 June 1760: "La garnison de québec ne peut cacher le fond de tristesse qui l'a rongé."

53. TNA, CO 5/64, fol. 111: Murray to Amherst, 13 July 1760.

54. TNA, CO 5/64, fol. 127: Murray to Amherst, 7 Oct. 1760.

55. TNA, CO 5/64, fols. 14–15: Murray to Amherst, 30 Apr. 1760.

56. TNA, CO 5/64, fol. 19: Murray's Journal, introductory letter to Pitt, 25 May 1760.

57. TNA, CO 5/64, fol. 46: Murray's Journal, 10 Apr. 1760.

58. Knox, *Journal*, 2:344.

59. Ibid., 2:354.

60. TNA, CO 5/64, fol. 43: Murray's Journal, 29 Feb. 1760.

61. Knox, *Journal*, 2:355.

62. Lind, *Scurvy* (1772), 269–70.

63. Ibid., 514.

64. Ibid., 514–15.

65. Pringle MS, 4:179, Cuthbert, 1757.

66. Pringle MS, 5:259, Huck, 2 Oct. 1762.

67. Pringle MS, 7:169, Temple, July 1763. See also Kopperman, introduction to *Regimental Practice*, for evidence of dissections in the army during the 1740s.

68. Harrison, *Medicine in an Age of Commerce and Empire*, 3.

69. Kopperman has identified 828 British military medical officers who served in North America and the West Indies alone, over the period 1755–83. Kopperman, introduction to *Regimental Practice*, 1.

70. Bynum and Porter, *Medical Fringe & Medical Orthodoxy*; Porter, *Health for Sale*; Porter, *Patients and Practitioners*; Bynum and Porter, *William Hunter*. See also Pelling, *Common Lot*, pt. 3, esp. chap. 10; Lawrence, *Charitable Knowledge*; Digby, *Making a Medical Living*; Brown, *Performing Medicine*; Jenner and Wallis, *Medicine*

and the Market; Harrison, *Medicine in an Age of Commerce and Empire*. See more on this in chapters 3 and 5 below.

71. TNA, WO 34/64, fol. 40: Memorial of James Napier, New York, 10 Nov. 1761. On Monro's appointment and subsequent difficulties in having it recognized, see LO 6333, Napier to Loudoun, 11 Apr. 1763; LO 6334, Munro to Loudoun, 12 Apr. 1763; LO 5994, Munro petition to George II, 1763.

72. On Huck's degree, see LO 6043, Huck to Loudoun, 20 Feb. 1759. For more on Huck, see Webb, "Richard Huck Saunders."

73. See also chapter 5 below.

74. Kopperman, "Medical Services in the British Army," 443–47.

75. Stevenson, "Relation of Military Service to Licensing"; Clark, *History of the Royal College of Physicians*, 553–69; Butterton, "William Smellie."

76. Bell, *John Morgan*, chap. 2.

77. Kopperman, "Medical Services in the British Army," 444–46; Kopperman, introduction to *Regimental Practice*, 1–45; see also Kopperman, "British Army in North America and the West Indies."

78. Buchanan, *"Regimental Practice,"* 202.

79. Marshall, "Surgeons Reconsidered."

80. KHLC, U1350/Z9A, James Miller, Memoirs of an Invalid, fol. 72.

81. Devine, *Scotland's Empire*.

82. Reid, "Simon Fraser"; Brumwell, *Redcoats*, chap. 8; Devine, *Scotland's Empire*, chap. 6; Thomson, *Memoirs of the Life and Gallant Exploits*; Clyde, *Rebel to Hero*; Lenman, *Jacobite Risings in Britain*.

83. James Boswell recorded how their distinctive dress occasioned cries of "No Scots! No Scots! Out with them!" when two Highland officers in full dress just back from service went to the opera at Covent Garden in 1762. Boswell, *Boswell's London Journal*, 71–72. These responses demonstrated anti-Bute sentiment, rife in the 1760s.

84. TNA, WO 1/973, p. 956: Henry Seton to Barrington, 29 Nov. 1757.

85. Fraser, "Capture of Quebec," 161.

86. Fraser, "Capture of Quebec," 161n.

87. On "irregular" warfare and regiments, see, e.g., Brumwell, *White Devil*; Steele, *Guerillas and Grenadiers*; Chet, *Conquering the American Wilderness*. Provincial regiments varied in terms of their composition and structure: British officials often referred to both militias and independent companies, for example, as "provincial regiments." Moreover, many provincials joined British regular forces, while many provincial regiments had a high proportion of British or Irish-born soldiers: see, e.g., Ward, *Breaking the Backcountry*, appendix, "Composition of the Provincial Regiments," 263–64. Here, I follow the usage of British contemporaries, in which "provincial" indiscriminately described colonial American soldiers.

88. TNA, CO 5/64, fols. 90–103; the rates of morbidity among Hazzan's Rangers range from 34 percent to 52 percent while the rates of morbidity among British regular troops range from 22 percent to 32 percent during the siege. On comments, see, e.g., Holden, *Journal*; Anderson, *People's Army*, 95–107, 116; Brumwell, *Redcoats*, chap. 4.

89. Pringle MS, 2:216–18, Huck to Pringle, 5 Dec. 1760.

90. Pringle MS, 3:10–11, Kirkpatrick to Pringle.

91. Lind, *Scurvy* (1753), 285, 65; see Lawrence, "Disciplining Disease," for more on the relationship between scurvy and discipline.

92. J. M., "Letter," *The Gentleman's Magazine*, London, Sept. 1756, 420.

93. J. M., "Letter"; although the magazine printed a reply not fully agreeing with this claim, it also does not fully disagree.

94. NAC, MG18-L4 (Amherst's Journal), 9 Sept. 1759.

95. Jenks, *Diary*, 7 Sept. 1760, 28.

96. Jenks, *Diary*, 26 Sept. 1760, 33.

97. Jenks, *Diary*, 27 Sept. 1760, 33.

98. See chapter 3 below for more on diseases of army camps.

99. Anderson, *People's Army*, pt. 1.

100. Jenks, *Diary*, 3 Sept. 1760, 26.

101. Jenks, *Diary*, 19 Sept. 1760, 31; 7 Oct. 1760, 35, mentioning infectious air.

102. Jenks, *Diary*, 20 Sept. 1760, 30.

103. Holden, *Journal*, 23.

104. Loudoun to Cumberland, 22 Nov.–26 Dec. 1756, in Cumberland, *Military Affairs in North America*, 280.

105. Brocklesby, *Oeconomical and Medical Observations*, 231.

106. There is still debate over whether a variety of types exist: for a clear discussion, see Meier, "Smallpox in Stuart London." More generally, see Hopkins, *Greatest Killer*; Dixon, *Smallpox*, chaps. 1–2; Carmichael and Silverstein, "Smallpox in Europe."

107. Miller, *Adoption of Inoculation*; Razzell, *Conquest of Smallpox*, chaps. 3–6.

108. Scott, Duncan, and Duncan, "Dynamics of Smallpox Epidemics"; Scott, Duncan, and Duncan, "Periodicity of Smallpox Epidemics."

109. Although some historians have assumed that recruits were inoculated upon joining, there is no archival evidence of such procedures. Moreover, inoculation among the lower ranks in Britain was unusual until the later 1770s: see Miller, *Adoption of Inoculation*, 170–71; Razzell, *Conquest of Smallpox*, chap. 4; Brunton, "Smallpox Inoculation."

110. Steppler, "Common Soldier," 32, 11; Conway, "Mobilization of Manpower."

111. Brocklesby, *Oeconomical and Medical Observations*, 231.

112. Duffy, *Epidemics*, 101–6; Reynolds, "Inoculation for the Smallpox"; Blake, "Smallpox Inoculation."

113. Duffy, *Epidemics*, 109.

114. M. de Doreil to M. de Paulmy, 25 Oct. 1757, in New York State, *Documents*, 10:653.

115. Heagerty, *Medical History in Canada*, 41–42; Brumwell, *Redcoats*, 42.

116. "La petite vérole qui n'est regardée en Canada comme une maladie populaire qui prend tous les vingt ans, fait du ravage cette année, quoiqu'on l'ait eue il y a deux ans. Elle a été communiqué par les Acadiens et les Anglois pris au fort Guillame-Henry." Entry for 13 Nov. 1757 in Montcalm, *Journal*, 317.

117. MacLeod, "Microbes and Muskets."

118. Ibid., 51; on blaming the British for spreading smallpox during the American

War of Independence, see Fenn, *Pox Americana*, chaps. 2–3; Fenn, "Biological Warfare"; see also Lewy, "Victims of Genocide?"; Charters, "Military Medicine and Ethics of War."

119. "Les sauvages ont perdu plusieurs d'entre eux de la petite vérole; c'est fâcheux; ils seront dégoutés de venir en guerre de nos côtés, et il en coûtera d'autant plus cher au Rois, pour couvrir les morts et autres cérémonies accoutumées, que les commandants des postes auront une belle occasion pour faire des *Mémoires*." Entry of 26 Feb. 1758 in Montcalm, *Journal*, 333–34.

120. Although one study on measles has suggested that the overall genetic homogeneity of Amerindians may have contributed to the virulence of an epidemic striking an early Native American settlement, it is questionable whether this can be applied to eighteenth-century smallpox outbreaks. See Black, "Explanation of High Death Rates"; Black, "Why Did They Die?"

121. Loudoun to Cumberland, 25 Apr. 1757–3 June 1757, in Cumberland, *Military Affairs in North America*, 361.

122. Knox, *Journal*, 254.

123. Rogers, *Reminiscences of the French War*, 42.

124. TNA, WO 34/30, fol. 15: Amherst to De Lancy, 21 May 1758.

125. Loudoun mentions inoculation in a letter to Cumberland, 22 Nov.–26 Dec. 1756, in Cumberland, *Military Affairs in North America*, 280, but only as something he will do.

126. On inoculations among militia regiments, see Brocklesby, *Oeconomical and Medical Observations*, 231–32.

127. HRO, W/B/26, fol. 1: 15 February 1758 (and see fols. 2–4).

128. Becker, "Smallpox in Washington's Army," 387.

129. On inoculation among British forces, see Marshall, "Health of the British Soldier in America," 102–3; on inoculation in the Continental Army, see Becker, "Smallpox in Washington's Army"; Fenn, *Pox Americana*, chap. 3.

130. Duffy points out: "The long intervals between smallpox outbreaks in the colonies resulted in the growth of a large body of nonimmunes, few of whom escaped the infection during an epidemic. This high case incidence brought many deaths and led to the popular colonial misconception that smallpox was peculiarly fatal to Americans. In actuality the death rate in the colonies was, if anything, slightly lower than that in England." Duffy, *Epidemics*, 22.

131. TNA, CO 5/50, fol. 168: Abercromby to Pitt, 29 June 1758.

132. TNA, WO 34/24, fol. 1: Amherst to Wentworth, 22 Oct. 1756.

133. TNA, WO 34/24, fols. 142–43: Amherst to Hopkin, 5 Nov. 1756.

134. TNA, WO 34/90, fol. 235: Walker to Amherst, Virginia, 23 June 1762.

135. Benjamin Franklin and Thomas Jefferson are among the best-known contributors to this debate; see Gerbi, *Dispute of the New World*; Glacken, *Traces on the Rhodian Shore*; Cañizares-Esguerra, *Histories, Epistemologies, and Identities.*

136. Brocklesby, *Oeconomical and Medical Observations*, 232.

137. James De Lancey to Pitt, 25 Mar. 1759, in Pitt, *Correspondence*, 1:7.

138. NAC, MG18-L4 (Amherst's Journal), 14 Nov. 1759.

139. TNA, WO 34/30, fol. 103: Amherst to Delancey, 23 June 1759.

140. Cited in Anderson, *Crucible of War*, 372; see problems with ill-disciplined provincials in Ward, *Breaking the Backcountry*, 107–13.

141. Leach, *Roots of Conflict*; Shy, *Toward Lexington*.

142. Steppler, "Common Soldier"; Conway, "Mobilization of Manpower."

143. Anderson, *People's Army*, pt. 1; Anderson, "Contractual Principles and Military Conduct." Not all provincial regiments were alike; the Virginia and Pennsylvania regiments that Ward studied in detail greatly differ in social composition; see Ward, *Breaking the Backcountry*, 115–17 and appendix.

144. Duffy, *Epidemics*, chap. 2; Krebsbach, "Charlestown Smallpox Epidemic," 32–33.

145. Gale, "Historical Memoirs," 195.

146. Becker notes that smallpox was "instrumental to the American defeat in Canada." Becker, "Smallpox in Washington's Army," 382.

147. Fenn, *Pox Americana*, chaps. 2–3; Fenn, "Biological Warfare." For a differing interpretation applying the context of the Seven Years' War, see Charters, "Military Medicine and the Ethics of War."

148. On negotiated empire, see, e.g., Greene, *Peripheries and Center*; Greene, *Creating the British Atlantic*, esp. chap. 8; Daniels and Kennedy, *Negotiated Empires*.

149. McConnell, *Army and Empire*, see esp. chaps. 1, 6, 7, and the conclusion.

150. Colley, *Britons*; on the development of American identity during an earlier war, see Harkness, "Americanism and Jenkins' Ear"; Harding, "Anglo-American Alienation."

CHAPTER TWO

1. TNA, CO 5/41, fol. 315: "A Journal of the Expedition that sailed from Spithead to the West Indies."

2. TNA, CO 5/41, fol. 109: Cathcart to Harrington, 13 Aug. 1740.

3. On its origins, see Kiple and Higgins, "Yellow Fever"; McNeill, *Mosquito Empires*, esp. chap. 2.

4. McNeill, "Ecological Basis of Warfare," 27; see also McNeill, *Mosquito Empires*, esp. chap. 5; Guerra, "Influence of Disease on Race, Logistics and Colonization"; O'Shaughnessy, "Redcoats and Slaves."

5. Gardiner, *Account of the Expedition*, 90.

6. Harding, *Amphibious Warfare*, esp. the conclusion; see also Harding, *Emergence of Britain's Global Naval Supremacy*.

7. Syrett, *Shipping and Military Power*, chap. 5.

8. For a recent discussion of mercantilism, see Pincus, "Rethinking Mercantilism"; see also Coleman, "Mercantilism Revisited."

9. Peters, *Pitt and Popularity*, esp. the introduction; Gauci, *William Beckford*.

10. Rodger, *Command of the Ocean*, 276.

11. Harris, *Politics and the Nation*, chap. 3; Harris, "War, Empire, and the 'National Interest'."

12. Burke, *Examination of the Commercial Principles*, 36; for a review of the pamphlet debate, see Grant, "Canada versus Guadeloupe."

13. Burke, *Remarks*, 28.

14. *Detection of the False Reasons and Fact*, 43.

15. The classic summary of the West Indies in this period is Pares, *War and Trade in the West Indies*; for a recent overview of the role of disease in West Indian warfare, see McNeill, *Mosquito Empires*.

16. Lind, *Hot Climates*, 8–9.

17. Worboys, "Tropical Diseases"; Worboys, "Emergence of Tropical Medicine"; Harrison, *Medicine in an Age of Commerce and Empire*, esp. chap. 3.

18. Lind, *Hot Climates*, 18.

19. Ibid., 68.

20. Ibid., 69.

21. Ibid., 146.

22. Ibid., 2–3.

23. Ibid., 2, 113. More generally, see Kupperman, "Fear of Hot Climates," 177–78, 199–201; Burnard, "White Mortality"; Harrison, "'The Tender Frame of Man'"; Curtin, "'The White Man's Grave'"; and see chapter 5 below. On British eighteenth-century theories of fevers, see Bynum, "Cullen and the Study of Fevers in Britain."

24. Lind, *Hot Climates*, 188.

25. Pringle MS, 4:200, Munro to Pringle, 2 July 1757.

26. Hillary, *Observations on the Changes of the Air*, 146.

27. Pringle MS, 5:249, Huck to Pringle, 2 Oct. 1762.

28. Cooper and Kiple, "Yellow Fever"; also see Hirsch, *Handbook of Geographical and Historical Pathology*, 1:343–71, for a much later work that still emphasizes the role of location and climate for yellow fever. On so-called differential immunity, see McNeill, "Epidemics, Environment and Empire"; McNeill, *Mosquito Empires*, 40–46; Burnard, "White Mortality."

29. See the analyses by Crewe, *Yellow Jack and the Worm*; Buchet, *Lutte pour l'espace caraïbe*, vol. 2, chaps. xvii-xviii, along with his more concise "Quantification des pertes."

30. Guy, introduction.

31. Guy, introduction, 10–11; see also Smelser, *Campaign for the Sugar Islands*; and Corbett, *England in the Seven Years' War*, vol. 1, chaps. 15–16, and vol. 2, chaps. 7–9, for basic summaries of the campaigns.

32. Gardiner, *Account of the Expedition*, 4n.

33. Durant never published his journal; see the modern publication: Durant, "George Durant's Journal," ed. Guy.

34. Hopson to Pitt, 30 Jan. 1759, in Pitt, *Correspondence*, 2:24–25.

35. BL, Add. MS 73730, no. 38/13: Memorandum Relative to the Sick, 25 Feb. 1759.

36. BL, Add. MS 73730, no. 35/1: Council of War, 28 Feb. 1759.

37. Guy, introduction; Smelser, *Campaign for the Sugar Islands*.

38. Barrington to Pitt, 2 Mar. 1769, in Pitt, *Correspondence*, 2:46–47.

39. BL, Add. MS 73730, no. 35/5: Barrington to Barrington, 3 Mar. 1759.

40. BL, Add. MS 73730, no. 38/154.

41. TNA, ADM 1/307, fol. 141: Moore to Admiralty, 6 Mar. 1759.

42. Barrington to Pitt, 6 March 1759, in Pitt, *Correspondence*, 2:53; Pitt to Barrington, 9 March 1759, ibid., 2:59; Pitt to Moore, 6 March 1759, ibid., 2:63.

43. BL, Add. MS 73731, no. 38/81: An Account of Live Stock Sent; see also correspondence in BL, Add. MSS 73730 and 73731 regarding difficulties in raising men from nearby islands.

44. Guy, introduction.

45. BL, Add. MS 73732, no. 35/9: Barrington to Barrington, 9 May 1759; Barrington to Pitt, 9 May 1759, in Pitt, *Correspondence*, 2:100.

46. Crump to Pitt, 4 Oct. 1759, in Pitt, *Correspondence*, 2:175.

47. Ibid.

48. See the papers concerning the military establishment on Guadeloupe: TNA, WO 24/366, WO 24/382, and WO 24/396. This price may have included the cost of building barracks: O'Shaughnessy, "Redcoats and Slaves," 108.

49. Crump to Pitt, 4 Oct. 1759, in Pitt, *Correspondence*, 2:175. This also applied at an individual level: paymaster Durant acquired enough wealth to buy Tong Castle in Shropshire and establish himself as MP for Evesham in 1768, while suffering constantly from sickness throughout the campaign. See Guy, introduction, 13–14; Durant, "George Durant's Journal," 57.

50. McNeill, *Mosquito Empires*, 169–75.

51. For details of Havana in this period, see McNeill, *Atlantic Empires of France and Spain*, 85–92, 97–104.

52. Corbett, *England in the Seven Years' War*, vol. 2, chap. 9; Buchet, *Lutte pour l'espace caraïbe*, vol. 1, chap. xiv.

53. Syrett, *Siege and Capture of Havana*, xxx.

54. Lloyd and Coulter, *Medicine and the Navy*, 3:119.

55. Kuethe, *Cuba*, 16.

56. McNeill, *Mosquito Empires*, 188.

57. TNA, CO 117/1, fol. 150: Albemarle to Egremont, 7 Oct. 1762.

58. BL, Add. MS 73730, no. 35/5: Barrington to Barrington, 3 Mar. 1759.

59. TNA, WO 34/90, fol. 29: Barré to Amherst, 13 Feb. 1762.

60. SRO, HA 67/969/HI, Egremont to Amherst, 13 Jan. 1762.

61. TNA, CO 166/2, fols. 4–6: Egremont to Monckton, 5 Feb. 1762.

62. TNA, CO 117/1, fol. 28: Egremont to Albemarle, 18 Feb. 1762.

63. Leach, "Cartagena Expedition."

64. TNA, CO 5/42, fol. 19: Wentworth to Newcastle, 2 June 1741.

65. Knowles, *Account of the Expedition to Carthagena*, 38n.

66. Leach, "Cartagena Expedition," 55; Harkness, "Americanism and Jenkins' Ear," 89.

67. Harding, "Anglo-American Alienation"; Shy, *Toward Lexington*.

68. TNA, CO 5/41, fol. 227: Blakeney to Newcastle, 21 Aug. 1740.

69. SRO, HA 67/969/HI, Egremont to Amherst, 13 Jan. 1762.

70. TNA, CO 117/1, fol. 32: Egremont to Albemarle, 18 Feb. 1762.

71. TNA, WO 34/24, fol. 108: Wentworth to Amherst, 25 Mar. 1762.

72. TNA, CO 5/62, fol. 148; and SRO HA 67/969/H47, Colden to Amherst, 20 May 1762.

73. TNA, CO 5/62, fol. 150: Amherst to Colden, 20 May 1762.

74. See, e.g., TNA, CO 5/62, fol. 156: Amherst to Fitch, 1 June 1762.

75. For details of the disastrous sailing of the provincials, see Syrett, "American Provincials."

76. SRO, HA 67/969/HI, Egremont to Amherst, 13 Jan. 1762.

77. See note 24 above.

78. TNA, CO 117/1, fol. 98: Albemarle to the governor of Jamaica, 16 July 1762. On West Indian assemblies' reluctance to provide manpower, see O'Shaughnessy, "Redcoats and Slaves."

79. Lind, *Hot Climates*, 37.

80. TNA, ADM 1/237, fol. 58: Pocock to Cleveland, 14 July 1762.

81. BL, Add. MSS 73730, no. 35/5: Barrington to Barrington, 3 Mar. 1759.

82. Prado to V. S., 13 May 1762, in Archivo Nacional de Cuba, *Nuevos papeles*, 37: "viruelas, como de Matlazagua." McNeill and Parcero Torre suggest that this was the result of the arrival of unseasoned Spanish regiments: McNeill, *Mosquito Empires*, 177–78; Parcero Torre, *La pérdida de La Habana*, chap. 2.

83. Acuna-Soto, "Large Epidemics of Hemorrhagic Fever," 733–34.

84. Duro, *Armada Española*, 42–43. For a comprehensive account of the problems facing Prado in his defense against the British, see Parcero Torre, *La pérdida de La Habana*.

85. Mayor de la Plaza de Bayamo to Francisco de la Torre, 19 and 29 May 1762, in Archivo Nacional de Cuba, *Nuevos papeles*, 155.

86. SRO, HA 67/969/E15.

87. SRO, HA 67/969/H53. Returns recorded various categories, including how many men were absent, on command, and held prisoner by the enemy: these last three categories make up the remainder of the total rank and file.

88. See, e.g., TNA, WO 34/55, fols. 139–40: Albemarle to Amherst, 6 May 1762; NAC, MG23-K34, Order Books, fol. 81.

89. TNA, ADM 50/12, 22 June 1762.

90. NLS, MS 3850, fol. 8: Memorandum of the Operations of the Havana Expedition of 1762.

91. TNA, CO 117/1, fol. 96: Albemarle to Egremont, 17 July 1762.

92. SRO, HA 67/969/E8; see the similar return in TNA, CO 117/1, fols. 94–95.

93. SRO, HA 67/969/E12.

94. KHLC, U1350/Z9A, fol. 65: James Miller, Memoirs of an Invalid.

95. Lind, *Hot Climates*, 169, 126.

96. NAC, MG18-N21, Extract of a letter from an officer to Colonel Howe, 15 July 1762.

97. NAC, MG18-N21, fol. 71: Extracts of other letters relative to the siege, 29 July 1762.

98. NAC, MG23-K34, fol. 107: Order Books.

99. *Authentic Journal of the Siege*, 36–38.

100. TNA, CO 117/1, fols. 116–17: Patrick McKellar's Journal, 6 Aug. 1762.

101. TNA, ADM 50/12, 6 Aug. 1762.

102. SRO, HA 67/969/E9.

103. See the daily tallies of dead and wounded in Prado, "El diario."

104. Prado, "El diario," 14 Aug. 1762, 120.

105. TNA, CO 117/1, fols. 107–8. See also the return of killed, wounded, and missing, 13 July 1762: TNA, CO 117/1, fol. 81.

106. *Authentic Journal of the Siege*, 41.

107. TNA, CO 117/1, fol. 136: Albemarle to Egremont, 21 Aug. 1762.

108. TNA, WO 34/55 fol. 193: Return of 16 Aug 1762.

109. NAC, MG18-N21, Extracts of other letters relative to the siege, by A. W., 29 July.

110. KHLC, U1350/Z9A, fols. 70–71: James Miller,Memoirs of an Invalid.

111. SRO, HA 67/969/E5.

112. TNA, WO 34/55, fol. 185: Albemarle to Amherst, 18 Aug. 1762.

113. Amherst, *Journal*, 293.

114. TNA, WO 34/99, fol. 192: Amherst to Calcraft, 21 Sept. 1762.

115. TNA, CO 5/62, fol. 320: A Report on the State of the Men of the 17th, two Battalions of the 42d, and 77th Regiments, 18 Sept. 1762.

116. TNA, WO 34/64, fol. 55.

117. SRO, HA 67/969/E25.

118. TNA, CO 117/1, fol. 149: Albemarle to Egremont, 7 Oct. 1762.

119. SRO, HA 67/969/E17.

120. SRO, HA 67/969/E7.

121. TNA, CO 117/1, fol. 176: Albemarle to Amherst, 19 Oct. 1762.

122. Mante, *History of the Late War*, 464.

123. NAC, MG23-K34, Journal 1758–1765, entry for 4 Nov. 1762.

124. See, e.g., Stein and Stein, *Apogee of Empire*, chaps. 2–3.

125. BL, Add. MS 32942, fol. 427: Newcastle to Hardwicke, 30 Sept. 1762, reprinted in Archivo Nacional de Cuba, *Nuevos papeles*, 194.

126. See, e.g., the *London Gazette Extraordinary*, 30 Sept. 1762.

127. See, e.g., the *London Evening Post*, 30 Sept.–2 Oct. 1762; the letter appears in most London newspapers.

128. *Annual Register . . . of the Year 1762*, 39.

129. See, e.g., the *London Evening Post*, 22–24 June 1762 and 24–26 June 1762; *General Evening Post*, 22–25 May 1762, 17–19 June 1762.

130. *London Evening Post*, 24–26 June 1762.

131. Ibid., 20–22 July 1762.

132. *General Evening Post*, 17–20 July 1762.

133. *London Evening Post*, 16–18 Sept. 1762.

134. *Williamson's Liverpool Advertiser*, as a paper produced in an alternate key English port, also contains hardly a reference to the sickness at Havana.

135. *Boston Evening-Post*, 2 Aug. 1762.

136. Ibid., 30 Aug. 1762; and see the *Boston Gazette*, *New-York Gazette*, and *New-York Mercury* of similar dates.

137. *Boston Gazette*, 6 Sept. 1762.

138. Ibid., 20 Sept. 1762.

139. Ibid., 8 Nov. 1762.

140. *Boston Evening-Post*, 6 Dec. 1762, with similar reports printed in the *Boston Gazette* and the *New-York Gazette*.

141. *Providence Gazette*, 25 Dec. 1762.

142. Watts, *Letter Book*, 100: Watts to Baker, 30 Nov. 1762 (references to Watts's letters from Brumwell, *Redcoats*, 47).

143. TNA, WO 34/5, fol. 242: Gage to Amherst, 17 Nov. 1762.

144. Copeland, "'Join, or Die,'" quotation on 113.

145. Heyd, *Reading Newspapers*; Barker and Burrows, *Press, Politics and the Public Sphere*. On America, see Copeland, "America"; on Britain, see Barker, "England"; Barker, *Newspapers, Politics and English Society*.

146. TNA, WO 34/30, fol. 230: Amherst to Colden, 26 May 1762.

147. Rush, *Account of the Bilious Remitting Yellow Fever*, 13–15. While Rush, a staunch anticontagionist, would hardly admit that the fever originated in the West Indies, a contemporaneous account reports that sailors from the West Indies were considered the most likely source; see Duffy, *Epidemics*, 161–62.

148. NAC, A-1826 014, personal journal, entry for 9 May 1763.

149. Shy, *Toward Lexington*, 108–23. Americanists consider the weak British reaction, in part because of recurring tropical illnesses (likely malaria), as contributing to British-provincial friction over responses to Amerindian issues and as a key reason for the infamous Bouquet-Amherst smallpox incident. See, e.g., Duffy, *Epidemics*, 192–96; Richter, *Facing East from Indian Country*, 200–201. On the Bouquet-Amherst incident, see Charters, "Military Medicine and Ethics of War." For the broader context, see Middleton, *Pontiac's War*.

150. For a measured and persuasive overview of the tensions caused by the British Army in the colonies, see Shy, *Toward Lexington*.

151. Harding, "Anglo-American Alienation," 178–80; Leach, *Roots of Conflict*, chap. 5.

152. Greene, "Seven Years' War and the American Revolution," 99; see also Anderson, *People's Army*, for a detailed examination of the extent and nature of provincial military contributions.

153. Marshall, "Thirteen Colonies in the Seven Years' War," 72.

154. Harris, *Politics and the Nation*, chap. 3; Barker, "England"; Marshall, "Thirteen Colonies in the Seven Years' War," 69–92.

155. Gardiner, *Account of the Expedition*, 78.

156. See note 29 above.

157. Leach, "Cartagena Expedition," 43–48.

158. See, e.g., Barrett and Higgs, "Yellow Fever"; Monath, "Yellow Fever"; Tomori, "Recurring Plague"; Gardner and Ryman, "Reemerging Threat"; Downs, "Known and the Unknown in Yellow Fever"; Mathai and Vasanthan, "State of the Globe." For a study of the present-day risk of yellow fever to armed forces, see Izurieta et al., "Assessing Yellow Fever Risk."

159. For Spanish forces, see Massons, *Historia de la sanidad militar española*; Hernández-Sáenz, "Seamen, Surgeons and Empire"; Archer, "Health and Hospital Care in the Army of New Spain"; Lafuente and Sala Catalá, "Militarización de las actividades científicas." These provide useful overviews of the structure of military medicine and its broader influence, but little detail on rates of disease or levels of care during campaigns; indeed, Massons notes the difficulty in pinning down rates of morbidity

and mortality in Spanish America (473–74). There are no detailed analyses of medical care in French Caribbean campaigns, although Pluchon, *Histoire des médecins et pharmaciens*, and McClellan and Regourd, *Colonial Machine*, provide overviews of military medicine and colonial medical practice, while Buchet, *Lutte pour l'espace caraïbe*, analyzes the operations of French and British campaigns in detail, noting their relationship to rates of sickness and death, but does not examine the influence of medical care.

160. Kopperman, "British Army in North America and the West Indies," 59.

161. Buchet, *Lutte pour l'espace caraïbe*; Buchet, *Marine, économie et société*, introduction.

162. Harrison, *Medicine in an Age of Commerce and Empire*, 64.

163. Manderson, *Sickness and the State*, 10; Stepan, "Tropical Medicine and Public Health in Latin America," (pathology of the tropics); more generally, see Worboys, "Tropical Diseases"; Worboys, "Emergence of Tropical Medicine"; Arnold, *Warm Climates and Western Medicine*; MacLeod and Lewis, *Disease, Medicine and Empire*.

CHAPTER THREE

1. For details of the European campaigns of the Seven Years' War, see Corbett, *England in the Seven Years' War*, vol. 1, chaps. 6, 10, and vol. 2, chaps. 1–2; Savory, *His Britannic Majesty's Army in Germany*; Szabo, *Seven Years War in Europe*; Schumann and Schweizer, *Seven Years War*; Marston, *Seven Years' War*; Baugh, *Global Seven Years War*, esp. chaps. 8–9.

2. Simms, *Three Victories*, 451. British campaigns against the French took place in the region of Westphalia, which contemporaries simply referred to as "Germany."

3. Wilson, *Sense of the People*; Harris, *Politics and the Nation*; Rogers, *Whigs and Cities*; Brewer, *Party Ideology and Popular Politics*; Barker and Burrows, *Press, Politics and the Public Sphere*, esp. the introduction and chap. 4. On debates and wartime policy, see Simms, *Three Victories*; Wilson, *Sense of the People*, chap. 3; Peters, *Pitt and Popularity*; Black, *America or Europe?*; Black, *Continental Commitment*; Birke et al., *England and Hanover*; Pares, "American versus Continental Warfare"; Cardwell, *Arts and Arms*; Danley, "British Political Press and Military Thought."

4. Hotham to Charles Hotham, 1755, in Danley, "British Political Press and Military Thought," 364.

5. For a comprehensive overview of policy and action in Europe, see Szabo, *Seven Years War in Europe*.

6. Savory, *His Britannic Majesty's Army in Germany*, 1–4.

7. Shebbeare, *Letter to the People of England*, 29.

8. Gould, *Persistence of Empire*, chap. 2; for political details regarding the theft of the handkerchief, see BL, Egerton MS 3440.

9. For more details on specific regiments, see Savory, *His Britannic Majesty's Army in Germany*, Appendix II, 450–57.

10. For more on Cumberland, see Whitworth, *William Augustus*.

11. CP, MFR 682 (reel 75), box 50/131: Diary of Andrew Mitchell, 21–29 Apr. 1757.

12. CP, MFR 684 (reel 77), box 51/75: Cumberland to Mitchell, 13 May 1757.

13. CP, MFR 685 (reel 78), box 51/352: Cressener to Cumberland, 29 May 1757.

14. NAM, 1975-10-61, Webb to Wilson, Aug. 1761.

15. CP, MFR 685 (reel 78), box 52/71: Yorke to Cumberland, 4 June 1757.

16. "Il y a déjà beaucoup de soldats malades, et une cinquantaine de soldats blessés, en diverses petites Escarmouches." CP, MFR 686 (reel 79), box 52/159: Avis reçus de la Frontière, 9 Juin 1757.

17. For a detailed account of the structure and efficiency of the British Commissariat in Germany during the Seven Years' War, see Little, "Supply of the Combined Army"; on the British Army and contractors during this period, see Bannerman, *Merchants and the Military*; on the structure of military finances and administration, see Guy, *Oeconomy and Discipline*.

18. NAM, 2001-05-105, Henry Hulton, Letterbook, fol. 21. Hulton's account is not beyond doubt, as he himself was accused of bad dealings and inflated accounting: see Newcastle to Granby, 6 May 1760, in RCHM, *Rutland*, Appendix, pt. 5, 2:213; and notes from a May 1761 Cabinet meeting: entry for 11 May 1761, in Cavendish, *Devonshire Diary*, 97.

19. Modern-day definitions of "corruption" are unhelpful when applied to eighteenth-century military pay systems. See Ritchie and Ritchie, "Troubles of a Commissary"; Little, "Supply of the Combined Army," 2.

20. See, e.g., Lynn, "How War Fed War."

21. Townshend to Loudoun, 9 Aug. 1762, LO Add. MS 52, 1762–63, Portugal. For more on the British campaign in Portugal, see Charters, "Caring Fiscal-Military State," 927–30; Baugh, *Global Seven Years War*, 590–98.

22. Oughton, *Labour and Perseverance*, 42.

23. Oughton, *Labour and Perseverance*, entry for 6 Sept. 1758, 52; see also BL, Add. MS 17493, fol. 41: Calcraft to Stanwix, 25 Oct. 1758.

24. Munro, *Account of the Diseases*, 57.

25. Ibid., 57–58.

26. Bland, *Military Discipline*, 248.

27. BL, Add. MS 28855, fol. 23: Standing Orders for the Campaign, 16 Oct. 1760.

28. *Soldier's Journal*, 8.

29. See, e.g., BL, Add. MS 28855, fol. 31: Standing Orders for the Campaign, 2 Feb. 1761.

30. BL, Add. MS 28855, fols. 31–32: Standing Orders for the Campaign, 2 Feb. 1761.

31. CP, MFR 707 (reel 100), box 8/123: Order Book, 16 Aug. 1761.

32. Pringle, *Diseases of the Army*, 24.

33. DuPont, "Diarrheal Diseases (Acute)."

34. Harden, "Typhus, Epidemic"; Snyder, "Typhus Fever Rickettsiae," 1075 and 1060 (reference to the Serbian typhus epidemic of 1915 with 70 percent mortality).

35. Harden, "Typhus, Epidemic"; Topley, Smith, and Easman, *Principles of Bacteriology, Virology and Immunology*, 674–76; Holtom and Leedom, "Rickettsial Infections," 647.

36. Hardy, "Typhus in the Victorian City," 406; Harden, "Typhus, Epidemic."

37. Zinsser, *Rats, Lice, & History*; Weiss, "Role of Rickettsioses"; Prinzing, *Epidemics Resulting from Wars*, chaps. 4–5; Kiple and Ornelas, "Typhus, Ships and Soldiers"; Snyder, "Typhus Fever," 1060.

38. Weiss, "Role of Rickettsioses," 3.

39. Brocklesby, *Oeconomical and Medical Observations*, 200.

40. Hoffman, *Dissertation on Endemial Diseases*, 260–61.

41. Pringle MS, 9:329, Knox to Pringle, Mar. 1771.

42. Munro, *Account of the Diseases*, 8, 91.

43. Pringle, *Diseases of the Army*, 291–92, viii.

44. Ibid., 26–27.

45. See, e.g., Lettsom, *Reflections*; Day, *Removing Confined and Infectious Air.*

46. See, e.g., Pringle, *Hospital and Jayl-Fevers*, 4; Howard, *State of the Prisons*, 13; Lind, *Health of Seamen*, 82–83; Priestley, *Experiments and Observations*; Arbuthnot, *Effects of Air.*

47. Arbuthnot, *Effects of Air*, 17. More generally, see Riley, *Eighteenth-Century Campaign.*

48. Munro, *Account of the Diseases*, 355–56.

49. Brocklesby, *Oeconomical and Medical Observations*, 27.

50. Munro, *Account of the Diseases*, 356–71; see also CP, MFR 708 (reel 101), OB Ex2/147: 19 May–15 July, mostly likely for 1761.

51. See, e.g., BL, Add. MS 28855, fol. 31: Standing Orders for the Campaign 1760–61, 2 Feb. 1761.

52. See, e.g., CP, MFR 707 (reel 100), OB 8/3: Paderborn, 8 Apr. 1761.

53. Munro, *Observations on Diseases*, 389; on malingerers, see, e.g., CP, MFR 707 (reel 100), OB 9/82: Orderly Book, 9 Dec. 1761.

54. CP, MFR 707 (reel 100), OB 9/31: Orderly Book, Wilhelmsdahl, 29 Sept. 1761.

55. Bland, *Military Discipline*, 191.

56. Kopperman, "Medical Services in the British Army," 443–47.

57. On medical practice in eighteenth-century Britain, see Bynum and Porter, *William Hunter*; Lane, *Health, Healing and Disease in England*; Jewson, "Medical Knowledge and the Patronage System"; Porter and Porter, *Patient's Progress*; Digby, *Making a Medical Living*; Loudon, *Medical Care and the General Practitioner.*

58. Heberden, "Richard Brocklesby"; Herrick, "Donald Monro."

59. Lawrence, *Charitable Knowledge*, 263.

60. Hanway, *Account*, dedication page.

61. Lawrence, *Charitable Knowledge*, 224, 189.

62. Munro, *Letters and Essays*, preface; Munro, *Account of the Diseases*, 71, 77.

63. BL, Add. MS 6861, fol. 187: Pringle to Mitchell, Ghent, 31 Jan. 1743.

64. BL, Add. MS 6861, fol. 187: Pringle to Mitchell, Ghent, 31 Jan. 1743.

65. See, e.g., CP, MFR 701 (reel 94), box 67/X:32:8: Orders, 24 May 1758; Brocklesby, *Oeconomical and Medical Observations*, 96.

66. Munro, *Account of the Diseases*, 378, 273.

67. Brocklesby, *Oeconomical and Medical Observations*, 136, 309.

68. On hospitals in general during this period, see Berry, "Patronage, Funding and the Hospital Patient"; Fissell, *Patients, Power and the Poor*; Lawrence, *Charitable Knowledge*; Risse, *Hospital Life in Enlightenment Scotland*; Porter and Granshaw, *Hospital in History*, esp. Porter, "Gift Relation"; Bynum "Physicians, Hospitals and Career Structures"; Lane, *Health, Healing and Disease in England*, chap. 5; Woodward,

British Voluntary Hospital System; for a European context to hospital medicine, see Keel, "Politics of Health"; Keel, *L'avènement de la medicine clinique*.

69. Fissell, *Patients, Power, and the Poor*, 148.

70. Lawrence, *Charitable Knowledge*.

71. Munro, for example, indiscriminately mixed civilian and military hospital cases in his publications. Here I follow Ulrich Tröhler's excellent and innovative analysis. My focus on an earlier period, however, leads me to see the use of quantitative data as compatible with mainstream medicine, whereas Tröhler identifies it as a challenge to traditional medical authority by the later eighteenth century. See Tröhler, *"To Improve the Evidence of Medicine."*

72. Heberden, "Richard Brocklesby"; Herrick, "Donald Monro."

73. On the development of military medical expertise during the later eighteenth and early nineteenth centuries, see Kelly, *War and Militarization*.

74. BL, Add. MS 73554, fol. 18: Barrington to Granby, 2 Jan. 1761.

75. Little, "Supply of the Combined Army," 300–301.

76. Cantlie, *History of the Army Medical Department*, vol. 1, chap. 5; Fortescue, *History of the British Army*, vol. 2, bks. 8–10, on Continental campaigns; Savory, *His Britannic Majesty's Army in Germany*, 306–8.

77. Cook, "Practical Medicine and the British Armed Forces"; von Arni, *Hospital Care and the British Standing Army*; Kopperman, "Medical Services in the British Army"; Kelly, *War and Militarization*: Hudson, *British Military and Naval Medicine*; Harrison, *Medicine in an Age of Commerce and Empire*.

78. See, e.g., Cantlie, *History of the Army Medical Department*, vol. 1, chap. 7. Kopperman details and praises military medicine during this period, but criticizes political officials for involving themselves with military medical departments only to save money. Kopperman, "Medical Services in the British Army," 448–50, 452, 455.

79. TNA, WO 4/63, pp. 69–70: Barrington to Granby, 9 Jan. 1761.

80. BL, Add. MS 73554, fol. 22: Wintringham and Burlton to Barrington, 23 Jan. 1761.

81. BL, Add. MS 73554, fol. 22: Wintringham and Burlton to Barrington, 23 Jan. 1761.

82. BL, Add. MS 73554, fol. 22: Wintringham and Burlton to Barrington, 23 Jan. 1761.

83. BL, Add. MS 73554, fol. 20: Barrington to Granby, 10 Feb. 1761.

84. A Cabinet meeting discussing the ill management of hospitals in Germany (at which Barrington would have been present) did not take place until the middle of May 1761: entry for 11 May 1761, in Cavendish, *Devonshire Diary*, 97.

85. Barrington to Drummond, 21 Nov. 1766, in Barrington, *Secretary at War*, 334–35; see also BL, Add. MS 73632, regarding Barrington on ending the selling of surgeon posts during the 1770s.

86. Barrington to Newcastle, Feb. 1761, in Barrington, *Secretary at War*, 202.

87. Ibid.

88. Guy, *Oeconomy and Discipline*, 22–23.

89. *New Manual Exercise*, verso of title page.

90. For civilian matters, see, e.g., Gray, *Considerations on Several Proposals*, 15. On parliamentary requests, see below.

91. Guy, *Oeconomy and Discipline*, esp. chap. 3.

92. Houlding, *Fit for Service*, 293–317.

93. Parliament, *State of His Majesty's Land Forces and Marines*, 61; Guy notes the political context of this inquiry and resulting report; see Guy, *Oeconomy and Discipline*, 78–79.

94. NAM, 1968–06–41, Howard to Townshend, 2 June 1761; see also 23 May 1761.

95. Marshall, "Health of the British soldier in America," appendix A.1.

96. Returns are likely German in origin; Peter H. Wilson notes that German forces used returns since the period of the Thirty Years' War (1618–48). Peter H. Wilson, personal communication, 12 Sept. 2013.

97. Fournier, Projet Montcalm, and Société généologique canadienne-française, *Combattre pour la France*.

98. Hospital records, for example, track admissions, and thus one case of illness would be counted multiple times. Curtin has also noted this trend for nineteenth-century French military records; see Curtin's notes regarding the statistical tables, in *Death by Migration*, 162–65.

99. BL, Add. MS 32918, fol. 60: Peirson to Newcastle, Uslar, 25 Jan. 1761.

100. TNA, WO 1/5, fol. 133: Amherst to Barrington, 18 Oct. 1760.

101. TNA, WO 34/55, fol. 246: Albemarle to Amherst, 19 Oct. 1762.

102. See, e.g., BL, Add. MS 73730, no. 35/1: Council of War, 28 Feb. 1759; ibid., no. 38/53: Brooke to Barrington, 23 March 1759.

103. Brewer, *Sinews of Power*, 181–89; Innes, *Inferior Politics*, chap. 4; Buck, "People Who Counted"; Hoppit, "Political Arithmetic in Eighteenth-Century England." On the development of quantitative methodology more broadly, see Poovey, *History of the Modern Fact*; Hacking, *Taming of Chance*, chaps. 3–4; Porter, *Trust in Numbers*; Tröhler," *To Improve the Evidence of Medicine*."

104. Brewer, *Sinews of Power*, 183–84.

105. Cited in Hoppit, "Political Arithmetic," 517.

106. 8 February 1757, in Parliament, *Journals of the House of Commons*, 27:687.

107. Parliament, *Parliamentary Register*, 2 Dec. 1777, 10:56; for the duke's requests, see, e.g., ibid., 10:57–88, 66, 136–37.

108. Parliament, *Parliamentary Register*, 26 Jan. 1778, 10:137.

109. Blane, *Diseases Incident to Seamen*, vi.

110. For the use of military data in the nineteenth century, see Curtin, *Death by Migration*.

111. Tröhler, "*To Improve the Evidence of Medicine*"; on structures of medical recording in this period, see Hess and Mendelsohn, "Case and Series"; Delbourgo and Müller-Wille, "Introduction: Listmania."

112. Brewer, *Sinews of Power*, 187. See also Stewart and Jacob, *Practical Matter*; Mokyr, *Gifts of Athena*; Gascoigne, *Science in the Service of Empire*.

113. Mokyr, *Gifts of Athena*; Jacob, *Scientific Culture and the Making of the Industrial West*.

114. Innes, *Inferior Politics*, 112. See also Porter, "Statistics and the Career of Public Reason."

115. Hoppit, "Political Arithmetic," 528, on medical "arithmetic" or statistics; see also Rusnock, *Vital Accounts*; Innes, *Inferior Politics*, chap. 4.

116. England, Wales, and Scotland had a population of roughly 7.5 million in 1750, whereas France's population was close to 22 million. At the same time, Britain's population was more urban and increasing faster than that of France: see Grigg, *Population Growth*, chaps. 13 (England) and 14 (France). Given that population figures were a state secret in eighteenth-century France, and that exact numbers were a matter of debate, contemporaries would not have known these figures, although it was accepted that France's population greatly exceeded that of Britain.

117. Brown, *Estimate of Manners*, 181–82.

118. Ibid., 187–89, 213–20.

119. Rusnock, *Vital Accounts*, 181.

120. See Glass, *Numbering the People*, on debates over methods of enumeration; and Riley, *Population Thought*, on the conceptual framework surrounding the growth of population-related political arithmetic.

121. Bellers, *Improvement of Physick*.

122. Munro, *Account of the Diseases*, ix.

123. Cited in Andrew, *Philanthropy and Police*, 99. See also chapter 6 below.

124. Pietsch, "Urchins for the Sea."

125. Hanway, *Account*, 17, 18.

126. Ibid., 44–45.

127. Baugh, "Maritime Strength and Atlantic Commerce"; Gould, *Persistence of Empire*, chap. 2.

128. Baugh, "Great Britain's 'Blue-Water' Policy," 41.

129. For more on Britain's foreign policy and public opinion, see Peters, *Pitt and Popularity*; Wilson, *Sense of the People*, chap. 3; Harris, *Politics and the Nation*; Black, *America or Europe?*; Black, *Continental Commitment*; Birke et al., *England and Hanover*; Pares, "American versus Continental Warfare." For a convincing revision of the history of Britain's Continental policy during the eighteenth century, see Simms, *Three Victories*.

130. [Mauduit], *Considerations*, 67–68; on the popularity and influence of Mauduit's pamphlet, see Black, *Continental Commitment*, 5; Simms, *Three Victories*, 469–70.

131. *Letter from a British Officer*, 28–31.

132. See, e.g., *Anecdotes Relative to Our Affairs*, 183.

133. [Mauduit], *Occasional Thoughts*, 23–24.

134. *Annual Register . . . of the Year 1760*, 51.

135. BL, Add. MS 32917, fol. 273: Newcastle to Granby, 13 Jan. 1761.

136. BL, Add. MS 32918, fol. 234: Memoranda, 3 Feb. 1761. Simms notes that, by the beginning of 1761, "supporters of the German war were now under constant assault." Simms, *Three Victories*, 471.

137. BL, Add. MS 32922, fols. 292–93: Memorandum, 1 May 1761; also in BL, Add. MS 73655, fols. 84–85.

138. See BL, Add. MS 73654, for detailed correspondence.

139. See, e.g., BL, Add. MS 32923, fol. 218: Newcastle to Mansfield, 22 May 1761.

140. Little, "Supply of the Combined Army," chap. 1; Middleton, *Bells of Victory*, chaps. 7–8, refers to the Commissariat and its problems.

141. Middleton, *Bells of Victory*, 181; see also BL, Add. MS 32923, fol. 183: Newcastle to Kinnoul, 19 May 1761.

142. BL, Add. MS 32923, fol. 302: Newcastle to Ferdinand, [30 May 1761].

143. Historians of the eighteenth-century British press have tended to focus on its relative freedom, with few details on the extent of censorship or control. On the English press in the eighteenth century, see Barker, *Newspapers, Politics and English Society*, chap. 4, on the relationship between politicians and the press; Barker, "England, 1760–1815"; Black, *English Press*, chap. 6, on press control; on the press and politics in an earlier period of warfare, see Harris, *Patriot Press*; on the London press during the war, see Peters, *Pitt and Popularity*, introduction.

144. On public controversy regarding Byng and the ministry, see Rogers, *Whigs and Cities*, chap. 3; and Wilson, *Sense of the People*, chap. 3. For details regarding Byng and Minorca, see Tunstall, *Admiral Byng*; Pope, *Mr. Byng*; Baugh, *Global Seven Years War*, 182–95. For more on Byng and the recording of sickness, see chapter 4 below.

145. *Case of British Troops*, 63, 60–61.

146. Rodney to Grenville, 13 Oct. 1757, in Temple, *Grenville Papers*, 1:214.

147. Sir John Irwine to Sackville, 21 Sept. 1758, in RCHM, *Stopford-Sackville*, 1:297, 296; see also 297–301, on failed landing.

148. Jenkinson to Grenville, 20 June 1761, in Temple, *Grenville Papers*, 1:370.

149. Clark, *Iron Kingdom*, chap. 7 and specifically 210, on population loss; see also note 16 in the conclusion below.

CHAPTER FOUR

1. Harding, *Amphibious Warfare*, esp. chap. 4; for logistical details of amphibious operations during the Seven Years' War, see Syrett, *Shipping and Military Power*, esp. 88–100; and Syrett, "Methodology of British Amphibious Operations." Even Continental campaigns relied on naval power: Baugh, "War on Water"; see also Baugh, *Global Seven Years War*, 8–9, 13, 623–25. For a useful overview of logistics, particularly victualing, for the Royal Navy throughout its operations during the war, see Buchet, *Marine, économie et société*.

2. Rodger, "Le scorbut dans la Royal Navy"; Rodger, "Medicine and Science."

3. Rodger, "La mobilisation navale."

4. Middleton, "Naval Administration," 122–23; Rodger, "La mobilisation navale"; Rodger, *Command of the Ocean*, chap. 19.

5. Gradish, *Manning of the British Navy*, chaps. 2 and 3; Baugh, *British Naval Administration*, chap. 4.

6. Rodger, *Wooden World*, 104–5, observes that this is one reason why rates of death and disease are difficult to calculate.

7. See, e.g., Byng's questioning of Vice Admiral West, Captains Everitt, Cornwall, and Young, and Lieutenant Bishop, in TNA, ADM 7/946.

8. For details of these operations, see also Gradish, *Manning of the British Navy*, chaps. 2, 5, and 6; on operations during 1759, see Marcus, *Quiberon Bay*.

9. TNA, ADM 1/89, Hawke to Admiralty, 7 Sept. 1755, and accompanying returns, 29 Sept. 1755 and 30 Sept. 1755.

10. See, e.g., TNA, ADM 1/89, Hawke to Admiralty, 9 Oct. 1755.

11. In the eighteenth-century, the term "scurvy" covered a broad swath of diseases and was often used in a general sense, in part because observation showed that one disease often gave rise to another, and in part because "scurvy" itself was not easily distinguished from other diseases. See, e.g., "The Water-Dock," in *Medical Museum*, 1:50, 51. Modern medical science too finds few diseases that are caused by only one factor and that are not notably influenced by an individual's constitution or exacerbated by environmental circumstances. As a consequence, distinguishing between scurvy and other prevalent ship diseases such as fevers in this period is difficult, as well as ahistorical, not only because contemporary observers claimed these diseases were not always distinct, but also because remedies for scurvy and fever were often the same. With miasma and putrefaction considered the root causes of ill health, prevention and cure came in the form of fresh air, ventilation, fumigation, and a diet of fresh provisions supplemented with acidic foodstuffs (in eighteenth-century terminology); all were recommended to maintain the health of seamen against both fevers and scurvy.

12. Lind, *Scurvy* (1753), 272–73.

13. Although most naval historians, such as Rodger, recognize this reading of Lind, there is still a surprising number who credit Lind with observing that lemon juice or fresh vegetables alone would cure scurvy. See, e.g., Harvie, *Limeys*.

14. Lind, *Scurvy* (1753), 53.

15. Ibid., 64, 65, 67; see an excellent summary of Lind's theory of scurvy in McBride, "British Treatment of the Sea Scurvy, 1753–75," 160–63; more broadly, see Carpenter, *Scurvy*; for a reinterpretation of scurvy and sea voyages, see Chaplin, "Earthsickness."

16. Rodger estimates that ships usually spent more than half their time in port during this period. See Rodger, *Wooden World*, 37–39, and Appendix II: "Sea Time," 352.

17. Duffy, "Western Squadron," 67–68.

18. See, e.g., chapter 1 above; Lind, *Scurvy* (1772), 232.

19. The sending out of fresh provisions to ships in the Western Squadron was briefly attempted in 1705: Duffy, "Western Squadron," 69.

20. Ryan, "Blockade of Brest," 176, 181.

21. Ibid., 181; Duffy, "Western Squadron." On the squadron's role in the Seven Years' War, see Middleton, "British Naval Strategy"; Rodger, *Command of the Ocean*, chap. 18; Baugh, *Global Seven Years War*, chap. 12, on the 1759 British victory at sea and its implications for France.

22. Rodger, *Command of the Ocean*, 279–81.

23. Ryan, "Blockade of Brest," 182; Lind, *Health of Seamen*, 18–19; Baugh notes that "sea warfare's greatest challenge concerned health." Baugh, *Global Seven Years War*, 9.

24. Harding, *Seapower and Naval Warfare*, 216.

25. On the limitations of British naval capability during the first part of the eighteenth century, see Harding, *Emergence of Britain's Global Naval Supremacy*; Harding, "Royal Navy in the West Indies." On the Royal Navy's ability to deal with the logistical demands of the Seven Years' War, see Buchet, *Marine, économie et société*.

26. Ryan, "Blockade of Brest," 183–85. On limitations of the Royal Navy during

the American War of Independence more generally, see Gwyn, "Royal Navy in North America"; Baugh, "Why Did Britain Lose Command of the Sea"; Mackesy, *War for America.*

27. TNA, ADM 1/90, fol. 528: Anson to Admiralty, 27 May 1758, and turn-over-note of 30 May 1758; TNA, ADM 1/90, fols. 581–82: Anson to Admiralty, 27 Aug. 1758, and turn-over-note of 1 Sept. 1758.

28. Rodger, *Command of the Ocean,* 281.

29. Ibid., 308; see also Rodger, *Wooden World,* 102.

30. Baugh, *Seven Years War,* 430 n. 12.

31. Gradish, *Manning of the British Navy,* chap. 6.

32. Rodger, "Le scorbut dans la Royal Navy," 455–62; Rodger, "Medicine and Science," 341. On the efficiency of naval administration more broadly, see Baugh, *British Naval Administration*; Middleton, "Naval Administration," 109–27; Middleton, "Pitt, Anson and the Admiralty." For an even broader perspective, see Glete, *Navies and Nations.*

33. NMM, ADM/L/P/3, entries of Lieutenant Richard Phillip Shewan, Sept. and Oct. 1759, regarding the cutting up of bullocks and sheep; regarding live cattle sent out, see Rodger, "Victualling of the British Navy." Whether these units correspond to modern-day weights is debatable, as even sheep listed weigh at least half the weight of present-day sheep, assuming the units are the same. Weights and measurements at the time were not standardized; see Hoppit, "Reforming Britain's Weights and Measures"; livestock was also smaller in this period; see Turner, Beckett, and Afton, *Farm Production,* chap. 6. On the victualing and supply of fresh meat during the war, see Buchet, *Marine, économie et société,* chap. 8.

34. NMM, ADM/L/P/4; ADM/L/P/3.

35. TNA, ADM 2/526, fols. 332–33: Admiralty to Hawke, 5 Oct. 1759. As beer was widely regarded as an antiscorbutic, see the extensive attempts to remedy bad beer: Gradish, *Manning,* 156–57; on Admiralty efforts to remedy bad beer, see NMM, HWK/11, Aug.–Oct. 1759; HWK/14, Aug.–Oct. 1759.

36. TNA, ADM 111/49, 3 Aug. 1759. Syrett, *Shipping and Military Power,* 47–53, details the logistics of this development through the use of merchant shipping.

37. TNA, ADM 30/44, fol. 170.

38. On standard victualing procedures during this period, see Macdonald, "New Myth of Naval History"; Morris, *Foundations of British Maritime Ascendancy,* chap. 7; Buchet, *Marine, économie et société.*

39. TNA, ADM 2/526, fols. 65–66: Admiralty to Hawke, 7 Aug. 1759; ADM 2/82, fol. 257: Admiralty to Victualling Board, 2 Aug. 1759; NMM, HWK/5, Hawke to Captains, 6 Aug. 1759.

40. TNA, ADM 1/92, fol. 103: Hawke to Admiralty, 28 Aug. 1759.

41. NMM, HWK/14, Hawke to Pett, 31 Aug. 1759.

42. See, e.g., NMM, HWK/14, Hawke to Pett, 31 Aug. 1759; HWK/11, Tyrrell to Hawke, 3 Oct. 1759.

43. TNA, ADM 36/6354. I have followed Rodger, *Wooden World,* and Crewe, *Yellow Jack and the Worm,* in using muster books to establish sick rates, although there are discrepancies between these and the few existing monthly and weekly returns.

44. NMM, HWK/14, Hawke to Admiralty, 16 Dec. 1759.

45. TNA, ADM 1/92, fol. 296: Hawke to Admiralty, 7 Jan. 1760.

46. TNA, ADM 1/90, fol. 168: Boscawen to Admiralty, 24 Feb. 1760, and turn-over-note, 27 Feb. 1760; Boscawen reported sickness throughout February–May 1760. He reports "remarkable good health" among the squadron on 8 June 1760 after he had sent four ships to Plymouth containing all of the sick crew (TNA, ADM 1/90, fol. 253: Boscawen to Admiralty, 8 June 1760); see also Syrett, *Shipping and Military Power*, 52–54, on the continued use of shipments.

47. TNA, ADM 1/91, fol. 492: Keppel to Admiralty, 6 Nov. 1761; and fol. 445: 26 Sept. 1761, regarding sheep mortality.

48. TNA, ADM 1/90, fol. 255: Boscawen to Admiralty, 15 June 1760. For more on riots and provisions during the war, see Bohstedt, *Politics of Provisions*, 110.

49. Duffy, "Western Squadron," 68–69. Vegetables were widely available by the mid-eighteenth century but were not part of the common diet except when there was a shortage of grain. The general population also did not eat meat regularly because of its cost. Although Macdonald convincingly argues that naval victualing did not significantly disrupt domestic markets, it is clear that the diet supplied to the Western Squadron over 1759–60 was unusual compared with, and more expensive than, the common diet; see Macdonald, "New Myth of Naval History"; on vegetables, see Thick, "Market Gardening," esp. 508; prices: Bowden, "Agricultural Prices," esp. 43; meat and vegetables in Irish diets: Clarkson and Crawford, *Feast and Famine*, esp. 181–82. As the fresh provisions were supplied centrally, via the Victualling Board, cost would have been determined according to domestic markets. See note 38 above on standard victualing procedures.

50. NMM, HWK/15, Hawke to Admiralty, 13 Jan. 1761.

51. NMM, AGC/5/8, Hawke to Lady Kingston, 9 Feb. 1760.

52. NMM, HWK/15, Hawke to Admiralty, 11 Oct. 1760.

53. Crimmin, "Sick and Hurt," 4. On salaries, see *Court and City Kalendar*, 209.

54. Lloyd and Coulter, *Medicine and the Navy*, 3:7; Crimmin, "Sick and Hurt," 6–7.

55. James Maxwell was a physician with hospital experience, and Henry Tom a former naval ship and hospital surgeon: Gradish, *Manning of the British Navy*, 21; the quotation: Rodger, "Medicine and Science," 335.

56. NMM, ADM/F/17, Sick and Hurt to Admiralty, enclosure in 4 Jan. 1758. See also NMM, ADM/F/19, Sick and Hurt to Admiralty, enclosure in 24 Jan. 1759.

57. For instructions on its use, see NMM, ADM/F/17, Sick and Hurt to Admiralty, 3 Feb. 1758; on standardization, see NMM, ADM/F/18, Sick and Hurt to Admiralty, 12 Oct. 1758.

58. NMM, ADM/F/19, Sick and Hurt to Admiralty, 24 Feb. 1759.

59. Lind, *Health of Seamen*, viii; Gradish, *Manning of the British Navy*, 160.

60. NMM, ADL/M/2, Hawke to Young, 12 Aug. 1757; NMM, HWK/5, Hawke to Fergussone, 16 Nov. 1757; NMM, HWK/4, Hawke to Hobbs, 13 Aug.1757.

61. NMM, ADM/F/16, Sick and Hurt to Admiralty, 5 Aug. 1757.

62. NMM, ADM/F/16, Sick and Hurt to Admiralty, 5 Dec. 1757.

63. NMM, ADM/F/17, Sick and Hurt to Admiralty, 27 Mar. 1758.

64. NMM, ADM/F/19, Sick and Hurt to Admiralty, 24 May 1759.

65. NMM, ADM/F/19, Sick and Hurt to Admiralty, 11 Apr. 1759.

66. NMM, ADM/F/17, Sick and Hurt to Admiralty, 14 Apr. 1758.

67. NMM, ADM/F/21, Sick and Hurt to Admiralty, 21 July 1760.

68. NMM, ADM/F/21, Sick and Hurt to Admiralty, 22 Apr. 1761.

69. NMM, ADM/F/23, Sick and Hurt to Admiralty, 1 July 1762.

70. NMM, ADM/F/22, Sick and Hurt to Admiralty, 27 Aug. 1761.

71. NMM, ADM/E/1, fol. 258: Admiralty to Sick and Hurt, 29 April 1703. On trials in earlier periods, see also Crimmin, "Sick and Hurt," 11–12.

72. NMM, ADM/E/13, Admiralty to Sick and Hurt, 27 Sept. 1752.

73. NMM, ADM/E/9, Admiralty to Sick and Hurt, 8 Jan. 1741, 22 Apr. 1742, and 1 Oct. 1742.

74. NMM, ADM/F/11, 6 Mar. 1754, copy of Hill's responses.

75. For earlier periods and empiricism, see Shapin and Schaffer, *Leviathan and the Air-Pump*; Shapin, *Social History of Truth*; Licoppe, *La formation de la pratique scientifique*; Daston and Lunbeck, *Histories of Scientific Observation*, although these forms of empirical practice are somewhat different from the medical "trials" of the navy. See also Cook, "Practical Medicine and the British Armed Forces"; and for the eighteenth century, Maehle, *Drugs on Trial*; Hilaire-Pérez, *L'invention technique*, esp. 59–65 and 85–95.

76. Stewart, "Experimental Spaces," "experimental enthusiasm" on 165, 167, and 171; see also Stewart, *Rise of Public Science*; Stewart and Jacob, *Practical Matter*, esp. chap. 3.

77. Within the voluntary hospitals that were established throughout urban areas in Britain, discussed in chapter 3, clinical observations and clinical trials were sporadically practiced, and by the 1780s and 1790s they appear to have been common. Only in the 1770s and 1780s were they extended to groups of patients in hospital care: see Risse, *Hospital Life in Enlightenment Scotland*, esp. chap. 4 and epilogue; Lawrence, *Charitable Knowledge*; Maehle, *Drugs on Trial*. In eighteenth-century France clinical trials also appeared first at military and naval hospitals and then in civilian hospitals: Brockliss and Jones, *Medical World of Early Modern France*, chap. 11.

78. Tröhler, *"To Improve the Evidence of Medicine."*

79. On the transmission and translation of naval and military medical works, see Charters, "Colonial Disease, Translation, and Enlightenment."

80. Pluchon, *Histoire des médecins et pharmaciens*; Sardet, *L'École de chirurgie*; McClellan and Regourd, *Colonial Machine*, esp. pt. 1.

81. Baugh, *Seven Years War*, esp. 306, suggests that this was also the case for French naval administration more generally; Buchet, *Marine, économie et société*, also concludes that British naval capability, compared with France's, during the Seven Years' War owed much to financial and administrative ability; Jonathan R. Dull, *Ship of the Line*, also broadly compares French and British naval structure (e.g., 18–19). The papers of France's Ministry of the Marine contain a wide-ranging collection of medical suggestions and innovations, but archival material is not clear as to whether these were trialed or implemented: see the correspondence in ANF, MAR/G/178–179 (1749–88). It should be noted that conclusions are difficult to draw, given that none of the secondary works cited provides full-scale, detailed comparisons of French and British naval medicine.

82. Pritchard, "Le problème de l'Amérique du Nord"; for a nuanced comparison of British and French scientific activity in the eighteenth century, see Hilaire-Pérez, *L'invention technique.*

83. Rodger, *Command,* 409. See also Pritchard, "From Shipwright to Naval Constructor."

84. Higher rates of scurvy in the Royal Navy may also be explained by longer time spent at sea, given British naval dominance and its use of convoys; Baugh, *Global Seven Years War,* 10, notes, "Potentially, health was a greater problem for the Royal Navy because it was a cruising navy and a ship's time at sea could last for months, thus introducing the deficiency disease of scurvy."

85. Pritchard, *Louis XV's Navy,* 71. For more details on disease in the French Navy during the war, see Pritchard, *Louis XV's Navy,* chap. 5; Dull, *French Navy,* 80–88, 104–6.

86. Rodger, *Wooden World,* 346; also chaps. 1, 6, and the conclusion.

87. BL, Add. MS 73632, fols. 1–2: Maxwell to Barrington, 16 Mar. 1756.

88. Stevenson, *Medicine and Magnificence,* chaps. 2–3.

89. See, e.g., Schaffer, "Self-Evidence"; and notes 75–78 above.

90. BL, Add. MS 35895, fol. 326.

91. BL, Add. MS 35895, fol. 326.

CHAPTER FIVE

1. Wills, *Adventures and Sufferings,* 2.

2. Prior, "John Zephaniah Holwell"; Crawford, *Indian Medical Service,* vol. 1, chap. 11, 155–77.

3. For useful surveys of Franco-British fighting within the context of local conflict, see Bryant, "War in the Carnatic" and "War in Bengal." For a broader context, see Bayly's seminal *Indian Society and the Making of the British Empire,* esp. chap. 1.

4. Marshall, *Making and Unmaking of Empires,* 128, and more generally, chap. 4. See also Lawson, *East India Company,* esp. chap. 5; Marshall, *Problems of Empire,* chap. 1; Bowen, "Mobilising Resources for Global Warfare." For an examination of the early period of the East India Company that refines the traditional narrative of a private corporation transformed into political power, see Stern, *Company-State.*

5. Arnold, *Colonizing the Body,* 4. See also Harrison, *Medicine in an Age of Commerce and Empire*; Harrison, *Public Health in British India*; Arnold, *Science, Technology and Medicine in Colonial India*; Arnold, "India's Place in the Tropical World"; Arnold, *Imperial Medicine*; MacLeod and Lewis, *Disease, Medicine, and Empire*; Kumar, *Medicine and the Raj*; Peers, "Colonial Knowledge and the Military in India"; Pande, *Medicine, Race and Liberalism.*

6. Marshall, *East India Fortunes,* esp. chaps. 7–8; Sutherland, *East India Company,* chap. 3; Bowen, *Business of Empire*; on financial opportunities specifically during the Seven Years' War, see Marshall, *Making and Unmaking of Empires,* 131–35.

7. APAC, IOR/H/359/1, p. 196: Campbell to Board, 22 Oct. 1777.

8. APAC, IOR/H/78, fol. 131: List of Allowances to the Company's Covenant Servants in the East Indies.

9. APAC, IOR/H/359/1, pp. 199–200: Campbell to Board, 22 Oct. 1777.

10. APAC, MSS Eur/Orme OV 197, fols. 13–17: Memorial of James Ellis.

11. Consultation, 28 Dec. 1756, in Madras Record Office, *Diary and Consultation Book, Public*, 85:375–76.

12. APAC, IOR/H/359/1, p. 331: General Consultation, 3 May 1771; see also responses, ibid., pp. 327–38.

13. On the history of India as a tropical climate, see Arnold, "India's Place in the Tropical World."

14. The Bengal, Madras, and Bombay Medical Services were reformed in 1763, 1767, and 1779, respectively: Ghosh, *Armed Forces Medical Services*, 17–18.

15. Committee to Fort St. George, 13 Feb. 1756, in Madras, *Diary and Consultation, Military*, 5:84. See more on the relationship between the council and settlement hospitals in APAC, MSS Eur/G37/24 (Clive's Papers), Company's General Letter to Bengal, 3 Mar. 1757, point 85.

16. Hill, *Bengal*, 2:415n.

17. Summary of a list of inhabitants, &c., who bore arms at late siege of Calcutta, 1 July 1756, in Hill, *Bengal*, 2:415; Crawford, *Indian Medical Services*, 1:163.

18. Richard Owen Cambridge, *Account of the War*, xvi, boldly claims that Indian princes "have an implicit faith in the abilities of the European physicians." For the use of company medical personnel by rulers, see, e.g., Crawford, *Indian Medical Services*, vol. 1, chaps. 2 and 5, who explodes the claim that Gabriel Boughton's medical services established the East India Company's trading rights in Bengal. Regardless of its mythical origin, the story demonstrates the expected priorities of medical practitioners.

19. Cambridge, *Account of the War*, xvi; see also APAC, MSS Eur/Orme India XIII, fol. 74: St. George to Caillaud, 9 Feb. 1757; Crawford, *Indian Medical Services*, 1:165.

20. APAC, MSS Eur/Orme India V, fol. 51: Committee at Fulta, 22 Dec. 1756. On Forth's activities, see, e.g., APAC, MSS Eur/Orme India V, fol. 56: Fort William Committee, 16 Jan. 1757.

21. Sutton, *Lords of the East*, 79. Clive, for example, suggested that his friend and fellow military officer T. Hancock be made a company surgeon in 1759, in order to help Hancock recover financially: APAC, MSS Eur/G37/26, Jan. 1759.

22. On diversity within medical occupations more broadly during the early modern period, see Pelling, *Common Lot*, pt. 3, esp. chap. 10.

23. Court of Directors to Fort William, 1 Apr. 1760, in National Archives of India and East India Company, *Fort William-India House Correspondence*, 3:20.

24. See, e.g., APAC, IOR/H/359/1, pp. 228–29: Proceedings of the Board of Inspection, 18 Nov. 1772; Chakrabarti, "Medicine amidst War and Commerce"; and more broadly, Chakrabarti, *Materials and Medicine*. For the view that the Indian environment—cultural and physical—encouraged its own kind of medical practice, see Harrison, "Disease and Medicine in British India," as well as Harrison, *Medicine in the Age of Commerce and Empire*.

25. Ives, *Voyage*, 43–45.

26. Crawford, *Indian Medical Services*, 1:175; Sutherland, *East India Company*, 67–69.

27. Holwell, *Manner of Inoculating*, 20.

28. Ibid., 21.

29. Ibid.

30. See esp. Harrison, *Climates and Constitutions*, chaps. 1–2; Harrison, "Medicine and Orientalism"; Pearson, "Thin Edge of the Wedge."

31. Anderson, "Immunities of Empire"; Harrison, "'The Tender Frame of Man'"; Arnold, *Colonizing the Body*; Arnold, *Imperial Medicine*.

32. Harrison, *Climates and Constitutions*, 3. The most comprehensive summary of this shift is Harrison, *Climates and Constitutions*; see also Harrison, "'The Tender Frame of Man'"; Anderson, "Immunities of Empire"; Hannaford, *Race*; Hudson, "From 'Nation' to 'Race'."

33. On the penetration of state structures, see Marshall, *Making and Unmaking of Empire*, 134–36.

34. See, e.g., APAC, MSS Eur/G37/24, Company to Fort William, 8 Mar. 1758, point 26.

35. Marshall, *East-India Fortunes*, 14; Wickremesekera, *"Best Black Troops,"* 86–95.

36. London to Fort William, 23 January 1759, in National Archives of India and East India Company, *Fort William-India House Correspondence*, 2:123; evidence of Captain Brereton and Eyre Coote in Hill, *Bengal*, 3:320–23.

37. Marshall, *East Indian Fortunes*, 14–15.

38. Hill, *Bengal*, 3:15–16.

39. Cadell, *History of the Bombay Army*, 43–45.

40. Clive and Becher to Directors, 31 Dec. 1758, in National Archives of India and East India Company, *Fort William-India House Correspondence*, 2:358.

41. Directors to Fort William, 15 Feb. 1760, in National Archives of India and East India Company, *Fort William-India House Correspondence*, 3:35.

42. Steppler, "Common Soldier"; Guy, *Oeconomy and Discipline*; Conway, *War, State, and Society*, chap. 3.

43. Marshall, *East India Fortunes*, 16–18.

44. Spavens, *Seaman's Narrative*, 68.

45. *Soldier's Journal*, 182.

46. Brumwell, "Home from the Wars"; see also Hudson, "Disabled Veterans."

47. Lloyd and Coulter, *Medicine and the Navy*, vol. 3, chaps. 14–17; see also Hudson, "Internal Influences."

48. Sutton, *Lords of the East*, 81.

49. Directors to Fort William, 31 Dec. 1760, in National Archives of India and East India Company, *Fort William-India House Correspondence*, 3:61.

50. Bryant, "Indigenous Mercenaries," 15–16.

51. Lincoln, *Representing the Royal Navy*, 88.

52. NMM, ADM F/23, Sick and Wounded Commissioners to Admiralty, 24 Dec. 1762.

53. See the order of 1742 in Ghosh, *Armed Forces Medical Services*, 17.

54. Sutton, *Lords of the East*, 94; see the rest of the book for details on British East India Company ships.

55. Ives, *Voyage*, 5. For a recent revised interpretation of scurvy and long voyages during this period, see Chaplin, "Earthsickness."

56. APAC, IOR/L/MAR/B/602 J, log of the *Marlborough*.

57. Sutton, *Lords of the East*, 94–105.

58. See chapter 1 above for detailed discussion on scurvy and food storage, and chapter 4 above on food storage and scurvy on board ships. On dried fruit, see Lind, *Health of Seamen*, 31–32; Çağlarirmak, "Sun-Dried Grapes and Sultanas."

59. Lind, *Scurvy* (1772), 45, 231.

60. Holwell, *Manner of Inoculating*, 9, 10–11. Calling this fever the "genuine putrid nervous fever of Bengall," Holwell further emphasized the significance of location and climate for the disease (13).

61. Lind, *Hot Climates*, 79.

62. Ibid., 87–88.

63. J. M., "Of the Inflammation of the Liver," in *Medical Museum*, 67:611–12.

64. Ibid., 611; Harrison, "Disease and Medicine in British India"; Harrison, "Racial Pathologies." Such liver disease was most probably a hepatitis virus, spread by infected water or blood.

65. Lind, *Hot Climates*, 80.

66. Wilson, "Fevers"; Bynum, "Cullen and the Study of Fevers in Britain"; Dunn, "Malaria"; Packer, *Making of a Tropical Disease*, esp. chap. 1.

67. Bynum, "Cullen and the Study of Fevers in Britain."

68. Harrison, "Disease and Medicine in British India," esp. 92–94; Wilson, "Fevers," 398–99; Worboys, "Tropical Diseases."

69. Pringle MS, 3:1, Stevenson to Pringle, 10 Dec. 1754.

70. See, e.g., Lind, *Hot Climates*, 90–91n.

71. Worboys, "Emergence of Tropical Medicine," 75.

72. Lind, *Hot Climates*, 80–87.

73. Defoe, *Robinson Crusoe*, 1:68.

74. Clark, *Observations*, 57.

75. Ibid., 59.

76. Lind, *Hot Climates*, 76.

77. APAC, MSS Eur/Orme India VI, fol. 85.

78. Lind, *Hot Climates*, 8.

79. See, e.g., APAC, MSS Eur/Orme India XII, fol. 57: Caillaud to Fort William, 4 Aug. 1760.

80. APAC, MSS Eur/Orme India VI, fol. 87: "Plans of the means to conquer Bengal."

81. APAC, IOR/L/MIL/10/130, pts. II–IV; rate is for legible year 1767.

82. Harrison, "Disease and Medicine in British India," 90–92.

83. See, e.g., Campbell to Pigot, 23 July 1756, in Madras Record Office, *Diary and Consultation, Military*, 5:249, on the state of troops upon news of approaching war with the French.

84. Narrative by Governor Drake in Hill, *Bengal*, 2:160.

85. For the long-term significance of this event, see Barrow, "Many Meanings"; Teltscher, "'Fearful Name of the Black Hole'"; Travers, "Death and the Nabob." Some

contemporaries were aware of what had really happened and how it was being represented; see BL, Add. MS 15956, fol. 313: Vice Admiral George Pocock to George Anson, 8 Oct. 1756. Locking up prisoners in black holes, and thereby suffocating them, appears to have been a common trope about despotic leaders during this period; see similar accusations leveled against the French in Stokes, *Narrative of the Many Unparallel'd Hardships*, 14–16.

86. Jean Law, in Hill, *Bengal*, 3:171.

87. Fort William to Directors, 31 Jan. 1757, in Hill, *Bengal*, 2:192.

88. Kilpatrick to Fort St. George, in Madras Record Office, *Diary and Consultation, Military*, 5:5, Aug. 1756, 294.

89. APAC, IOR/L/MAR/B/322 C, *Delaware* log, 13 Aug. 1756.

90. See, e.g., Watson to Consultation, 26 Aug. 1756, in Madras Record Office, *Diary and Consultation, Public*, 85:257.

91. Consultation, 26 Aug. 1756, in Madras Record Office, *Diary and Consultation, Public*, 85:258.

92. APAC, IOR/L/MAR/B/322 C, *Delaware* log; see list of officers and seamen and list of dead.

93. APAC, MSS Eur/Orme India VII, fol. 123: "Journal of the Expedition to Bengal . . . kept by one of Colonel Clive's Family," 8 Dec. 1756.

94. Watson to Clevland, 31 Jan. 1757, in Hill, *Bengal*, 2:200; Clive to Fort St. George, 28 Jan. 1757, ibid., 2:275.

95. APAC, MSS Eur/Orme India X, fol. 6: Clive to Watson, 20 Jan. 1757.

96. Watson to Clive, 21 Jan. 1757, in Hill, *Bengal*, 2:127.

97. APAC, MSS Eur/Orme India XIII, fols. 94–95: Weekly return of the Honble Company's Troops near Barnagore in Camp January 21st 1757.

98. APAC, MSS Eur/Orme India X, fol. 9: Clive to Secret Committee, 1 Feb. 1757.

99. APAC, MSS Eur/Orme India IV, fol. 135: Account of the Siege at Calcutta by R.O.

100. APAC, MSS Eur/F190/1, fols. 1–19: Journal in India of Sir Eyre Coote.

101. APAC, MSS Eur/F190/1, fol. 15: 14 Mar. 1757.

102. See, e.g., APAC, MSS Eur/Orme India V, fols. 63–64: Watson to Fort William, 14 Feb. 1757.

103. Clive to Nawab, 30 Mar. 1757 and 4 May 1757, in Hill, *Bengal*, 2:305 and 376.

104. Clive to Fort St. George, 30 Mar. 1757, in Hill, *Bengal*, 2:308.

105. APAC, MSS Eur/Orme India XIII, fols. 96–97: Return of 10 Apr. 1757; ibid., fol. 98: Return of 12 June 1757.

106. Military historians generally credit British naval gunnery for British success; see, e.g., Lenman, "Transition to European Military Ascendancy," 114–20; for general surveys of events, see Fortescue, *History of the British Army*, vol. 2, bk. 8, and 425–30; Gupta, *Sirajuddaullah*; Marshall, *Bengal*, chap. 3; and note 3 above.

107. APAC, MSS Eur/F190/1, fols. 87–88: Coote to Clive, 25 July 1757.

108. APAC, MSS Eur/F/190, fols. 75–76: Council of War, 4 Aug. 1757.

109. APAC, MSS Eur/G37/5, Coote to Clive, 17 Aug. 1757.

110. APAC, MSS Eur/G37/5, Coote to Clive, 10 Sept. 1757.

111. APAC, MSS Eur/Orme India X, fol. 94: Clive to Directors, 22 Aug. 1757.

112. APAC, MSS Eur/Orme India X, fol. 93: Clive to Secret Committee, 22 Aug. 1757.

113. APAC, MSS Eur/Orme India X, fol. 68: Clive to Drake, 17 Oct. 1757.

114. APAC, MSS Eur/G37/23, Grant to Clive, 2 Oct. 1757.

115. Fort William to Secret Committee, 13 Jan. 1758, in National Archives of India and East India Company, *Fort William-India House Correspondence*, 2:299. See also, e.g., APAC, MSS Eur/Orme India V, fol. 118: Bengal to Pigot, 15 Nov. 1757; APAC, MSS Eur/Orme India X, fol. 61: Clive to Fort William, 6 Dec. 1757.

116. See, e.g., APAC, MSS Eur/Orme India XIII, fols. 103–5: Returns, 16 Dec. 1757.

117. Black, *Warfare in the Eighteenth Century*, 173–74.

118. APAC, MSS Eur/Orme India V, fols. 43–44: Wynch to Pigot, 6 Sept. 1758.

119. APAC, MSS Eur/F/128/82, fol. 11: Journal of the Siege of Fort St. David, 16 May 1758.

120. APAC, MSS Eur/Orme India V, fol. 42: Wynch to Pigot, 21 May 1758. On his surrender, Wynch listed 500 in the garrison, including Topasses but not sepoys. See APAC, MSS Eur/F/128/82, fol. 21: 2 June 1758.

121. APAC, MSS Eur/F/128/82, fol. 21: 2 June 1758; see also ibid., fol. 18: 28 May 1758.

122. APAC, MSS Eur/Orme India XIII, fols. 111–12: 16 Oct. 1758.

123. APAC, MSS Eur/G37/26, as reported in Brereton to Clive, 3 June 1759.

124. APAC, MSS Eur/F190/2, fol. 253: Coote Journal, 5 Aug. 1760.

125. APAC, MSS Eur/F190/2, fols. 272–73: Coote Journal, 23 Sept. 1760; Orme, *History of the Military Transactions*, 2:656.

126. APAC, MSS Eur/F190/2, fol. 273: Coote Journal, 26 Sept. 1760.

127. Ward to Hastings, 5 Feb. 1761, in RHMC, *Hastings*, 3:141.

128. APAC, MSS Eur/F190/2, fol. 294: Coote Journal, 28 Nov. 1760.

129. APAC, MSS Eur/F190/2, fol. 307: Coote Journal, 11 Jan. 1761.

130. Orme, *History*, 2:714.

131. APAC, MSS Eur/Orme India VI, fol. 14: Turner to Maskelyne, 5 Feb. 1761.

132. On military medicine and conventions of war, see Charters, "Military Medicine and the Ethics of War."

133. APAC, MSS Eur/F190/3, fols. 378–79: Lally to Coote, 15 May 1760.

134. Knott, "Sensibility and the American War for Independence"; Van Buskirk, *Generous Enemies*, chap. 3; Conway, "British Perceptions of the Americans." Attitudes toward the French also varied according to social rank, with the aristocracy adopting French styles while the lower classes considered the French as effeminate enemies; see Colley, *Britons*; Newman, *Rise of English Nationalism*; Williams, "Encountering the French"; see also chapter 6 below, on the range of British attitudes toward the French.

135. Kennedy, *Magic Mountains*.

136. APAC, MSS Eur/F128/27, Mrs. Clive to Carnac, 6 May 1761.

137. Ives, *Voyage*, 90.

138. APAC, MSS Eur/G37/26, Johnson to Latham, 7 Feb. 1759.

139. Harrison, *Medicine in an Age of Commerce and Empire*, pt. 3; Johnson, *Influence of Tropical Climates*; Trotter, *Nervous Temperament*; Trotter, *Medicina Nautica*. On sensibility and nervous disease during this period, see Beatty, *Nervous Disease*.

140. Bryant, "Military Imperative."

141. See, e.g., Marshall, *Bengal*; Travers, *Ideology and Empire*, esp. chap. 1; Wilson, *Domination of Strangers*; Bowen, *Business of Empire*. For broader approaches, including historiographical debates, see Marshall, *Eighteenth Century in Indian History*; Alavi, *Eighteenth Century in India*; Bayly, *Indian Society*, esp. chap. 1.

142. Robert Clive's wife, for example, criticized how English ladies no longer followed native customs: APAC, MSS Eur/F128/27, Lady Clive to Carnac, 5 May 1763.

143. Wickremesekera, *"Best Black Troops,"* chaps. 3–4.

144. Bryant, "Indigenous Mercenaries," 5–6.

145. APAC, MSS Eur/Orme India XIII, fol. 98, 103–4.

146. APAC, MSS Eur/Orme India XIII; see returns in ff. 103–4, 115–20; Wickremesekera, *"Best Black Troops,"* makes no mention of disease concerns in sepoy recruitment.

147. For example, the incidence of sickle-cell traits ranges from 9 to 22 percent in India, higher than the European average: Awasthy et al., "Sickle Cell Disease"; Dhumne and Jawade, "Sickle Cell Anemia and Morbidity"; Shukla and Solanki, "Sickle-Cell Trait in Central India"; more generally on sickle cell and its global prevalence, see Rees, Williams, and Gladwin, "Sickle-Cell Disease."

148. APAC, MSS Eur/Orme India X, fol. 93: Clive to Secret Committee, 22 Aug. 1757.

149. Bryant, "Indigenous Mercenaries"; Wickremesekera, *"Best Black Troops,"* chaps. 2–3.

150. For a convincing critique of the role of discipline in explaining British military superiority in India, see Peers, "Revolution, Evolution, or Devolution."

151. APAC, MSS Eur/Orme India XIII, fol. 166: "Of the Military Establishment," Col. Caillaud.

CHAPTER SIX

1. Smith, *Wealth of Nations*, 2:920.

2. See, e.g., Wilson, *Sense of the People*; Harris, *Politics and the Nation*; Rogers, *Whigs and Cities*; Colley, *Britons*.

3. Le Goff, "L'impact des prises," 106.

4. *Public Ledger or the Daily Register of Commerce and Intelligence*, 29 April 1760.

5. A notable exception is Morieux, "Patriotisme humanitaire," who details the role of public opinion and prisoner treatment during the Napoleonic Wars.

6. On prisoners during the first part of the eighteenth century, see Morieux, "French Prisoners of War"; Le Goff, "L'impact des prises"; Le Goff, "Problèmes de recrutement"; Scouller, *Armies of Queen Anne*, 310–21;. Wilson, "Prisoners in Early Modern European Warfare." Studies on prisoners during the American War of Independence tend to focus on the role of British cruelty in fostering American identity: Cogliano, "'We all Hoisted the American Flag'"; Cohen, *Yankee Sailors in British Gaols*; Burrows, *Forgotten Patriots*. For contrasting interpretations, see Ranlet, "Prison Ships of the American Revolution"; Anderson, "Treatment of Prisoners of War"; Bowman, *Captive Americans*. Even where narratives of British cruelty are not emphasized,

the nature of imprisonment during the American war is further decontextualized by the tendency to start histories on prisoner treatment with the American war: see, e.g., Springer, *America's Captives*. On Napoleonic prisoners in Britain, see Crimmin, "French Prisoners of War on Parole"; Gavin Daly, "Napoleon's Lost Legions," considers eighteenth-century precedents, but suggests that prisoners were always regularly exchanged through cartels, thus concluding that long detention during the Napoleonic Wars was unusual. For a revisionist account of American Civil War prisoner-of-war welfare, see Marvel, *Andersonville*.

7. On the treatment of prisoners after the 1715 Jacobite rebellion, see Sankey, *Jacobite Prisoners*; on Native American captivity, see Steele, "Surrendering Rites"; studies on the American War of Independence could also fall under the category of rebellion; on the significance of prisoner conventions as a part of war negotiations, see Anderson, "Treatment of Prisoners of War."

8. Walpole, *Memoirs*, 3:58.

9. Stott, *Hannah More*, 11. I am indebted to Hannah Smith for this reference.

10. Le Goff, "L'impact des prises," 106.

11. See NMM, ADM/F/15, Account of Prisoners of War in Great Britain and Ireland, 22 June 1757; NMM, ADM/F/17, Account of Prisoners of War in England, 1 May 1758; NMM, ADM/F/21, Sick and Hurt to Admiralty, 28 May 1761.

12. *London Chronicle*, 1 July 1760; this somewhat exaggerated number was also reprinted in the *Public Ledger*, 2 July 1760.

13. Le Goff, "L'impact des prises," 106.

14. On captures up to 1707, see PA, HL/PO/JO/10/3/196aj2, An Acct of ye Exch. of Engl & Fren Prison of Warr, Dec. 1707 [OS]; on exchanges from 1707, see Le Goff, "L'impact des prises," 106; for conventions on prisoners during the War of Spanish Succession, see Scouller, *Armies of Queen Anne*, 310–21.

15. Anderson, "Impact on the Fleet"; Wilson, "Prisoners in Early Modern European Warfare."

16. See, e.g., Savory, "Convention of Écluse"; on negotiations, see TNA, SP 87/41, fols. 10–13. On European practices during the war, see Anklam, *"Battre l'estrade,"* 231–36.

17. On the composition of French prisoners held in Britain, see Le Goff, "L'impact des prises," 110–14; on difficulties regarding exchanges, see Le Goff, "Problèmes de recrutement"; on exchange conventions, see Anderson, "Treatment of Prisoners of War."

18. Whereas accommodation and food rations were provided by the host, clothing and other "additionals" were to be obtained through extra money, as was the case for provisioning on campaign.

19. Walpole, *Memoirs*, 3:38.

20. See, e.g., NMM, ADM/F/20, 22 Sept. 1759, letter from doctor and agent James Walker at Edinburgh; TNA, T 1/381/1, 25 Nov. 1757, memorial of James Dickson, surgeon and agent at Minorca; TNA, ADM 106/1017/146, 27 Aug. 1745, Henry Thomson, agent and surgeon formerly at Woolwich and now at Kinsale; *Authentick List* lists John Marsh as surgeon and agent for prisoners of war.

21. Devon Heritage Centre, Z 19/46/4, Account Book of Matthew Limbrey, 1756–1762.

22. Norris, "Administration of Prisoners of War," esp. chap. 3. On merchants and contractors in general, see Bannerman, *Merchants and the Military*; Conway, *War, State, and Society*, esp. chap. 4.

23. See, e.g., NMM, ADM/F/16, Joseph Knight to Sick and Hurt, 22 July 1757, enclosed in Sick and Hurt to Admiralty, 5 Aug. 1757; ADM/F/15, Sick and Hurt to Admiralty, 11 June 1757; for the French regulation, see ANF, MAR/B/4/97, fols. 184–85.

24. NMM, ADM M/387, item 31, Admiralty to Sick and Hurt, 10 May 1744.

25. In Winchester, over £1,000 was spent converting and maintaining the King's House: Derbyshire Record Office, D3155/C3386, 9 Sept. 1763.

26. Heath, *Case of the County of Devon*, 10.

27. For details of the administration of prisoners in Winchester during the war, see Charters, "Administration of War and French Prisoners," 110–14.

28. See, e.g., Bodleian Library, MS Carte 222, 24 July 1666, fols. 107–8; Plymouth and West Devon Record Office, MS 129, Plymouth Hospital Collection, folder 2, Complaint to the Admiralty.

29. Truxes, *Defying Empire*, chap. 5. For a later period, see Crimmin, "Alternative Roles."

30. On social problems caused by the prisoners, see Morieux, "French Prisoners of War"; Williams, "Encountering the French," chap. 3.

31. NMM, ADM/F/18, Sick and Hurt to Cleveland, 6 Nov. 1758.

32. TNA, ADM 106/1130, fol. 23: 31 Jan. 1763; ibid., fol. 102: 3 May 1763.

33. TNA, SP 89/43, fol. 60: John Barnaby Parker to Newcastle, 25 June 1742.

34. Sick and Hurt to Taylour, 21 Aug 1712, in Public Record Office, *Calendar of Treasury Papers*, CLI no. 20, 4:418–19.

35. *Considerations on the Exchange*, 14.

36. On the general history of laws of war, see Howard, Andreopoulos, and Shulman, *Laws of War*; Neff, *War and the Law of Nations*; Tuck, *Rights of War and Peace*; specifically on the role of noncombatants within the history of laws of war, see McKeogh, *Innocent Civilians*; Charters, Rosenhaft, and Smith, *Civilians and War in Europe*.

37. Vattel, *Law of Nations*, 2:49.

38. Ibid, 2:54–55.

39. TNA, SP 42/119, 28 Sept. 1704, fol. 297.

40. BL, Add. MS 61595, no. 2/13 April 1709, fol. 83; see also fols. 84, 86, on long confinement as itself a reason for petition.

41. PA, HL/PO/JO/10/6/62, 1985, pt. 3, February 1704, fol. 61: Extract of an Ord. to One of the Masters of the Transport Ships. This is notable, given that the historian Le Goff, "Problèmes de recrutement," 219–22, describes such a policy as part of a deliberate British strategy to weaken French naval power during the Seven Years' War.

42. Beattie, *Crime and the Courts in England*, esp. chaps. 9–10; Ignatieff, *Just Measure of Pain*.

43. *Considerations on the Exchange*, 51.

44. Sick and Hurt to Chateauneuf, 12 July 1705, in RCHM, *Manuscripts of the House of Lords*, 7:155.

45. PA, HL/PO/JO/10/6/62, fol. 137: 13 March 1704.

46. PA, HL/PO/JO/10/6/62, Copy of an order from the Comm. for Sick and Wounded

Seamen, and Exchange of Prisoners at War to their Marshall at Plymouth, Southampton, Farnham & Dover, 18 March 1703, fol. 144, on the French practice, and fol. 146, on directions to their agents. On prisoner negotiations during the 1700s, see Anderson, "Establishment of British Supremacy," 83–86.

47. TNA, SP 78/227A, fol. 97: Newcastle to Thompson, 3 April 1742.

48. TNA, SP 78/225, fol. 59: Thompson to Newcastle, 15 Feb 1741 NS.

49. 9 March 1704, in RCHM, *Manuscripts of the House of Lords*, 5:534–35.

50. "La détention dans les Iles britanniques fut surtout décisive pendant la guerre de Sept Ans," Le Goff, "L'impact des prises," 116; see also Le Goff, "Problèmes de recrutement."

51. Rodney to Grenville, 4 Dec. 1762, in Temple, *Grenville Papers*, 20.

52. Vattel was clear that prisoners could be detained for the duration of a war either so that "they may not return again to the enemy, or else for obtaining from their sovereign a just satisfaction, as the price of their liberty." Vattel, *Law of Nations*, 2:55.

53. ANF, MAR B/4/97, fol. 165: Belle-Isle to le Duc D'Aiguillon, 22 Sept. 1758.

54. ANF, MAR B/4/97, fol. 177: Nov. 1758, Mémoire sur la correspondance du Ministère de la marine avec les commissaires anglois au sujet de l'Echange des prisonniers respectifs.

55. ANF, MAR B/4/97, fol. 210: 9 Oct. 1759, from the Sick and Hurt Board.

56. Letter published 8 Oct. 1759, reprinted in *Letter from a Gentleman in Town*, 22 (quotation), 23 (Sissinghurst).

57. *Proceedings of the Committee Appointed to Manage the Contributions.*

58. See the list of "several public and private collections" in Appendix IV, in *Proceedings of the Committee Appointed to Manage the Contributions.*

59. Andrew, *Philanthropy and Police*, esp. chaps. 3 and 4.

60. *Proceedings of the Committee Appointed to Manage the Contributions*, v.

61. *Conduct of the Sovereign.*

62. *Letter from a Gentleman in Town*, 5, 10, 33.

63. Ibid., 24.

64. *Proceedings of the Committee Appointed to Manage the Contributions*, ix, i.

65. *Conduct of the Sovereign*, 3.

66. *London Chronicle*, 19–22 Jan. 1760.

67. Ibid., on Jacobites; on religious groups, see the letter signed JF, *London Chronicle*, 5–8 Jan. 1760.

68. *London Chronicle*, 19–22 Jan. 1760.

69. Letter signed JF, *London Chronicle*, 5–8 Jan. 1760.

70. *Proceedings of the Committee Appointed to Manage the Contributions*, second page of the introduction.

71. Innes, "Mixed Economy of Welfare"; Cunningham and Innes, *Charity, Philanthropy and Reform*, esp. Cunningham, introduction, and Innes, "State, Church and Voluntarism"; Andrew, *Philanthropy and Police.*

72. Letter from W. Sandys, at Cornwall, 28 Feb. 1760, in *Proceedings of the Committee Appointed to Manage the Contributions*, Appendix IV.

73. Hanway, *Account*, 9.

74. See chapter 3 above.

75. *Owen's Weekly Chronicle or Universal Journal*, 9–16 Sept. 1758; reprinted in *Lloyd's Evening Post*, 11–13 Sept. 1758.

76. [Goldsmith], *Citizen of the World*, 88.

77. Hanway, *Account*, 14n. Williams, "Encountering the French," chap. 3, identifies a growing association between humanitarianism and British identity over the course of the eighteenth century; Morieux, "Patriotisme humanitaire," sees a similar use of humanitarianism tied to discourses of patriotism and political legitimacy in both Britain and France.

78. For prisoners and public opinion during the later period, see Morieux, "Patriotisme humanitaire."

79. Le Goff, "L'impact des prises," 114.

80. Le Goff, "L'impact des prises," 114 and n. 40, finds evidence of British refusals to release numbers, and calculates French prisoner deaths during the Seven Years' War at 9,000. The refusal of the British authorities did not last: ANF MAR/F/93 has a British list of French prisoners who died in British prisons during the war, dated 1764. This appears complete, as its total of 11,147 dead is notably higher than the 9,000 that Le Goff calculates.

81. Andrews, preface to Lesuire, *Savages of Europe*, iii.

82. Lesuire, *Les sauvages de l'Europe*, 19: "Dépouiller les prisonniers, les charger de fers, les accabler d'outrages, c'est l'usage de tous les Peuples sauvages." The 1764 English translation renders it as follows: "Every savage nation has made it a law, from time immemorial, to plunder their prisoners; to load them with fetters; to heap all kinds of insults upon them." Lesuire, *Savages of Europe*, 27.

83. *London Chronicle*, 29–31 Jan. 1760, cited in Charters, "Administration of War," 97.

84. *London Chronicle*, 24–26 Jan. 1760.

85. TNA, SP 78/262, fol. 228: Hertford to Halifax, 1 Aug. 1764.

86. Grenville to Hertford, 20 July 1764, in Temple, *Grenville Papers*, 398.

87. *Gazetteer and New Daily Advertiser*, 8 Jan. 1765; Felix, "Finances, opinion publique et diplomatie."

88. TNA, SP 78/256, fols. 284, 287; SP 78/262, fols. 33, 144, 169–83, 217–34.

89. PA, HL/PO/JO/10/7/183, fol. 5010, 15 Jan. 1765.

90. See, e.g., *Annual Register . . . of the Year 1765*, 62.

91. Carvin, *Prisoners of America's Wars*, 43.

92. Regarding the American War of Independence, Anderson long ago recognized that "the evidence in British archives has never been systematically consulted nor the 'tales' of the survivors subjected to critical examination." Anderson, "Treatment of Prisoners of War," 82. Marvel's *Andersonville* demonstrates how administrative and political analysis challenges traditional prisoner-of-war narratives. For examples of histories of prisoners during the American war, see note 6 above.

EPILOGUE

1. Brown, *Foul Bodies*, 189, and more generally, chap. 5. On shifts in sensibility during this period, see Langford, *Polite and Commercial People*, chap. 10; Barker-Benfield, *Culture of Sensibility*; Knott, *Sensibility and the American Revolution*.

2. Siena, "Investigating Westminster Prison Deaths." See also Ignatieff, *Just Measure of Pain*, esp. chap. 3; Beattie, *Crime and the Courts in England*, chap. 10.

3. In his study of French prisoners of war in Britain over the second half of the eighteenth century, Williams, "Encountering the French," points out that by the 1800s there was "much wider expression among the British public of concerns at the treatment of the French and the conditions in which they were held" (164), but notes that this "does not prove that this marked a new development in the standards of treatment of prisoners of war by the British" (184). See also note 2 above.

4. On the pattern of American captivity narratives, see Doyle, *Voices from Captivity*. On shifts in narratives, particularly the role of personal passions during this period, see Eustace, *Passion Is the Gale*; Knott, *Sensibility and the American Revolution*.

5. Morgan, "John Howard."

6. On numbers serving during the war, see Conway, *War, State, and Society*, chap. 3.

7. Foucault, *Discipline and Punish*, 144.

8. Cooper and Stoler, "Between Metropole and Colony."

9. Rublack, "Fluxes"; Koschorke, "Physiological Self-Regulation"; Vigarello, *Concepts of Cleanliness*; Brown, *Foul Bodies*; Kupperman, "Presentment of Civility"; Churchill, "Bodily Differences"; these views also underlie the debate outlined by Gerbi, *Dispute of the New World*. For a related shift in conceptual understandings of bodies, see Cody, *Birthing the Nation*.

10. Wahrman, *Making of the Modern Self*; Wheeler, *Complexion of Race*; for a focus on this period, see also Boulukos, *Grateful Slave*. This development maps onto the British shift toward imperial and global issues during the second half of the eighteenth century, as shown by Wilson, *Sense of the People*; Wilson, *Island Race*; Gould, *Persistence of Empire*; Bickham, *Savages within the Empire*.

11. Churchill, "Efficient, Efficacious and Humane Responses."

12. Hunt, *Inventing Human Rights*. This connection is made by Norberg, "Bodies in European and American Historiography." On the relationship between bodies and eighteenth-century identity, see also Cody, *Birthing the Nation*.

13. Historians have noted that not only is expertise about knowledge, but it also provides "tools for governing and a way to legitimize political powers." Laurence Dumoulin, cited in Rabier, "Introduction," 8.

14. On the development of the British medical profession during this period, see Jewson, "Medical Knowledge and the Patronage System"; Loudoun, *Medical Care and the General Practitioner*; Porter and Porter, *Patient's Progress*; Lawrence, *Charitable Knowledge*; Digby, *Making a Medical Living*; Brown, *Performing Medicine*. On medicine and medical practice during this period, see French and Wear, *British Medicine*; Tröhler, *"To Improve the Evidence of Medicine"*; Harrison, *Medicine in an Age of Commerce and Empire*; Cunningham and French, *Medical Enlightenment*; Riley, *Eighteenth-Century Campaign*.

15. Clark, *Iron Kingdom*, 210. Estimates of civilian deaths and deplacement vary; Speelman, "Conclusion," 525–26, suggests a 6 percent decline in Prussia, alongside a 15 percent decline in Austria.

16. The term "laboratories of modernity" is usually applied to later periods of sci-

ence and imperialism; influenced by Foucauldian studies, these works examine how disciplinary processes associated with modernity were first developed and applied in the colonies, often making use of scientific or medical practice. The phrase has, thereby, often become shorthand for modern Western imperialism. See, e.g., Dixon, *Prosthetic Gods*, chap. 1; Rabinow, *French Modern*; and Stoler, *Race and the Education of Desire*, 15–16, for explicit discussion.

17. An example of this view is Wootton, *Bad Medicine*.

18. One of the few detailed comparative studies of military strategy in this period that includes attention to disease is Buchet, *La lutte pour l'espace caraïbe*, in which he points out the difficulty of providing conclusive comparative evaluations of how disease was treated or prevented.

19. Fournier, Projet Montcalm, and Société généalogique canadienne-française, *Combattre pour la France*; Fournier, "Les soldats de la guerre."

20. Hacking, *Taming of Chance*, chaps. 3–4; Porter, *Trust in Numbers*; Tröhler, *"To Improve the Evidence of Medicine."*

21. On British concerns, see Harris, *Politics and the Nation*, esp. chap. 3.

22. Massie, "John Manners, Marquess of Granby."

23. Walpole, *Memoirs*, 4:161 and 162.

24. On the nature of early modern philanthropy, including its relationship to the state and utilitarianism, see Cavallo, "Motivations of Benefactors"; Ben-Amos, *Culture of Giving*; Slack, *Reformation to Improvement*; also see note 71 in chapter 6 above.

25. Glete, *Navies and Nations*, 1:16.

26. On layering and the growth of mass, see Conway, *War, State, and Society*; Cookson, *British Armed Nation*.

BIBLIOGRAPHY

MANUSCRIPTS AND ARCHIVAL SOURCES

Archives Nationales de la France, Paris

MAR/B/4. Marine. Campaigns.

MAR/F/93. Marine. Captures: Prisoners of War.

MAR/G/178–179. Marine. Diverse Documents Relating to Medicine, Naval Hospitals, Naval Hygiene, 1728–1831.

Asia, Pacific and Africa Collections, British Library, London

India Office Records

H/78. Papers concerning Civilians in India; Revenue Matters.

H/359. Orders concerning New Offices, Salaries, Remission of Debts, and Civil Establishments in Bengal.

L/MAR/B. Ships' Journals, Logs and Related Records.

L/MIL/10/130. Bengal Army Muster Rolls and Casualty Returns.

Private Papers (European Manuscripts)

MSS Eur/E1. A Narrative of the Several Transactions of the French in Their Attack on Fort St. George.

MSS Eur/F128. Sutton Court Collection (Papers of Brig-Gen John Carnac and Sir Henry Strachey).

MSS Eur/F190. Sir Eyre Coote Papers.

MSS Eur/G37. The Clive Collection.

MSS Eur/Orme India. Robert Orme Papers.

MSS Eur/Orme OV. Robert Orme Manuscripts.

Bodleian Library, University of Oxford, Oxford

MS Carte 222. Carte Papers.

British Library, London

Add. MS 6861. Miscellaneous Correspondence of Andrew Mitchell.

Add. MSS 15956–15957. Private and Official Correspondence of Admiral George, Lord Anson, 1744–1762.

Add. MSS 17493–17495. Register of Private Letters of John Calcraft, Army Agent.

Add. MSS 28551, 28552, 28855. Journal of the Campaigns of the Anglo-Hanoverian Army in Germany.

Add. MSS 32867–32870, 32893–32895, 32910–32928. Official Correspondence of Thomas Pelham Holles, Duke of Newcastle.

Add. MSS 35357, 35895. Hardwick Papers (Philip Yorke, 1st Earl of Hardwick with His Son Sir Joseph Yorke).

Add. MSS 44070–44071, 44076. Loudoun Papers (General Correspondence of Lord Loudoun).

Add. MS 61595. Blenheim Papers (Correspondence and Papers Relating to English, French, and Spanish Prisoners of War).

Add. MSS 73554–73732. Correspondence and Papers of William Wildman Barrington, 2nd Viscount Barrington.

CP, MFR 608–710. The Cumberland Papers, Microform Research Collections (The Papers of William Augustus, Duke of Cumberland, from the Royal Archives, Windsor Castle).

Egerton MS 3440, 3442–3444. Holderness Papers (Correspondence and Papers of Robert Darcy, 4th Earl of Holdernesse, Secretary of State).

Derbyshire Record Office, Matlock, UK

D3155. Wilmot-Horton of Osmaston and Catton Papers.

Devon Heritage Centre, Exeter, UK

Z 19/46/4. Account Book of Matthew Limbrey, 1756–1762.

Hampshire Record Office, Winchester, UK

W/B. Winchester City Administrative Records.

Huntington Library, San Marino, CA

James Abercromby Papers, 1674–1787.

LO. Loudoun Papers. North America, 1682–1780.

Kent History and Library Centre, Maidstone, UK

U1350/Z9A. Amherst Papers. James Millar, Memoirs of an Invalid.

The National Archives, London

ADM 1. Admiralty, and Ministry of Defence, Navy Department. Correspondence and Papers.
ADM 2. Admiralty Board. Out-Letters.
ADM 7/946. Charles Fearne's Copy of John Byng's Court Martial.
ADM 30/44. Navy Board Pay Office. Precedents and Exceptions for Pursers' Accounts.
ADM 36. Admiralty. Royal Navy Ships' Musters.
ADM 50. Admiralty. Admirals' Journals.
ADM 106. Navy Board. Records.
ADM 111/49. Admiralty, Victualling Department. Board and Committees. Minutes.
CO 5. Board of Trade and Secretaries of State. America and West Indies.
CO 117. Secretary of State. Havana.
CO 166. Secretary of State for the Colonies and War and Colonial Department. Martinique.
SP 42. Secretaries of State. State Papers Naval.
SP 78. Secretaries of State. State Papers Foreign, France.
SP 87. Secretary of State. State Papers Foreign, Military Expeditions.
SP 89. Secretaries of State. State Papers Foreign, Portugal.
T 1/381. Treasury. Treasury Board Papers and In-Letters.
WO 1. Secretary-at-War. In-Letters.
WO 24. War Office. Papers concerning Establishments.
WO 34. War Office. Baron Jeffrey Amherst, Commander in Chief, Papers.

National Archives of Canada, Ottawa

MG18-L4, A-1826. Amherst Collection.
MG18-N21. George and Adam Williamson Papers.
MG23-K34. Frederick Mackenzie Collection.

National Army Museum, London

1968–06–41. Papers of George, 4th Viscount and 1st Marquess Townshend.
1968–07–191. Abstracts of General Orders in Germany, compiled by Thomas Downing.
1975–10–61. Maryon Wilson Papers.
1982–08–195. Journal of Edmund Cox.
1986–12–38. Major-General Alexander Dury Papers.
2001–05–105. Henry Hulton, Letterbook.

National Library of Scotland, Edinburgh

MS 3850. Papers of David Dundas.

National Maritime Museum, London

ADL/M. Royal Navy, Administration and Law.
ADM/D. Admiralty Board. In-Letters from the Victualling Board.
ADM/E. Sick and Hurt Board. In-Letters and Orders.
ADM/F. Admiralty Board. In-Letters from the Sick and Hurt Board.
ADM/G. Victualling Office Orders.
ADM/L/P. Navy Board. Lieutenants' Logs.
ADM/M. Sick and Hurt Board. In-Letters and Orders relating to Prisoners of War.
AGC/5. Hawke, Personal Letters.
HWK. Hawke Papers.

Parliamentary Archives, London

HL/PO/JO/10. House of Lords Papers.

Plymouth and West Devon Record Office, Plymouth, UK

MS 129. Plymouth Hospital Collection.

Royal College of Physicians of Edinburgh, Edinburgh

Pringle MS. John Pringle's Medical Annotations, 10 vols.

Service Historique de la Défense, Vincennes, France

A1 3624. Marine and Colonies, 1761–62.

Suffolk Record Office, Ipswich, UK

HA 67/969. Albemarle Papers.

PRINTED PRIMARY SOURCES

Books, Pamphlets, and Printed Collections

Amherst, Jeffery. *The Journal of Jeffery Amherst.* Edited by John Clarence Webster. Toronto: Ryerson Press, 1931.

Anecdotes Relative to Our Affairs in Germany: Carried back to the Debarking of the First British Regiment at Emden; and brought down to the present Critical Time:

in a series of letters to a noble lord in -shire. Authenticated by a Gentleman on the Spot, and confirmed by his Correspondents here, during the War. London, 1762.

Arbuthnot, John. *An Essay Concerning the Effects of Air on Human Bodies. By John Arbuthnot, M. D. Fellow of the Royal Colleges of Physicians of London and Edinburgh, and of the Royal Society.* London, 1733.

Archivo Nacional de Cuba. *Nuevos papeles sobre la toma de la Habana por los ingleses en 1762.* Edited by Rafael Nieto y Cortadellas. Havana: Archivo Nacional de Cuba, 1951.

———. *Papeles sobre la toma de la Habana por los ingleses en 1762.* Edited by Guillermo de Blanck. Havana: Archivo Nacional de Cuba, 1948.

An Authentic Journal of the Siege of the Havana. By an Officer. To which is prefixed, a Plan of the Siege of the Havana. London, 1762.

An Authentick List of all Names of the Members of the Society (or Corporation) of Great Yarmouth. London, 1762.

Barrington, William Wildman. *An Eighteenth-Century Secretary at War: The Papers of William, Viscount Barrington.* Edited by Tony Hayter. London: Bodley Head for the Army Records Society, 1988.

Bellers, John. *An Essay towards the Improvement of Physick. In Twelve Proposals. By which the Lives of many Thousands of the Rich, as well as of the Poor, may be Saved Yearly.* London, 1714.

Bland, Humphrey. *A Treatise of Military Discipline; in which is Laid Down and Explained the Duty of the Officer and Soldier, Thro' the Several Branches of the Service.* 5th ed. London, 1743.

Blane, Gilbert. *Observations on the Diseases Incident to Seamen.* London, 1785.

Boswell, James. *Boswell's London Journal, 1762–3.* Edited by Frederick A. Pottle. Harmondsworth, UK: Penguin Books, 1966.

Brocklesby, Richard. *Oeconomical and Medical Observations, in Two Parts. From the Year 1758 to the Year 1763, inclusive. Tending to the Improvement of Military Hospitals, and to the Cure of Camp Diseases, Incident to Soldiers.* London, 1764.

Brown, John. *An Estimate of the Manners and Principles of the Times. By the Author of Essays on the Characteristics, &c.* 5th ed. London, 1757.

Buchanan, John. *"Regimental Practice" by John Buchanan, M.D.: An Eighteenth-Century Medical Diary and Manual.* Edited by Paul E. Kopperman. Farnham, UK: Ashgate, 2012.

Burke, William. *An Examination of the Commercial Principles of the Late Negotiation between Great Britain and France in MDCCLXI. In which the System of that Negotiation with Regard to our Colonies and Commerce is Considered.* London, 1762.

———. *Remarks on the Letter Addressed to Two Great Men. In a Letter to the Author of that Piece.* London, 1760.

Cambridge, Richard Owen. *An Account of the War in India, between the English and French, on the Coast of Coromandel, from the Year 1750 to the Year 1760.* London, 1761.

Cartier, Jaqcues. *The Voyages of Jacques Cartier.* Edited by Ramsay Cook, originally translated and edited by Henry Percival Biggar. London: University of Toronto Press, 1993.

The Case of the British Troops serving in Germany. Humbly submitted to the Consideration of Parliament. London, 1761.

Cavendish, William. *The Devonshire Diary: Memoranda on State of Affairs, 1759–1762*. Edited by Peter D. Brown and Karl W. Schweizer. London: Offices of the Royal Historical Society, 1982.

Clark, John. *Observations on the Diseases in Long Voyages to Hot Countries, and Particularly on Those which Prevail in the East Indies*. London, 1773.

The Conduct of the Sovereign, Burgesses, and Principal Inhabitants of Belfast Vindicated; And, the Necessity and Propriety thereof, to procure Relief to the French Prisoners confin'd at Belfast fully shewn. [Belfast?] 1761.

Considerations on the Exchange of Seamen, Prisoners of War. London, 1758.

Cumberland, William Augustus, Prince, Duke of, et al. *Military Affairs in North America, 1748–1765: Selected Documents from the Cumberland Papers in Windsor Castle*. Edited by Stanley McCrory Pargellis. London: D. Appleton-Century, 1936.

Day, Thomas. *Some Considerations on the Different Ways of Removing Confined and Infectious Air; and the Means Adopted, with Remarks on the Contagion, in Maidstone Gaol*. Maidstone, UK, 1784.

Defoe, Daniel. *The Life and Adventures of Robinson Crusoe, of York, Mariner: Who Lived Eight and Twenty Years all Alone in an Uninhabited Island, on the Coast of America, near the Mouth of the Great River Oroonoque. With an Account of his Travels Round Three Parts of the Globe. Written by Himself*. 3 vols. London, 1790.

A Detection of the False Reasons and Facts, Contained in the Five Letters, (entitled, Reasons for Keeping Guadeloupe at a Peace, preferable to Canada; From a Gentleman in Guadaloupe to his Friend in London.) In which the Advantages of both Conquests are Fairly and Impartially Stated and Compared. By a Member of Parliament. London, 1761.

Durant, George. "George Durant's Journal of the Expedition to Martinique and Guadeloupe, October 1758-May 1759." In *Military Miscellany*, vol. 1, *Manuscripts from the Seven Years War, the First and Second Sikh Wars and the First World War*, edited by Alan J. Guy, 1–68. Stroud, UK: Sutton Publishing, 1996.

Fraser, Malcolm. "The Capture of Quebec: A Manuscript Journal relating to the Operations before Quebec from 8th May, 1759, to 17th May, 1760." Edited by R. O. Alexander. *Journal of the Society for Army Historical Research* 18 (1939): 135–68.

Gale, Benjamin. "Historical Memoirs, Relating to the Practice of Inoculation for the Small Pox, in the British American Provinces, Particularly in New England." *Philosophical Transactions* (1683–1775) 55 (1765): 193–204.

Gardiner, Richard. *An Account of the Expedition to the West Indies, Against Martinico, with the Reduction of Guadelupe, and other Leeward Islands*. 3rd ed. Birmingham, 1761.

[Goldsmith, Oliver.] *The Citizen of the World; or Letters from a Chinese Philosopher, Residing in London, to his Friends in the East*. London, 1762.

Gray, Charles. *Considerations on Several Proposals, lately made, for the better Maintenance of the Poor*. London, 1751.

Hadden, James Murray. *Hadden's Journal and Orderly Books: A Journal Kept in Canada and upon Burgoyne's Campaign in 1776 and 1777: Also Orders kept by Him and issued by Sir Guy Carleton, Lieut., General John Burgoyne, and Philips, in 1776, 1777 and 1778*. Edited by Horatio Rogers. Albany: J. Munsell, 1884.

Hanway, Jonas. *An Account of the Society for the Encouragement of the British Troops, in Germany and North America: with the Motives and the Making a Present to those Troops, also to the Widows and Orphans of such of them as have died in Defence of their Country, particularly at the Battles of Thonhausen, Quebec, &c.* London, 1760.

Heath, Benjamin. *The Case of the County of Devon: with Respect to the Consequences of the New Excise Duty on Cyder and Perry: Published by the Direction of the Committee appointed at a General Meeting of that County to Superintend the Application for the Repeal of that Duty*. London, 1763.

Hill, Samuel Charles, ed. *Bengal in 1756–1757: A Selection of Papers dealing with the Affairs of the British in Bengal during the Reign of Siraj-ud-Daula*. 3 vols. New York: AMS Press, 1905.

Hillary, William. *Observations on the Changes of the Air and the Concomitant Epidemical Diseases, in the Island of Barbadoes. To which is added a Treatise on the Putrid Bilious Fever, commonly called the Yellow Fever*. London, 1759.

Hoffman, Frederick. *A Dissertation on Endemial Diseases; or, Those Disorders which Arise from Particular Climates, Situations, and Methods of Living*. London, 1746.

Holden, David. *Journal Kept by Sergeant David Holden of Groton, Mass, During the Latter Part of the French and Indian War: February 20–November 29, 1760*. Edited by Samuel A. Green. Cambridge, MA: J. Wilson, University Press, 1889.

Holwell, John Zephaniah. *An Account of the Manner of Inoculating for the Small Pox in the East Indies. With some Observations on the Practice and Mode of Treating that Disease in those Parts*. London, 1767.

Howard, John. *The State of the Prisons in England and Wales, with Preliminary Observations, and an Account of some Foreign Prisons*. Warrington, UK, 1777.

Ives, Edward. *A Voyage from England to India, in the Year MDCCLIV, and an Historical Narrative of the Operations of the Squadron and Army in India, under the command of Vice-Admiral Watson and Colonel Clive, in the years 1755, 1756, 1757*. London, 1773.

Jenks, Samuel. *Diary of Captain Samuel Jenks, during the French and Indian War, 1760*. Cambridge, MA: J. Wilson, 1890.

Johnson, James. *The Influence of Tropical Climates more especially the Climate of India on European Constitutions: The Principal Effects and Diseases thereby induced, their Prevention or Removal, and the Means of Preserving Health in Hot Climates: Rendered Obvious to Europeans of every Capacity*. London: J. Callow, 1815.

"Journal of a Naval Surgeon, 1758–1763." In *Naval Yarns: Letters and Anecdotes; comprising Accounts of Sea Fights and Wrecks, Actions with Pirates and Privateers, &c., from 1616 to 1831*, edited by W. H. Long, 68–77. London: Gibbings and Col, 1899.

Knowles, Charles. *An Account of the Expedition to Carthagena, with Explanatory Notes and Observations*. London, 1743.

Knox, John. *An Historical Journal of the Campaigns in North America for the Years 1757, 1758, 1759, and 1760*. Edited by Arthur G. Doughty. 3 vols. Toronto: The Champlain Society, 1914.

Lacoursière, Jacques, and Hélène Quimper, eds. *Québec ville assiégée 1759–1760: D'après les acteurs et les témoins*. Quebec City: Septentrion, 2009.

Lesuire, Robert Martin. *Les sauvages de l'Europe*. 2nd ed. Berlin, 1762.

———. *Savages of Europe. From the French*. Translated and with a preface by James Pettit Andrews. London, 1764.

A Letter from a British Officer now in Germany: Containing Many Interesting Particulars Relative to the Considerations: Humbly recommended to the Perusal of the Legislature, and of every Free-Born Briton. London, 1761.

A Letter from a Gentleman in Town to his Friend in the Country, concerning the Cloathing of the French Prisoners now in the Castle of Edinburgh. Edinburgh, 1759.

Lettsom, John Coakley. *Reflections on the General Treatment and Cure of Fevers*. London, 1772.

Lind, James. *An Essay on Diseases Incidental to Europeans in Hot Climates*. London, 1768.

———. *An Essay on the Most Effectual Means of Preserving the Health of Seamen, in the Royal Navy*. 3rd ed. London, 1774.

———. *A Treatise of the Scurvy, in Three Parts*. 1st ed. Edinburgh, 1753.

———. *A Treatise on the Scurvy, in Three Parts*. 3rd ed. London, 1772.

Madras Record Office. *Diary and Consultation Book, Military Department*. Records of Fort St. George. 5 vols. Madras: Superintendent, Govt. Press, 1910–13.

———. *Diary and Consultation Book, Public Department*. Records of Fort St. George. 90 vols. Madras: Superintendent, Govt. Press, 1910–53.

Mante, Thomas. *The History of the Late War in North-America, and the Islands of the West-Indies, Including the Campaigns of MDCCLXIII and MDCCLXIV Against His Majesty's Indian Enemies*. London, 1772.

[Mauduit, Israel]. *Considerations on the Present German War*. London, 1760.

———. *Occasional Thoughts on the Present German War. By the Author of Considerations on the Same Subject*. 4th ed. London, 1762.

Mead, Richard. *The Medical Works of Richard Mead*. 2 vols. Edinburgh, 1763.

Montcalm de Saint-Véran, Louis-Joseph, Marquis de. *Journal du Marquis de Montcalm durant ses campagnes en Canada de 1756 à 1759*. Edited by H. R. Casgrain. Quebec City: L. J. Demers & frère, 1895.

Munro, Donald. *An Account of the Diseases which were most frequent in the British Military Hospitals in Germany, from January 1761 to the Return of the Troops to England in March 1763. To which is added, an Essay on the Means of Preserving the Health of Soldiers, and conducting Military Hospitals*. London, 1764.

———. *Letters and Essays on the Small-Pox and Inoculation, the Measles, the Dry Belly-Ache, the Yellow, and Remitting, and Intermitting Fevers of the West Indies . . . by different practitioners*. London, 1778.

National Archives of India and East India Company. *Fort William-India House Correspondence, and Other Contemporary Papers Relating Thereto*. 21 vols. Delhi: Published for the National Archives of India by the Manager of Publications, Government of India, 1949–85.

———. *Fort William-India House Correspondence, and Other Contemporary Papers Relating Thereto*. Vol. 2 (Public Series), 1757–1759, edited by H. N. Sinha. Delhi:

Published for the National Archives of India by the Manager of Publications, Government of India, 1957.

———. *Fort William-India House Correspondence, and Other Contemporary Papers Relating Thereto.* Vol. 3 (Public Series), 1760–63, edited by R. R. Sethi. Delhi: Published for the National Archives of India by the Manager of Publications, Government of India, 1960.

New Manual Exercise as Performed by His Majesty's Dragoons, Foot-guards, Foot, Artillery, Marines, and by the Militia. To which is added Two Copper Plates, and the New Forms of Encampments for Dragoons and Foot. 2nd ed. London, 1758.

New York State. *Documents Relative to the Colonial History of the State of New York, procured by J. R. Brodhead.* Edited by E. B. O'Callaghan. 15 vols. Albany: Weed, Parsons, 1856–87.

Orme, Robert. *A History of the Military Transactions of the British Nation in Indostan.* 2nd ed. 2 vols. London, 1775–78.

Oughton, James Adolphus. *—By Dint of Labour and Perseverance—: A Journal Recording Two Months in Northern Germany kept by Lieutenant-Colonel James Adolphus Oughton, commanding 1st Battalion 37th Regiment of Foot, 1758.* Edited by Stephen Wood. London: Society for Army Historical Research, 1997.

Parliament. *Journals of the House of Commons.* 1688–1834. Vol. 27, 31 May 1754–15 November 1757. London: H.S.M.O., 1803.

———. *The Parliamentary Register; or, History of the Proceedings and Debates of the House of Commons . . . of the fourteenth Parliament of Great Britain.* 17 vols. London, 1775–80.

———. *Report from the Committee, appointed to consider the State of His Majesty's Land Forces and Marines.* London, 1746.

Pitt, William, Earl of Chatham. *Correspondence of William Pitt when Secretary of State, with Colonial Governors and Military and Naval Commissioners in America.* Edited by Gertrude Stein Kimball. 2 vols. New York: Kraus Reprint, 1969.

Prado, Juan. "El diario de Juan de Prado." In *Cinco diarios del sitio de La Habana,* edited by Amalia A. Rodriguez, 65–120. Havana: Dep. de col. cubana, 1963.

Priestley, John. *Experiments and Observations on Different Kinds of Air.* London, 1774.

Pringle, John. *Observations on the Diseases of the Army.* 5th ed. London, 1765.

———. *Observations on the Nature and Cure of Hospital and Jayl-Fevers.* London, 1750.

Proceedings of the Committee Appointed to Manage the Contributions begun at London Dec XVII MDCCLVIII for Cloathing French Prisoners of War. London, [1760].

Public Record Office. *Calendar of Treasury Papers: Preserved in Her Majesty's Public Record Office,* vol. 4: 1708–1714. Edited by Joseph Redington. London: H.M.S.O., 1879.

RCHM. *The Manuscripts of His Grace the Duke of Rutland, G.C.B., preserved at Belvoir Castle.* 4 vols. London: H.M.S.O, 1888–1905.

———. *The Manuscripts of the House of Lords.* Vol. 5: *1702–1704.* Vol. 7: *1706–1708.* London: H.M.S.O., 1887–1977.

———. *Report on the Manuscripts of the Late Reginald Rawdon Hastings, Esq., of the Manor House, Ashby de la Zouche.* 4 vols. London: H.M.S.O., 1928–47.

———. *Report on the Manuscripts of Mrs. Stopford-Sackville, of Drayton House, Northamptonshire.* 2 vols. London: H.M.S.O., 1904–10.

Rogers, Robert. *Reminiscences of the French War; containing Rogers' Expeditions. To which is added an Account of the Life and Military Services of Maj. Gen. John Stark.* Edited by Caleb Stark. Concord, NH: Luther Roby, 1831.

Rush, Benjamin. *An Account of the Bilious Remitting Yellow Fever, as It Appeared in the City of Philadelphia, in the Year 1793.* Philadelphia, 1794.

Shebbeare, John. *A Letter to the People of England, on Foreign Subsidies, Subsidiary Armies, and their Consequences to this Nation.* 2nd ed. London, 1755.

Smith, Adam. *An Inquiry into the Nature and Causes of the Wealth of Nations.* Edited by R. H. Campbell and A. S. Skinner. 2 vols. 1976. Reprint, Indianapolis: Liberty Classics, 1981.

A Soldier's Journal, Containing a Particular Description of the Several Descents on the Coast of France last War, with an Entertaining Account of the Islands of Guadeloupe, Dominique, &c. And also for the Isles of Wight and Jersey. To which are Annexed, Observations on the Present State of the Army of Great Britain. London, 1770.

Spavens, William. *The Seaman's Narrative; Containing an Account of a Great Variety of Such Incidents as the Author met with in the Sea Service.* London, 1796.

St. Paul, Horace. *1757: The Defence of Prague: The Journal of Horace St Paul from 7th May to 28th June including the Campaign of Marshal Daun.* Translated and edited by Neil Cogswell. Guisborough, UK: Gralene Books, 1998.

Stokes, Samuel. *An Narrative of the Many Unparallel'd Hardships, and Cruel Sufferings, while in France; of the Crew of the Terrible Privateer, commanded by Captain William Death.* [London, 1757?].

Temple, Richard Grenville-Temple, Earl. *The Grenville Papers: Being the Correspondence of Richard, Grenville, Earl Temple, K.G., and the Right Hon: George Grenville, their Friends and Contemporaries.* Edited by William James Smith. 4 vols. London: John Murray, 1852–53.

Trotter, Thomas. *Medicina Nautica: An Essay on the Diseases of Seamen.* London, 1797–1803.

———. *A View of the Nervous Temperament.* London, 1807.

Vattel, Emer de. *The Law of Nations; or, Principles of the Law of Nature: Applied to the Conduct and Affairs of Nations and Sovereigns. By M. de Vattel. A Work Tending to Display the True Interest of Powers. Translated from the French.* 2 vols. London, 1759.

Walpole, Horace. *Memoirs of King George II.* Edited by John Brooke. 3 vols. New Haven, CT: Yale University Press, 1985.

Watts, John. *Letter Book of John Watts, Merchant and Councillor of New York.* Edited by Dorothy C. Barck. New York: Printed for the Society, 1928.

William, Thomson, D. *Memoirs of the Life and Gallant Exploits of the Old Highlander, Serjeant Donald Macleod (1688–1791).* Edited by James Gabriel Fyfe. London: Blackie & Son Limited, 1933.

Wills, William. *A Narrative of the Very Extrarodinary [sic] Adventures and Sufferings of Mr. William Wills, Late Surgeon on Board the Durrington Indiaman, Captain*

Richard Crabb, in her Late Voyage to the East-Indies, under the Convoy of Admiral Boscawen. London, 1750/1.

Periodicals

American Colonial Newspapers

Boston Evening-Post. Boston, 1760–63.
Boston Gazette. Boston, 1759–63.
New-York Gazette. New York, 1760–63.
New-York Mercury. New York, 1760–63.
Providence Gazette. Providence, 1762–63.

British Periodicals

Annual Register: A view of the History, Politicks and Literature of the Year. London, 1758–67.
The Court and City Kalendar: Or, Gentleman's Register, for the Year 1762. London, 1762.
Gazetteer and London Daily Advertiser. London, 1756–64.
Gazetteer and New Daily Advertiser. London, 1764–65.
General Evening Post. London, 1756–65.
The Gentleman's Magazine. London, 1754–65.
Lloyd's Evening Post. London, 1757–65.
London Chronicle. London, 1757–65.
London Evening Post. London, 1756–65.
London Gazette. London, 1756–65. With *London Gazette Extraordinary*. London, 1759, 1762.
The Medical Museum: or, a Repository of Cases, Experiments, Researches, and Discoveries, Collected at Home and Abroad. 3 vols. London, 1763–64.
Owen's Weekly Chronicle or Universal Journal. London, 1758–62.
Public Ledger or the Daily Register of Commerce and Intelligence. London, 1760–61.
Williamson's Liverpool Advertiser. Liverpool, 1756–63.

SECONDARY SOURCES

Published Works

Acuna-Soto, R. "Large Epidemics of Hemorrhagic Fever in Mexico, 1545–1815." *American Journal of Tropical Medical Hygiene* 62:6 (2000): 733–39.
Alavi, Seema, ed. *The Eighteenth Century in India*. New Delhi: Oxford University Press, 2002.
Anderson, Fred. *The Crucible of War: The Seven Years' War and the Fate of Empire in North America, 1754–1766*. New York: Alfred A. Knopf, 2000.

———. *A People's Army: Massachusetts Soldiers and Society in the Seven Years' War.* Chapel Hill: University of North Carolina Press, 1984.

———. *The War That Made America: A Short History of the French and Indian War.* New York: Penguin Books, 2005.

———. "Why Did Colonial New Englanders Make Bad Soldiers? Contractual Principles and Military Conduct during the Seven Years' War." *William and Mary Quarterly,* 3rd ser., 38 (July 1981): 395–417.

Anderson, M. S. *War and Society in Europe of the Old Regime, 1618–1789.* London: Fontana, 1988.

Anderson, Olive. "The Establishment of British Supremacy at Sea and the Exchange of Naval Prisoners of War." *English Historical Review* 75:294 (1960): 77–89.

———. "The Impact on the Fleet of the Disposal of Prisoners of War in Distant Waters, 1689–1783." *Mariner's Mirror* 45 (1959): 243–49.

———. "The Treatment of Prisoners of War in Britain during the American War of Independence." *Bulletin of the Institute of Historical Research* 28:77 (1955): 63–88.

Anderson, Warwick P. "Immunities of Empire: Race, Disease, and the New Tropical Medicine." *Bulletin of the History of Medicine* 70:1 (1996): 94–118.

———. "Where Is the Postcolonial History of Medicine?" *Bulletin of the History of Medicine* 72:3 (1998): 522–30.

Andrew, Donna T. *Philanthropy and Police: London Charity in the Eighteenth Century.* Princeton, NJ: Princeton University Press, 1989.

Anklam, Ewa. "*Battre l'estrade*: Military Reconnaissance in the German Theatre of War." Translated by Charlotte Massemann. In *The Seven Years' War: Global Views,* edited by Mark H. Danley and Patrick J. Speelman, 213–41. Leiden: Brill, 2012.

Archer, Christon I. "Combatting the Invisible Enemy: Health and Hospital Care in the Army of New Spain, 1760–1810." *New World* 2:1–2 (1987): 49–92.

Arnold, David. *Colonizing the Body: State Medicine and Epidemic Disease in Nineteenth-Century India.* Berkeley: University of California Press, 1993.

———, ed. *Imperial Medicine and Indigenous Societies.* Manchester: Manchester University Press, 1988.

———. "India's Place in the Tropical World, 1770–1930." *Journal of Imperial and Commonwealth History* 26:1 (1998): 1–21.

———. *Science, Technology and Medicine in Colonial India, 1760–1947.* New Cambridge History of India 3.5. Cambridge: Cambridge University Press, 2000.

———. *Warm Climates and Western Medicine: The Emergence of Tropical Medicine, 1500–1900.* Amsterdam: Rodopi, 1996.

Ash, Eric H., ed. *Expertise: Practical Knowledge and the Early Modern State.* Osiris Series. Chicago: University of Chicago Press, 2010.

———. "Expertise: Practical Knowledge and the Early Modern State." *Osiris* 25:1 (2010): 1–24.

———. *Power, Knowledge and Expertise in Elizabethan England.* Baltimore: Johns Hopkins University Press, 2004.

Awasthy, Neeraj, et al. "Sickle Cell Disease: Experience of a Tertiary Care Center in a Nonendemic Area." *Annals of Tropical Medicine and Public Health* 1 (2008): 1–4.

Bannerman, Gordon. *Merchants and the Military in Eighteenth-Century Britain: Brit-*

ish Army Contracts and Domestic Supply, 1739–1763. London: Pickering & Chatto, 2008.

Barker, Hannah. "England, 1760–1815." In *Press, Politics and the Public Sphere in Europe and North America: 1760–1820*, edited by Hannah Barker and Simon Burrows, 93–112. Cambridge: Cambridge University Press, 2002.

———. *Newspapers, Politics and English Society, 1695–1855*. Harlow: Longman, 2000.

Barker, Hannah, and Simon Burrows, eds. *Press, Politics and the Public Sphere in Europe and North America: 1760–1820*. Cambridge: Cambridge University Press, 2002.

Barker-Benfield, G. J. *The Culture of Sensibility: Sex and Society in Eighteenth-Century Britain*. Chicago: University of Chicago Press, 1992.

Barrett, Alan D. T., and Stephen Higgs. "Yellow Fever: A Disease That Has Yet to Be Conquered." *Annual Review of Entomology* 52 (2007): 209–29.

Barrow, Ian J. "The Many Meanings of the Black Hole of Calcutta." In *Tall Tales and True: India, Historiography, and British Imperial Imaginings*, edited by Kate Brittlebank, 7–18. Clayton, AU: Monash University Press, 2008.

Baugh, Daniel. *British Naval Administration in the Age of Walpole*. Princeton, NJ: Princeton University Press, 1965.

———. *The Global Seven Years War, 1754–1763: Britain and France in a Great Power Contest*. Harlow: Longman, 2011.

———. "Great Britain's 'Blue-Water' Policy, 1689–1815." *International History Review* 10:1 (1988): 33–58.

———. "Maritime Strength and Atlantic Commerce." In *An Imperial State at War: Britain from 1689 to 1815*, edited by Lawrence Stone, 185–223. London: Routledge, 1994.

———. "Why Did Britain Lose Command of the Sea during the War for America?' In *The British Navy and the Use of Naval Power in the Eighteenth Century*, edited by Jeremy Black and Philip Woodfine, 149–70. Leicester: Leicester University Press, 1988.

Bayly, C. A. *Indian Society and the Making of the British Empire*. Cambridge: Cambridge University Press, 1988.

Beattie, Daniel J. "The Adaptation of the British Army to Wilderness Warfare, 1755–1763." In *Adapting to Conditions: War and Society in the Eighteenth Century*, edited by Maarten Ultee, 56–83. Tuscaloosa: University of Alabama Press, 1986.

Beattie, J. M. *Crime and the Courts in England, 1660–1800*. Princeton, NJ: Princeton University Press, 1986.

Beatty, Heather. *Nervous Disease in Late Eighteenth-Century Britain: The Reality of a Fashionable Disorder*. London: Pickering & Chatto, 2012.

Becker, Ann M. "Smallpox in Washington's Army: Strategic Implications of the Disease during the American Revolutionary War." *Journal of Military History* 68:2 (2004): 381–430.

Bell, David A. *The First Total War: Napoleon's Europe and the Birth of Modern Warfare*. London: Bloomsbury, 2007.

Bell, Whitfield J. *John Morgan, Continental Doctor*. Philadelphia: University of Pennsylvania Press 1965.

Ben-Amos, Ilana Krausman. *The Culture of Giving: Informal Support and Gift-Exchange in Early Modern England*. Cambridge: Cambridge University Press, 2008.

Berg, Maxine, ed. "Reflections on Joel Mokyr's *The Gifts of Athena*." Special issue, *History of Science* 45:2 (2007):123–221.

Bewell, Alan. *Romanticism and Colonial Disease*. Baltimore: Johns Hopkins University Press, 1999.

Bickham, Troy O. *Savages within the Empire: Representations of American Indians in Eighteenth-Century Britain*. Oxford: Clarendon Press.

Birke, Adolf M., et al., eds. *England und Hannover = England and Hanover*. Munich: Saur, 1986.

Black, F. L. "An Explanation of High Death Rates among New World Peoples When in Contact with Old World Diseases." *Perspectives in Biology and Medicine* 37:2 (1994): 292–307.

———. "Why Did They Die?' *Science*, n.s., 258:5089 (1992): 1739–40.

Black, Jeremy. *America or Europe? British Foreign Policy, 1739–63*. London: UCL Press, 1998.

———. *The Continental Commitment: Britain, Hanover and Interventionism, 1714–1793*. London: Routledge, 2005.

———. *Debating Foreign Policy in Eighteenth-Century Britain*. Farnham, UK: Ashgate, 2011.

———. *The English Press in the Eighteenth Century*. London: Croom Helm, 1987.

———. *European Warfare, 1660–1815*. London: UCL Press, 1994.

———. "A Military Revolution? A 1660–1792 Perspective." In *The Military Revolution Debate: Readings on the Military Transformation of Early Modern Europe*, edited by Clifford J. Rogers, 95–115. Boulder, CO: Westview, 1995.

———. *Warfare in the Eighteenth Century*. London: Cassell, 2003.

Blake, J. B. "Smallpox Inoculation in Colonial Boston." *Journal of the History of Medicine* 8 (1953): 284–300.

Blanning, T. C. W. *The Culture of Power and the Power of Culture: Old Regime Europe, 1660–1789*. Oxford: Oxford University Press, 2002.

Bohstedt, John. *The Politics of Provisions: Food Riots, Moral Economy, and Market Transition in England, c. 1550–1850*. Farnham, UK: Ashgate, 2010.

Bonney, Richard. Introduction to *The Rise of the Fiscal State in Europe, c. 1200–1815*, edited by Richard Bonney, 1–15. Oxford: Oxford University Press, 1999.

Boulukos, George. *The Grateful Slave: The Emergence of Race in Eighteenth-Century British and American Culture*. Cambridge: Cambridge University Press, 2008.

Bowden, Peter J. "Agricultural Prices, Wages, Farm Profits, and Rents." In *The Agrarian History of England and Wales*, vol. 5.2, *1640–1750: Agrarian Change*, edited by Jane Thirsk, 1–118. Cambridge: Cambridge University Press, 1985.

Bowen, H. V. *The Business of Empire: The East India Company and Imperial Britain, 1756–1833*. Cambridge: Cambridge University Press, 2006.

———. "Mobilising Resources for Global Warfare: The British State and the East India Company, 1756–1815." In *Mobilising Resources for War: Britain and Spain at Work during the Early Modern Period*, edited by H. V. Bowen and Augustín González Enciso, 81–110. Pamplona: EUNSA, 2006.

———. *Revenue and Reform: The Indian Problem in British Politics, 1757–1773*. Cambridge: Cambridge University Press, 1991..

Bowen, H. V., and Augustín González Enciso, eds. *Mobilising Resources for War: Britain and Spain at Work during the Early Modern Period*. Pamplona: EUNSA, 2006.

Bowman, Larry G. *Captive Americans: Prisoners during the American Revolution*. Athens, OH: Ohio University Press, 1976.

Braddick, Michael J. *State Formation in Early Modern England, c. 1550–1700*. Cambridge: Cambridge University Press, 2000.

Brewer, John. *Party Ideology and Popular Politics at the Accession of George III*. Cambridge: Cambridge University Press, 1976.

———. *The Sinews of Power: War, Money and the English State*. London: Unwin Hyman, 1989.

Brockliss, L. W. B., and Colin Jones. *The Medical World of Early Modern France*. Oxford: Clarendon Press, 1997.

Brown, Kathleen M. *Foul Bodies: Cleanliness in Early America*. New Haven, CT: Yale University Press, 2009.

Brown, Michael. *Performing Medicine: Medical Culture and Identity in Provincial England, c. 1760–1850*. Manchester: Manchester University Press, 2011.

Brumwell, Stephen. "Home from the Wars." *History Today* 52:3 (2002): 41–47.

———. *Redcoats: The British Soldier and War in the Americas, 1755–1763*. Cambridge: Cambridge University Press, 2002.

———. *White Devil: An Epic Story of Revenge from the Savage War That Inspired The Last of the Mohicans*. London: Weidenfeld & Nicolson, 2004.

Brunton, Deborah. "Smallpox Inoculation and Demographic Trends in Eighteenth Century Scotland." *Medical History* 36 (1992): 403–29.

Bryant, G. J. "Asymmetric Warfare: The British Experience in Eighteenth-Century India."*Journal of Military History* 68:2 (2004): 431–69.

———. "Indigenous Mercenaries in the Service of European Imperialists: The Case of the Sepoy in the Early British Indian Army, 1750–1800." *War in History* 7:1 (2000): 2–28.

———. "The Military Imperative in Early British Expansion in India, 1750–1785." *Indo-British Review* 21 (1996): 18–35.

———. "The War in Bengal." In *The Seven Years' War: Global Views*, edited by Mark H. Danley and Patrick J. Speelman, 399–427. Leiden: Brill, 2012.

———. "The War in the Carnatic." In Danley and Speelman, *The Seven Years' War*, 73–104. Leiden: Brill, 2012.

Buchet, Christian. *La lutte pour l'espace caraïbe et la façade atlantique de l'Amérique centrale et du sud (1672–1763)*. 2 vols. Paris: Librarie de l'Inde éditeur, 1991.

———. *Marine, économie et société: Un exemple d'interaction ; L'avitaillement de la Royal Navy durant la guerre de sept ans*. Paris: Honoré Champion, 1999.

———. "Quantification des pertes dans l'espace caraibe et retombées strategiques." In *L'homme, la santé et la mer: Actes du colloque international tenu à l'Institut catholique de Paris les 5 et 6 décembre 1995*, edited by Christian Buchet, 177–94. Paris: H. Champion, 1997.

Buck, Peter. "People Who Counted: Political Arithmetic in the Eighteenth Century." *Isis* 73:1 (1982): 28–45.

Burnard, Trevor. "'The Countrie Continues Sicklie': White Mortality in Jamaica, 1655–1780." *Social History of Medicine* 12 (1999): 45–72.

Burrows, Edwin G. *Forgotten Patriots: The Untold Story of American Prisoners during the Revolutionary War.* New York: Basic Books, 2008.

Butterton, J. R. "The Education, Naval Service, and Early Career of William Smellie." *Bulletin of the History of Medicine* 60 (1986): 1–18.

Bynum, W. F. "Cullen and the Study of Fevers in Britain, 1760–1820." *Medical History* Supplement No. 1 (1981): 135–47.

———. "Physicians, Hospitals and Career Structures in Eighteenth-Century London." In *William Hunter and the Eighteenth-Century Medical World*, edited by W. F. Bynum and Roy Porter, 105–28. Cambridge: Cambridge University Press, 1985.

Bynum, W. F., and Roy Porter, eds. *Medical Fringe & Medical Orthodoxy, 1750–1850.* London: Croon Helm, 1987.

———, eds. *William Hunter and the Eighteenth-Century Medical World.* Cambridge: Cambridge University Press, 1985.

Cadell, Patrick Robert. *History of the Bombay Army.* London: Longmans, Green, 1938.

Çağlarirmak, Necla. "Ochratoxin A, Hydroxymethylfurfural and Vitamin C Levels of Sun-Dried Grapes and Sultanas." *Journal of Food Processing and Preservation* 30 (2006): 549–62.

Cañizares-Esguerra, Jorge. *How to Write the History of the New World: Histories, Epistemologies, and Identities in the Eighteenth-Century Atlantic World.* Stanford, CA: Stanford University Press, 2001.

Cantlie, Neil. *A History of the Army Medical Department.* Edinburgh: Churchill Livingstone, 1974.

Cardwell, John. *Arts and Arms: Literature, Politics and Patriotism during the Seven Years War.* Manchester: Manchester University Press, 2004.

Carmichael, Ann G., and Arthur M. Silverstein. "Smallpox in Europe before the Seventeenth Century: Virulent Killer or Benign Disease?' *Journal of the History of Medicine and Allied Sciences* 42 (1987): 147–68.

Carpenter, Kenneth J. *The History of Scurvy and Vitamin C.* Cambridge: Cambridge University Press, 1986.

Carroll, Joy. *Wolfe & Montcalm: Their Lives, Their Times and the Fate of a Continent.* Richmond Hill, Ont.: Firefly Books, 2004.

Carvin, Stephanie. *Prisoners of America's Wars: From the Early Republic to Guantanamo.* New York: Columbia University Press, 2010.

Cavallo, Sandra. "The Motivations of Benefactors: An Overview of Approaches to the Study of Charity." In *Medicine and Charity before the Welfare State*, edited by Jonathan Barry and Colin Jones, 46–62. London: Routledge, 1991.

Chakrabarti, Pratik. *Materials and Medicine: Trade, Conquest and Therapeutics in the Eighteenth Century.* Manchester: Manchester University Press, 2010.

———. "'Neither of meate nor drinke, but what the Doctor alloweth': Medicine amidst War and Commerce in Eighteenth-Century Madras." *Bulletin of the History of Medicine* 80 (2006): 1–38.

Chaplin, Joyce E. "Earthsickness: Circumnavigation and the Terrestrial Human Body, 1520–1800." *Bulletin of the History of Medicine* 86:4 (2012): 515–42.

Charters, Erica. "The Administration of War and French Prisoners of War in Britain, 1756–1763." In *Civilians and War in Europe, 1618–1815*, edited by Erica Charters, Eve Rosenhaft, Hannah Smith, 87–99. Liverpool: Liverpool University Press, 2012.

———. "The Caring Fiscal-Military State during the Seven Years War, 1759–1763." *Historical Journal* 52:4 (2009): 921–41.

———. "Colonial Disease, Translation, and Enlightenment: Franco-British Medicine and the Seven Years' War." In *The Culture of the Seven Years' War: Empire, Identity, and the Arts*, edited by Frans de Bruyn and Shaun Regan, 77–101. Toronto: University of Toronto Press, 2014.

———. "Disease, Wilderness Warfare, and Imperial Relations: The Battle for Quebec, 1759–1760." *War in History* 16:1 (2009): 1–24.

———. "'The Intention is Certain Noble':The Western Squadron, Medical Trials, and the Sick and Hurt Board during the Seven Years War.' In *Health & Medicine at Sea, 1700–1900*, ed. David Boyd Haycock and Sally Archer, 19–37. Woodbridge, UK: Boydell Press, 2009.

———. "Military Medicine and Ethics of War: British Colonial Warfare during the Seven Years War (1756–63)." *Canadian Bulletin of Medical History* 27:2 (2010): 273–98.

Charters, Erica, Eve Rosenhaft, and Hannah Smith, eds. *Civilians and War in Europe, 1618–1815*. Liverpool: University of Liverpool Press, 2012.

Chartrand, René. *Québec: The Heights of Abraham 1759; The Armies of Wolfe and Montcalm*. Oxford: Osprey, 1999.

Chet, Guy. *Conquering the American Wilderness: The Triumph of European Warfare in the Colonial Northeast*. Amherst: University of Massachusetts Press, 2003.

Christiansen, David. "Colonial Warfare." In *Reader's Guide to Military History*, edited by Charles Messenger, 114–15. London: Fitzroy Dearborn, 2001.

Churchill, Wendy D. "Bodily Differences? Gender, Race, and Class in Hans Sloane's Jamaican Medical Practice, 1687–1688." *Journal of the History of Medicine and Allied Sciences* 60:4 (Oct. 2005): 391–444.

———. "Efficient, Efficacious and Humane Responses to Non-European Bodies in British Military Medicine, 1780–1815." *Journal of Imperial and Commonwealth History* 40:2 (2012): 137–58.

Clark, Christopher M. *Iron Kingdom: The Rise and Downfall of Prussia, 1600–1947*. London: Penguin, 2007.

Clark, G. N. *A History of the Royal College of Physicians of London*. Oxford: Clarendon Press for the Royal College of Physicians, 1966.

Clarkson, L. A., and E. Margaret Crawford. *Feast and Famine: A History of Food and Nutrition in Ireland, 1500–1920*. Oxford: Oxford University Press, 2001.

Clyde, Robert. *From Rebel to Hero: The Image of the Highlander, 1745–1830*. East Linton, UK: Tuckwell Press, 1995.

Cody, Lisa Forman. *Birthing the Nation: Sex, Science, and the Conception of Eighteenth-Century Britons*. Oxford: Oxford University Press, 2005.

Cogliano, Francis D. "'We All Hoisted the American Flag': National Identity among

American Prisoners in Britain during the American Revolution." *Journal of American Studies* 32 (1998): 19–37.

Cohen, Sheldon S. *Yankee Sailors in British Gaols: Prisoners of War at Forton and Mill, 1777–1783*. London: Associated University Presses, 1995.

Coleman, D. C. "Mercantilism Revisited." *Historical Journal* 23:4 (1980): 773–91.

Colley, Linda. *Britons: Forging the Nation, 1707–1837*. New Haven, CT: Yale University Press, 1992.

Contamine, Philippe, ed. *War and Competition between States*. Oxford: Clarendon, 2000.

Conway, Stephen. "From Fellow-Nationals to Foreigners: British Perceptions of the Americans, circa 1739–1783." *William and Mary Quarterly*, 3rd ser., 59:1 (2002): 65–100.

———. "The Mobilization of Manpower for Britain's Mid-Eighteenth-Century Wars." *Historical Research* 77:197 (2004): 377–404.

———. *War, State, and Society in Mid-Eighteenth-Century Britain*. Oxford: Oxford University Press, 2006.

Cook, Harold J. "Practical Medicine and the British Armed Forces after the 'Glorious Revolution.'" *Medical History* 34 (1990): 1–26.

Cookson, J. E. *The British Armed Nation, 1793–1815*. Oxford: Clarendon Press, 1997.

Cooper, Donald B., and Kenneth F. Kiple. "Yellow Fever." In *The Cambridge World History of Human Disease*, edited by Kenneth F. Kiple et al., 1100–1107. Cambridge: Cambridge University Press, 1993.

Cooper, Frederick, and Ann Laura Stoler. "Between Metropole and Colony: Rethinking a Research Agenda." In *Tensions of Empire: Colonial Cultures in a Bourgeois World*, edited by Frederick Cooper and Ann Laura Stoler, 1–58. Berkeley: University of California Press, 1997.

Cooter, Roger. "Discourses on War." *Studies in the History and Philosophy of Science* 26 (1995): 637–47.

———. "Medicine and the Goodness of War." *Canadian Bulletin for Medical History* 7 (1990): 147–59.

Copeland, David. "America, 1750–1820." In *Press, Politics and the Public Sphere in Europe and North America: 1760–1820*, edited by Hannah Barker and Simon Burrows, 140–58. Cambridge: Cambridge University Press, 2002.

———. "'Join, or Die': America's Press during the French and Indian War." *Journalism History* 24:3 (1998): 112–21.

Corbett, Julian Stafford. *England in the Seven Years' War: A Study in Combined Strategy*. 2 vols. London: Longmans, Green, 1907.

Crawford, D. G. *A History of the Indian Medical Service: 1600–1913*. 2 vols. London: W. Thacker, 1914.

Crewe, Duncan. *Yellow Jack and the Worm: British Naval Administration in the West Indies, 1739–1748*. Liverpool: Liverpool University Press, 1993.

Crimmin, P. K. "Alternative Roles: Fishermen as Smugglers, Agents of Escape, and Prisoners of War, 1793–1815." *Northern Seas Yearbook*, 1996, 53–62.

———. "French Prisoners of War on Parole, 1793–1815: The Welsh Border Towns." In

Guerres et paix 1660–1815, edited by France, Service historique de la marine, 61–71. Vincennes: Service historique de la Marine, 1987.

———. "The Sick and Hurt Board and the Health of Seamen, c. 1700–1806." *Journal for Maritime Research* 1:1 (1999): 48–65.

Cunningham, Andrew, and R. K. French. *The Medical Enlightenment of the Eighteenth Century*. Cambridge: Cambridge University Press, 1990.

Cunningham, Hugh. Introduction to *Charity, Philanthropy and Reform, from the 1690s to 1850*, edited by Hugh Cunningham and Joanna Innes, 1–14. Basingstoke, UK: Macmillan Press, 1998.

Cunningham, Hugh, and Joanna Innes, eds. *Charity, Philanthropy and Reform, from the 1690s to 1850*. Basingstoke, UK: Macmillan Press, 1998.

Curtin, Philip D. *Disease and Empire: The Health of European Troops in the Conquest of Africa*. Cambridge: Cambridge University Press, 1998.

———. "'The White Man's Grave': Image and Reality, 1780–1850." *Journal of British Studies* 1:1 (1961): 94–110.

Daly, Gavin. "Napoleon's Lost Legions: French Prisoners of War in Britain, 1803–1814." *History* 89:295 (2004): 361–80.

Damien, Robert, ed. *L'expertise*. Besançon: Presses universitaires franc-comtoises, 2001.

Daniels, Christine, and Michael V. Kennedy, eds. *Negotiated Empires: Centers and Peripheries in the Americas, 1500–1820*. London: Routledge, 2002.

Danley, Mark H. "The British Political Press and Military Thought during the Seven Years' War." In *The Seven Years' War: Global Views*, edited by Mark H. Danley and Patrick J. Speelman, 359–97. Leiden: Brill, 2012.

———. "Introduction: The 'Problem' of the Seven Years' War." In *The Seven Years' War: Global Views*, edited by Mark H. Danley and Patrick J. Speelman, xxiii-lvii. Leiden: Brill, 2012.

Daston, Lorraine, and Elizabeth Lunbeck, eds. *Histories of Scientific Observation*. Chicago: University of Chicago Press, 2011.

Delbourgo, James, and Staffan Müller-Wille. "Introduction: Listmania." *Isis* 103:4 (2012): 710–15.

Devine, T. M. *Scotland's Empire, 1600–1815*. London: Allen Lane, 2003.

Dhumne, Umesh L., and Aruna A. Jawade. "Sickle Cell Anemia and Morbidity in Rural Population of Chandrapur District, Maharashtra, India." *Anthropologist* 13:1 (2011): 61–63.

Dickson, P. G. M. *The Financial Revolution in England: A Study in the Development of Public Credit, 1688–1756*. London: Macmillan, 1967.

Digby, Anne. *Making a Medical Living: Doctors and Patients in the English Market for Medicine, 1720–1911*. Cambridge: Cambridge University Press, 1994.

Dixon, C. W. *Smallpox*. London: J. & A. Churchill, 1962.

Dixon, Robert. *Prosthetic Gods: Travel, Representation and Colonial Governance*. Brisbane: University of Queensland Press, 2001.

Doughty, Arthur G. *The Siege of Quebec and the Battle of the Plains of Abraham*. In collaboration with G. W. Parmelee. 6 vols. Quebec City: Dussault & Proulx, 1901.

Downing, B. M. *The Military Revolution and Political Change: Origins of Democracy and Autocracy in Early Modern Europe.* Princeton, NJ: Princeton University Press, 1992.

Downs, W. G. "The Known and the Unknown in Yellow Fever Ecology and Epidemiology." *Ecology of Disease* 1:2–3 (1982): 103–10.

Doyle, Robert C. *Voices from Captivity: Interpreting the American POW Narrative.* Lawrence: University Press of Kansas, 1994.

Drayton, Richard. "Knowledge and Empire." In *The Oxford History of the British Empire*, vol. 2, *The Eighteenth Century*, edited by P. J. Marshall, 231–52. Oxford: Oxford University Press, 2001.

———. *Nature's Government: Science, Imperial Britain, and the "Improvement" of the World.* New Haven, CT: Yale University Press, 2000.

Duffy, Christopher. *The Military Experience in the Age of Reason.* London: Routledge & Kegan Paul, 1987.

Duffy, John. *Epidemics in Colonial America.* Port Washington, NY: Kennikat Press, 1972.

Duffy, Michael. "The Establishment of the Western Squadron as the Linchpin of British Naval Strategy." In *Parameters of British Naval Power, 1650–1850*, edited by Michael Duffy, 60–81. Exeter: University of Exeter Press, 1992.

Dull, Jonathan R. *The Age of the Ship of the Line: The British & French Navies, 1650–1815.* Lincoln: University of Nebraska Press, 2009.

———. *The French Navy and the Seven Years' War.* Lincoln: University of Nebraska, 2005.

Dunn, Frederick L. "Malaria." In *The Cambridge World History of Human Disease*, edited by Kenneth F. Kiple et al., 852–55. Cambridge: Cambridge University Press, 1993.

DuPont, Herbert L. "Diarrheal Diseases (Acute)." In *The Cambridge World History of Human Disease*, edited by Kenneth F. Kiple et al., 676–80. Cambridge: Cambridge University Press, 1993.

Duro, Cesáreo Fernández. *Armada Española desde la Unión de los Reinos de Castilla y de Aragón.* 9 vols. Madrid: Museo Naval, 1972.

Eastwood, David. *Government and Community in the English Provinces.* Basingstoke, UK: Macmillan, 1997.

Ernst, Waltraud, and Bernard Harris, eds. *Race, Science and Medicine, 1700–1960.* London: Routledge, 1999.

Eustace, Nicole. *Passion Is the Gale: Emotion, Power, and the Coming of the American Revolution.* Chapel Hill: University of North Carolina Press, 2008.

Félix, Joël. "Finances, opinion publique et diplomatie: Le Committee of Canada Merchants et la question du remboursement par la France des 'billets du Canada' de propriété britannique 1763–1775." In *Le négoce de la paix : Les nations et les traités franco-britanniques (1713–1802)*, edited by Jean-Pierre Jessenne, Renaud Morieux, and Pascal Dupuy, 127–64. Paris: Société des études Robespierriestes, 2008.

Fenn, Elizabeth A. "Biological Warfare in Eighteenth-Century North America: Beyond Jeffery Amherst." *Journal of American History* 68:4 (2000): 1552–80.

———. *Pox Americana: The Great Smallpox Epidemic of 1775–82.* Stroud, UK: Sutton, 2004.

Fissell, Mary. *Patients, Power and the Poor in Eighteenth-Century Bristol.* Cambridge: Cambridge University Press, 1991.

Flavell, Julie, and Stephen Conway, eds. *Britain and America Go to War: The Impact of War and Warfare, 1754–1815.* Gainesville: University Press of Florida, 2004.

Fonck, Bertrand. "Une victoire inutile : Le rôle du corps expéditionnaire métropolitain dans la victoire de Sainte-Foy (28 avril 1760) et la défense de la Nouvelle-France." *Revue Historique des Armées* 258 (2010): 82–88.

Fordham, Douglas. *British Art and the Seven Years' War: Allegiance and Autonomy.* Philadelphia: University of Pennsylvania Press, 2010.

Fortescue, J. W. *A History of the British Army.* 2nd ed. 13 vols. London: Macmillan, 1910–30.

Foucault, Michel. *Discipline and Punish: The Birth of the Prison.* Translated by Alan Sheridan. New York: Random House, 1995.

Fournier, Marcel. "Les soldats de la guerre de Sept Ans en Nouvelle-France, 1755–1760." In *La guerre de Sept Ans en Nouvelle-France,* edited by Laurent Veyssière and Bertrand Fonck, 237–42. Paris: PUPS, 2011.

Fournier, Marcel, Projet Montcalm, and Société généologique canadienne-française. *Combattre pour la France en Amérique: Les soldats de la guerre de Sept Ans en Nouvelle-France 1755–1760.* Montreal: Société généologique canadienne-française, 2009.

Fowler, William M. *Empires at War: The French & Indian War and the Struggle for North America, 1745–1763.* New York: Walker, 2005.

Fox, Robert. "Science and Government." In *The Cambridge History of Science,* vol. 4, *Eighteenth-Century Science,* edited by Roy Porter, 107–24. Cambridge: Cambridge University Press, 2003.

French, Roger K. "Scurvy." In *The Cambridge World History of Human Disease,* edited by Kenneth F. Kiple et al., 1000–1005. Cambridge: Cambridge University Press, 1993.

French, Roger K., and Andrew Wear, eds. *British Medicine in an Age of Reform.* London: Routledge, 1991.

Frey, Sylvia R. *The British Soldier in America: A Social History of Military Life in the Revolutionary Period.* Austin: University of Texas Press, 1981.

Gallagher, Catherine, and Thomas Laqueur, eds. *The Making of the Modern Body: Sexuality and Society in the Nineteenth Century.* Berkeley: University of California Press, 1987.

Gardner, C. L., and K. D. Ryman. "Yellow Fever: A Reemerging Threat." *Clinics in Laboratory Medicine* 30:1 (2010): 237–60.

Gascoigne, John. *Science in the Service of Empire: Joseph Banks, the British State and the Uses of Science in the Age of Revolution.* Cambridge: Cambridge University Press, 1998.

Gauci, Perry. *William Beckford: First Prime Minister of the London Empire.* New Haven, CT: Yale University Press, 2013.

Gerbi, Antonello. *The Dispute of the New World: The History of a Polemic.* Translated by Jeremy Moyle. Rev. and enl. ed. Pittsburgh: University of Pittsburgh Press, 1973.

Ghosh, A. *History of the Armed Forces Medical Services, India*. Hyderabad: Orient Longman, 1988.

Glacken, Clarence J. *Traces on the Rhodian Shore: Nature and Culture in Western Thought from Ancient Times to the End of the Eighteenth Century*. Berkeley: University of California Press, 1967.

Glass, D. V. *Numbering the People: The Eighteenth-Century Population Controversy and the Development of Census and Vital Statistics in Britain*. Farnborough, UK: D. C. Heath, 1973.

Glete, Jan. *Navies and Nations: Warships, Navies and State Building in Europe and America, 1500–1860*. 2 vols. Stockholm: Almqvist & Wiksell International, 1993.

Gould, Eliga H. *The Persistence of Empire: British Political Culture in the Age of the American Revolution*. Chapel Hill: University of North Carolina Press, 2000.

Gradish, Stephen F. *The Manning of the British Navy during the Seven Years' War*. London: Royal Historical Society, 1980.

Grant, W. L. "Canada versus Guadeloupe, an Episode of the Seven Years' War." *American Historical Review* 17:4 (1912): 735–43.

Greene, Jack P. *Creating the British Atlantic: Essays on Transplantation, Adaptation, and Continuity*. Charlottesville: University of Virginia Press, 2013.

———. *Peripheries and Center: Constitutional Development in the Extended Polities of the British Empire and the United States, 1607–1788*. Athens, GA: University of Georgia Press, 1986.

———. "The Seven Years' War and the American Revolution: The Causal Relationship Reconsidered." *Journal of Imperial and Commonwealth History* 8:2 (1980): 85–105.

Grigg, David B. *Population Growth and Agrarian Change: An Historical Perspective*. Cambridge: Cambridge University Press, 1980.

Grove, Richard. *Green Imperialism: Colonial Expansion, Tropical Island Edens and the Origins of Environmentalism*. Cambridge: Cambridge University Press, 1995.

Guerra, F. "The Influence of Disease on Race, Logistics and Colonization in the Antilles." *Journal of Tropical Medicine and Hygiene* 69 (1966): 23–35.

Gunn, Steven, David Grummitt, and Hans Cools. "War and the State in Early Modern Europe: Widening the Debate." *War in History* 15:4 (2008): 371–88.

Gupta, Brijen K. *Sirajuddaullah and the East India Company, 1756–1757*. Leiden: Brill, 1962.

Guy, Alan J. Introduction to "George Durant's Journal of the Expedition to Martinique and Guadeloupe, October 1758–May 1759." In *Military Miscellany 1: Manuscripts from the Seven Years War*, edited by Alan J Guy, R. N. W Thomas, and Gerard J De Groot, 3–15. Stroud, UK: Sutton, 1997.

———. *Oeconomy and Discipline: Officership and Administration in the British Army, 1714–63*. Manchester: Manchester University Press, 1985.

Gwyn, Julian. "The Royal Navy in North America, 1712–1776." In *The British Navy and the Use of Naval Power in the Eighteenth Century*, edited by Jeremy Black and Philip Woodfine, 129–48. Leicester: Leicester University Press, 1988.

Habermas, Jürgen. *The Structural Transformation of the Public Sphere: An Inquiry into a Category of Bourgeois Society*. Translated by Thomas Burger with the assistance of Frederick Lawrence. 1962 ed. Cambridge: Polity, 2010.

Hacking, Ian. *The Taming of Chance*. Cambridge: Cambridge University Press, 1990.

Hannaford, Ivan. *Race: The History of an Idea in the West*. Washington, DC: Woodrow Wilson Center Press, 1996.

Hannaway, Caroline. "Environment and Miasmata." In *Companion Encyclopedia of the History of Medicine*, edited by W. F. Bynum and Roy Porter, 1:292–308. 2 vols. London: Routledge, 1993.

Harden, Victoria A. "Typhus, Epidemic." In *The Cambridge World History of Human Disease*, edited by Kenneth F. Kiple et al., 1080–84. Cambridge: Cambridge University Press, 1993.

Harding, Richard. *Amphibious Warfare in the Eighteenth Century: The British Expedition to the West Indies, 1740–1742*. London: Royal Historical Society, 1991.

———. *The Emergence of Britain's Global Naval Supremacy: The War of 1739–1748*. Woodbridge, UK: Boydell, 2010.

———. "The Growth of Anglo-American Alienation: The Case of the American Regiment, 1740–42." *Journal of Imperial and Commonwealth History* 17 (1989): 161–84.

———. *Seapower and Naval Warfare, 1650–1830*. London: UCL Press, 1999.

Hardy, Anne. "Urban Famine or Urban Crisis? Typhus in the Victorian City." *Medical History* 32:4 (1988): 401–25.

Harkness, Albert, Jr. "Americanism and Jenkins' Ear." *Mississippi Valley Historical Review* 37 (1950): 61–90.

Harling, Philip. *The Modern British State: An Historical Introduction*. Cambridge: Polity, 2001.

Harling, Philip, and Peter Mandler. "From 'Fiscal-Military' State to Laissez-Faire State, 1760–1850." *Journal of British Studies* 32:1 (1993): 44–70.

Harris, Bob. *A Patriot Press: National Politics and the London Press in the 1740s*. Oxford: Clarendon Press, 1993.

———. *Politics and the Nation: Britain in the Mid-Eighteenth Century*. Oxford: Oxford University Press, 2002.

———. "War, Empire, and the 'National Interest' in Mid-Eighteenth-Century Britain." In *Britain and America Go to War: The Impact of War and Warfare, 1754–1815*, edited by Julie Flavell and Stephen Conway, 13–40. Gainesville: University Press of Florida, 2004.

Harrison, Mark. *Climates & Constitutions: Health, Race, Environment and British Imperialism in India, 1600–1850*. New Delhi: Oxford University Press, 1999.

———. "Disease and Medicine in British India, 1750–1830: The Treatment of Fevers and the Emergence of Tropical Therapeutics." In *British Military and Naval Medicine, 1600–1830*, edited by Geoffrey L. Hudon, 87–119. Amsterdam: Rodopi, 2007.

———. "The Medicalization of War—the Militarization of Medicine." *Social History of Medicine* 9 (1996): 267–76.

———. "Medicine and the Management of Modern Warfare." *History of Science* 34 (1996): 379–410.

———. "Medicine and Orientalism: Perspectives on Europe's Encounter with Indian Medical Systems." In *Health, Medicine and Empire: Perspectives on Colonial India*, edited by Biswamoy Pati and Mark Harrison, 37–87. New Delhi: Orient Longman, 2001.

———. *Medicine in an Age of Commerce and Empire: Britain and Its Tropical Colonies, 1660–1830*. Oxford: Oxford University Press, 2010.

———. *Public Health in British India: Anglo-Indian Preventive Medicine, 1859–1914*. Cambridge: Cambridge University Press, 1994.

———. "Racial Pathologies: Morbid Anatomy in British India, 1770–1850." In *The Social History of Health and Medicine in Colonial India*, edited by Biswamoy Pati and Mark Harrison, 173–94. London: Routledge, 2009.

———. "'The Tender Frame of Man': Disease, Climate, and Racial Difference in India and the West Indies, 1760–1860." *Bulletin of the History of Medicine* 70:1 (1996): 68–93.

Harvie, David. *Limeys: The True Story of One Man's War against Ignorance, the Establishment and the Deadly Scurvy*. Stroud, UK: Sutton, 2002.

Haycock, David Boyd, and Sally L. Archer, eds. *Health & Medicine at Sea, 1700–1900*. Woodbridge, UK: Boydell Press, 2009.

Heagerty, John J. *Four Centuries of Medical History in Canada, and a Sketch of the Medical History of Newfoundland*. 2 vols. Bristol, UK: J. Wright, 1928.

Heberden, Ernest. "Richard Brocklesby (1722–1797)." In *Oxford Dictionary of National Biography*. Oxford University Press, 2004–. Accessed 9 Dec. 2006. doi:10.1093/ref:odnb/3475.

Hernández-Sáenz, Luz María. "Seamen, Surgeons and Empire: Spanish Naval Medical Reform and Mexican Medicine in the Late Colonial Period." *The Northern Mariner/Le Marin du nord* 10:1 (2000): 21–35.

Herrick, Claire E. J. "Donald Monro (1728–1802)." In *Oxford Dictionary of National Biography*. Oxford University Press, 2004–. Accessed 9 Dec. 2006. doi: 10.1093/ref:odnb/18969.

Hess, Volker, and Andrew J. Mendelsohn. "Case and Series: Medical Recording and Paper Technologies, 1750–1850." *History of Science* 48 (2010): 287–314.

Heyd, Uriel. *Reading Newspapers: Press and Public in Eighteenth-Century Britain and America*. Oxford: Voltaire Foundation, 2012.

Higginbotham, Don. "The Early American Way of War: Reconnaissance and Appraisal." *William and Mary Quarterly*, 3rd ser., 44:2 (1987): 230–73.

Hilaire-Pérez, Liliane. *L'invention technique au siècle des Lumières*. Paris: Albin Michel, 2000.

Hirsch, August. *Handbook of Geographical and Historical Pathology*. Translated by Charles Creighton. 2 vols. London: New Sydenham Society, 1883.

Hofstra, Warren R., ed. *Cultures in Conflict: The Seven Years' War in North America*. Lanham, MD: Rowman & Littlefield.

Holtom, Paul D., and John M. Leedom. "Rickettsial Infections." In *Current Therapy of Infectious Disease*, edited by David Schloisberg, 645–49. 2nd ed. London: Mosby, 2001.

Hoock, Holger. *Empires of the Imagination: Politics, War, and the Arts in the British World, 1750–1850*. London: Profile Books, 2010.

Hopkins, Donald R. *The Greatest Killer: Smallpox in History*. With a new introduction. Chicago: University of Chicago Press, 2002.

Hoppit, Julian. "Political Arithmetic in Eighteenth-Century England." *Economic History Review* 49:3 (1996): 516–40.

———. "Reforming Britain's Weights and Measures, 1660–1824." *English Historical Review* 108:426 (1993): 82–104.

Houlding, J. A. *Fit for Service: The Training of the British Army, 1715–1795*. Oxford: Clarendon Press, 1981.

Houston, C. S. "Scurvy and Canadian Exploration." *Canadian Bulletin of Medical History* 7:2 (1990): 161–67.

Howard, Michael, George J. Andreopoulos, and Mark R. Shulman, eds. *The Laws of War: Constraints on Warfare in the Western World*. New Haven, CT: Yale University Press, 1994.

Hudson, Geoffrey L., ed. *British Military and Naval Medicine, 1600–1830*. Amsterdam: Rodopi Press, 2007.

———. "Disabled Veterans and the State in Early Modern England." In *Disabled Veterans in History*, edited by David A. Gerber, 117–44. Ann Arbor: University of Michigan Press, 2000.

———. "Internal Influences in the Making of the English Military Hospital: The Early-Eighteenth-Century Greenwich." In *British Military and Naval Medicine, 1600–1830*, edited by Geoffrey L. Hudson, 253–72. Amsterdam: Rodopi Press, 2007.

Hunt, Lynn. *Inventing Human Rights: A History*. New York: W. W. Norton, 2007.

Ignatieff, Michael. *A Just Measure of Pain: The Penitentiary in the Industrial Revolution, 1750–1850*. London: Macmillan Press, 1978.

Innes, Joanna. "Central Government 'Interference': Changing Conceptions, Practices, and Concerns, c. 1700–1850." In *Civil Society in British History: Ideas, Identities, Institutions*, edited by Jose Harris, 39–60. Oxford: Oxford University Press, 2005.

———. "Forms of 'Government Growth', 1780–1830." In *Structures and Transformations in Modern British History*, edited by David Feldman and Jon Lawrence, 74–99. Cambridge: Cambridge University Press, 2011.

———. *Inferior Politics: Social Problems and Social Policies in Eighteenth-Century Britain*. Oxford: Oxford University Press, 2009.

———. "The Mixed Economy of Welfare in Early Modern England: Assessments of the Options from Hale to Malthus (1683–1803)." In *Charity, Self-Interest and Welfare in the English Past*, edited by M. J. Daunton, 139–80. London: UCL Press.

———. "State, Church and Voluntarism in European Welfare, 1690–1850." In *Charity, Philanthropy and Reform, from the 1690s to 1850*, edited by Hugh Cunningham and Joanna Innes, 15–64. Basingstoke, UK: Macmillan Press, 1998.

Izurieta, Ricardo O., et al. "Assessing Yellow Fever Risk in the Ecuadorian Amazon." *Journal of Global Infectious Diseases* 1:1 (2009): 7–13.

Jacob, Margaret C. *Scientific Culture and the Making of the Industrial West*. Oxford: Oxford University Press, 1997.

Jenner, Mark S. R., and Patrick Wallis, eds. *Medicine and the Market in England and Its Colonies*. Basingstoke, UK: Palgrave Macmillan, 2007.

Jewson, N. D. "Medical Knowledge and the Patronage System in Eighteenth-Century England." *Sociology* 8 (1974): 369–85.

Jones, Colin, and Roy Porter, eds. *Reassessing Foucault: Power, Medicine, and the Body*. London: Routledge, 1994.

Keel, Othmar. *L'avènement de la médicine clinique moderne en Europe 1750–1815*. Montreal: PUM, 2001.

———. "The Politics of Health and the Institutionalisation of Clinical Practices in Europe in the Second Half of the Eighteenth Century." In *William Hunter and the Eighteenth-Century Medical World*, edited by W. F. Bynum and Roy Porter, 207–58. Cambridge: Cambridge University Press, 1985.

Kelly, Catherine. *War and the Militarization of British Army Medicine, 1793–1830*. London: Pickering & Chatto, 2011.

Kennedy, Dane Keith. *The Magic Mountains: Hill Stations and the British Raj*. Delhi: Oxford University Press, 1996.

Kessel, A. *Air, the Environment and Public Health*. Cambridge: Cambridge University Press, 2005.

Kiple, Kenneth F., and Stephen V. Beck, eds. *Biological Consequences of the European Expansion, 1450–1800*. Aldershot, UK: Ashgate, 1997.

Kiple, Kenneth F., and Brian T. Higgins. "Yellow Fever and the Africanization of the Caribbean." In *Disease and Demography in the Americas*, edited by John W. Verano and Douglas H. Ubelaker, 227–48. London: Smithsonian Institution Press, 1992.

Kiple, Kenneth F., and Kriemhild Coneè Ornelas. "Typhus, Ships and Soldiers." In *Plague, Pox & Pestilence*, edited by Kenneth F. Kiple, 104–9. London: Weidenfeld & Nicolson, 1997.

Knott, Sarah. *Sensibility and the American Revolution*. Chapel Hill: University of North Carolina Press, 2009.

———. "Sensibility and the American War for Independence." *American Historical Review* 109:1 (2004): 19–40.

Kopperman, Paul E. "The British Army in North America and the West Indies, 1755–1783: A Medical Perspective." In *British Military and Naval Medicine, 1600–1830*, edited by Geoffrey L. Hudson, 51–86. Amsterdam: Rodopi Press, 2007.

———. Introduction to *Regimental Practice by John Buchanan, M.D.: An Eighteenth-Century Medical Diary and Manual*, 1–68. Farnham, UK: Ashgate, 2012.

———. "Medical Services in the British Army, 1742–1783." *Journal of the History of Medicine and Allied Sciences* 34:4 (1979): 428–55.

Koschorke, Albrecth. "Physiological Self-Regulation: The Eighteenth-Century Modernization of the Human Body." *MLN: Modern Language Notes* 123:3 (2008): 469–84.

Krebsbach, Suzanne. "The Great Charlestown Smallpox Epidemic of 1760." *South Carolina Historical Magazine* 97:1 (1996): 30–37.

Kuethe, Allan J. *Cuba, 1753–1815: Crown, Military, and Society*. Knoxville: University of Tennessee Press, 1986.

Kumar, Anil. *Medicine and the Raj: British Medical Policy in India, 1835–1911*. London: Sage, 1998.

Kupperman, Karen Ordahl. "Fear of Hot Climates in the Anglo-American Colonial Experience." *William and Mary Quarterly*, 2nd ser., 41:2 (1984): 213–40.

———. "Presentment of Civility: English Reading of American Self-Presentation in the

Early Years of Colonization." *William and Mary Quarterly*, 3rd ser., 54:1 (1997): 193–228.

Lafuente, Antonio, and José Sala Catalá. "Militarización de las actividades científicas en la Espana ilustrada (1726–1754)." In *La ciencia moderna y el nuevo mundo*, edited by José L. Peset, 127–47. Madrid: Consejo Superior de Investigaciones Cientificas, 1985.

Lane, Joan. *A Social History of Medicine: Health, Healing and Disease in England, 1750–1950*. London: Routledge, 2001.

Langford, Paul. *A Polite and Commercial People: England, 1727–1783*. Oxford: Clarendon Press, 1989.

———. *Public Life and the Propertied Englishman, 1689–1798*. Oxford: Clarendon Press, 1991.

LaPierre, Laurier L. *1759: The Battle for Canada*. Toronto: McClelland & Stewart, 1990.

Lawrence, Christopher. "Disciplining Disease: Scurvy, the Navy, and Imperial Expansion, 1750–1825." In *Visions of Empire: Voyages, Botany, and Representations of Nature*, edited by David Philip Miller and Peter Hanns Reill, 80–106. Cambridge: Cambridge University Press, 1996.

Lawrence, Susan C. *Charitable Knowledge: Hospital Pupils and Practitioners in Eighteenth-Century London*. Cambridge: Cambridge University Press, 1996.

Lawson, Philip. *The East India Company: A History*. London: Longman, 1993.

Leach, Douglas E. "The Cartagena Expedition, 1740–1742, and Anglo-American Relations." In *Adapting to Conditions: War and Society in the Eighteenth Century*, edited by Maarten Ultee, 43–55. Tuscaloosa: University of Alabama Press, 1986.

———. *Roots of Conflict: British Armed Forces and Colonial Americans, 1677–1763*. Chapel Hill: University of North Carolina Press, 1986.

Lee, Wayne E. "Early American Ways of War: A New Reconnaissance, 1660–1815." *Historical Journal* 44:1 (2001): 269–89.

Le Goff, T. J. A. "L'impact des prises effectuées par les anglais sur la capacité en hommes de la marine française au XVIIIe siècle." In *Les marines de guerre européennes XVII–XVIIIe siècles*, edited by Martine Acerra, José Merino, and Jean Meyer, 103–22. Paris: Presses de l'Université de Paris-Sorbonne, 1995.

———. "Problèmes de recrutement de la marine française pendant la Guerre de Sept Ans." *Revue Historique* 283, fasc. 2:574 (1990): 205–33.

Lenman, Bruce. *The Jacobite Risings in Britain, 1689–1746*. Aberdeen: Scottish Cultural Press, 1995.

———. "The Transition to European Military Ascendancy in India, 1600–1800." In *Tools of War: Instruments, Ideas, and Institutions of Warfare, 1445–1871*, edited by John A. Lynn, 100–130. Chicago: University of Illinois Press, 1990.

Lewy, Guenter. "Were American Indians the Victims of Genocide?" *Commentary* 118 (2004): 55–63.

Licoppe, Christian. *La formation de la pratique scientifique: Le discours de l'experience en France et en Angleterre (1630–1820)*. Textes à l'Appui. Paris: Découverte, 1996.

Lincoln, Margarette. *Representing the Royal Navy: British Sea Power, 1750–1815*. Aldershot, UK: Ashgate, 2002.

Lloyd, Christopher, and J. L. S. Coulter. *Medicine and the Navy, 1200–1900*. Vol. 3, *1714–1815*. Edinburgh: Livingstone, 1961.

Loudon, Irvine. *Medical Care and the General Practitioner, 1750–1850*. Oxford: Clarendon Press, 1986.

Lupton, Deborah. *Medicine as Culture: Illness, Disease and the Body in Western Societies*. London: Sage, 1994.

Lynn, John A. "How War Fed War: The Tax of Violence and Contributions during the *Grand Siecle*." *Journal of Modern History* 65 (1993): 286–310.

Macdonald, Janet. "A New Myth of Naval History? Confusing Magnitude with Significance in British Naval Victualling Purchases, 1750–1815." *International Journal of Maritime History* 21:2 (2009): 159–88.

Mackesy, Piers. *The War for America, 1775–1783*. London: Longmans, 1964.

Mackillop, Andrew. "The Political Culture of the Scottish Highlands from Culloden to Waterloo." *Historical Journal* 46 (2003): 511–32.

MacLeod, D. Peter. "Microbes and Muskets: Smallpox and the Participation of the Amerindian Allies of New France in the Seven Years' War." *Ethnohistory* 39:1 (1992): 42–64.

MacLeod, Roy M., and Milton James Lewis, eds. *Medicine and Empire: Perspectives on Western Medicine and the Experience of European Expansion*. London: Routledge, 1988.

Maehle, Andreas-Holger. *Drugs on Trial: Experimental Pharmacology and Therapeutic Innovation in the Eighteenth Century*. Amsterdam: Rodopi, 1999.

Manderson, Leonore. *Sickness and the State: Health and Illness in Colonial Malaya, 1870–1940*. Cambridge: Cambridge University Press.

Mapp, Paul W. *The Elusive West and the Contest for Empire, 1713–1763*. Chapel Hill: University of North Carolina Press, 2011.

Marcus, Geoffrey. *Quiberon Bay: The Campaign in Home Waters, 1759*. London: Hollis & Carter, 1960.

Marshall, P. J. *Bengal: The British Bridgehead; Eastern India, 1740–1828*. Cambridge: Cambridge University Press, 1987.

———. *East Indian Fortunes: The British in Bengal in the Eighteenth Century*. Oxford: Clarendon Press, 1976.

———, ed. *The Eighteenth Century in Indian History: Evolution or Revolution?* New Delhi: Oxford University Press, 2005.

———. *The Making and Unmaking of Empires: Britain, India, and America, c. 1750–1783*. Oxford: Oxford University Press, 2005.

———. *Problems of Empire: Britain and India, 1757–1813*. London: Allen and Unwin.

———. "The Thirteen Colonies in the Seven Years' War: The View from London." In *Britain and America Go to War: The Impact of War and Warfare, 1754–1815*, edited by Julie Flavell and Stephen Conway, 69–94. Gainesville: University Press of Florida, 2004.

Marshall, Tabitha. "Surgeons Reconsidered: Military Medical Men of the American Revolution." *Canadian Bulletin of Medical History* 27:2 (2010): 299–319.

Marston, Daniel. *The Seven Years' War*. Oxford: Osprey, 2001.

Marvel, William. *Andersonville: The Last Depot*. Chapel Hill: University of North Carolina Press, 1994.

Massie, Alastair W. "John Manners, Marquess of Granby (1721–1770)." In *Oxford Dictionary of National Biography*. Oxford University Press, 2004–. Accessed 20 Dec. 2010. doi:10.1093/ref:odnb/17958.

Massons, José Maria. *Historia de la sanidad militar española*. 4 vols. Barcelona: Pomares-Corredor, 1994.

Mathai, Dilip, and A. George Vasanthan. "State of the Globe: Yellow Fever Is Still Around and Active!' *Journal of Global Infectious Diseases* 1:1 (2009): 4–6.

Mathias, Peter. "Swords into Ploughshares: The Armed Forces, Medicine and Public Health in the Late Eighteenth Century." In *War and Economic Development: Essays in Memory of David Joslin*, edited by J. M. Winter, 73–90. Cambridge: Cambridge University Press, 1975.

Mathias, Peter, and Patrick O'Brien. "Taxation in Great Britain and France, 1715–1810." *Journal of European Economic History* 5 (1976): 601–50.

McBride, William. "'Normal' Medical Science and British Treatment of the Sea Scurvy, 1753–75." *Journal of the History of Medicine and Allied Sciences* 46 (1991): 158–77.

McClellan, James E., and François Regourd. *The Colonial Machine: French Science and Overseas Expansion in the Old Regime*. Turnhout: Brepols, 2012.

McConnell, Michael N. *Army and Empire: British Soldiers on the American Frontier, 1758–1775*. Lincoln: University of Nebraska Press, 2004.

———. *A Country Between: The Upper Ohio Valley and Its Peoples, 1724–1774*. Lincoln: University of Nebraska Press, 1992.

McKeogh, Colm. *Innocent Civilians: The Morality of Killing in War*. Basingstoke, UK: Palgrave, 2002.

McLynn, Frank. *1759: The Year Britain Became Master of the World*. London: Jonathan Cape, 2004.

McNairn, Alan. *Behold the Hero: General Wolfe and the Arts in the Eighteenth Century*. Montreal: McGill-Queen's University Press, 1997.

McNeill, John Robert. *Atlantic Empires of France and Spain: Louisbourg and Havana, 1700–1763*. Chapel Hill: University of North Carolina Press, 1985.

———. "The Ecological Basis of Warfare in the Caribbean, 1700–1804." In *Adapting to Conditions: War and Society in the Eighteenth Century*, edited by Maarten Ultee, 26–42. Tuscaloosa: University of Alabama Press, 1986.

———. "Epidemics, Environment and Empire: Yellow Fever and Geopolitics in the American Tropics, 1650–1825." *Environment and History* 5 (1999): 175–84.

———. *Mosquito Empires: Ecology and War in the Greater Caribbean, 1620–1914*. Cambridge: Cambridge University Press, 2010.

Middleton, Richard. *The Bells of Victory: The Pitt-Newcastle Ministry and the Conduct of the Seven Years' War, 1757–1762*. Cambridge: Cambridge University Press, 1985.

———. "British Naval Strategy, 1755–1762: The Western Squadron." *Mariner's Mirror* 75 (1989): 349–67.

———. "Naval Administration in the Age of Pitt and Anson, 1755–1763." In *The British*

Navy and the Use of Naval Power in the Eighteenth Century, edited by Jeremy Black and Philip Woodfine, 109–27. Leicester: Leicester University Press, 1988.

———. "Pitt, Anson and the Admiralty, 1756–1761." *History* 55:184 (1970): 189–98.

———. *Pontiac's War: Its Causes, Course and Consequences*. London: Routledge, 2007.

Miller, Genevieve. *The Adoption of Inoculation for Smallpox in England and France*. Philadelphia: University of Pennsylvania Press, 1957.

Mokyr, Joel. *The Gifts of Athena: Historical Origins of the Knowledge Economy*. Princeton, NJ: Princeton University Press, 2002.

Monath, Thomas P. "Yellow Fever: An Update." *Lancet Infectious Diseases* 1 (2001): 11–20.

Morgan, Rod. "John Howard (1726?–1790)." In *Oxford Dictionary of National Biography*. Oxford University Press, 2004–. Accessed 27 June 2011. doi: 10.1093/ref:odnb/13922.

Morieux, Renaud. "French Prisoners of War, Conflicts of Honour, and Social Inversions in England, 1744–1783." *Historical Journal* 56:1 (March 2013): 55–88.

———. "Patriotisme humanitaire et prisonniers de guerre en France et en Grande-Bretagne pendant la Révolution française et l'Empire." In *La politique par les armes: Conflits internationaux et politisation (XVe–XIXe siècle)*, edited by Laurent Bourquin et al., 299–314. Rennes: Presses universitaires de Rennes, 2014.

Morris, Roger. *The Foundations of British Maritime Ascendancy: Resources, Logistics and the State, 1755–1815*. Cambridge: Cambridge University Press, 2011.

Neff, Stephen C. *War and the Law of Nations: A General History*. Cambridge: Cambridge University Press, 2005.

Newman, Gerald. *The Rise of English Nationalism: A Cultural History, 1740–1830*. New rev. ed. Basingstoke, UK: Macmillan, 1997.

Norberg, Kathryn. "Bodies in European and American Historiography." *William and Mary Quarterly* 68:4 (2011): 686–89.

O'Brien, P. K. "The Political Economy of British Taxation, 1660–1815." *Economic History Review*, 2nd ser., 41 (1988): 1–32.

Olson, Donald W., et al. "Perfect Tide, Ideal Moon: An Unappreciated Aspect of Wolfe's Generalship at Quebec, 1759." *William and Mary Quarterly*, 3rd ser., 59:4 (2002): 957–74.

O'Shaughnessy, Andrew. "Redcoats and Slaves in the British Caribbean." In *The Lesser Antilles in the Age of European Expansion*, edited by Robert Paquette and Stanley Engerman, 105–27. Gainesville: University of Florida Press, 1996.

Packer, Randall M. *The Making of a Tropical Disease: A Short History of Malaria*. Baltimore: Johns Hopkins University Press, 2007.

Pande, Ishita. *Medicine, Race and Liberalism in British Bengal: Symptoms of Empire*. London: Routledge, 2010.

Parcero Torre, Celia María. *La pérdida de La Habana y las reformas borbónicas en Cuba*. Valladolid, Spain: Junta de Castilla y León, Consejería de Educación y Cultura, 1998.

Pares, Richard. "American versus Continental Warfare, 1739–1763." *English Historical Review* 51:203 (1936): 429–65.

———. *War and Trade in the West Indies, 1739–1763*. London: Frank Cass, 1963.

Pargellis, Stanley. *Lord Loudoun in North America.* New Haven, CT: Yale University Press, 1933.

Parkman, Francis. *Montcalm and Wolfe.* 2 vols. London: Macmillan, 1884.

Parrott, David. *The Business of War: Military Enterprise and Military Revolution in Early Modern Europe.* Cambridge: Cambridge University Press, 2012.

Pearson, M. N. "The Thin Edge of the Wedge: Medical Relativities as a Paradigm of Early Modern Indian-Europeans Relations." *Modern Asian Studies* 29:1 (1995): 141–70.

Peers, Douglas M. "Colonial Knowledge and the Military in India, 1780–1860." *Journal of Imperial and Commonwealth History* 33:2 (2005): 157–80.

———. "Revolution, Evolution, or Devolution: The Military and the Making of Colonial India." In *Empires and Indigenes: Intercultural Alliance, Imperial Expansion, and Warfare in the Early Modern World,* edited by Wayne E. Lee, 81–106. London: New York University Press, 2011.

Pelling, Margaret. *The Common Lot: Sickness, Medical Occupations and the Urban Poor in Early Modern England; Essays.* London: Longman, 1998.

———. "Contagion/Germ Theory/Specificity." In *Companion Encyclopedia of the History of Medicine,* edited by W. F. Bynum and Roy Porter, 1:309–34. London: Routledge, 1993.

Peters, Marie. *Pitt and Popularity: The Patriot Minister and London Opinion during the Seven Years' War.* Oxford: Clarendon Press, 1980.

Pietsch, Roland. "Urchins for the Sea: The Story of the Marine Society in the Seven Years War." *Journal for Maritime Research,* December 2000, 1–18.

Pincus, Steve. "Rethinking Mercantilism: Political Economy, the British Empire, and the Atlantic World in the Seventeenth and Eighteenth Centuries." *William and Mary Quarterly,* 3rd ser., 69:1 (2012): 3–34.

Pluchon, Pierre. *Histoire des médecins et pharmaciens de marine et des colonies.* Toulouse: Privat, 1985.

Poovey, Mary. *A History of the Modern Fact: Problems of Knowledge in the Sciences of Wealth and Society.* Chicago: University of Chicago Press, 1998.

Pope, Dudley. *At Twelve Mr. Byng Was Shot.* An Alison Press Book. London: Secker & Warburg, 1987.

Porter, Dorothy, and Roy Porter. *Patient's Progress: Doctors and Doctoring in Eighteenth-Century England.* Stanford, CA: Stanford University Press, 1989.

Porter, Roy, ed. *The Cambridge History of Science.* Vol. 4, *Eighteenth-Century Science.* Cambridge: Cambridge University Press, 2003.

———. *Disease, Medicine and Society in England, 1550–1860.* Basingstoke, UK: Macmillan Education, 1987.

———. *Doctor of Society: Thomas Beddoes and the Sick Trade in Late-Enlightenment England.* London: Routledge, 1992.

———. *Enlightenment: Britain and the Creation of the Modern World.* London: Allen Lane, 2000.

———. "The Gift Relation: Philanthropy and Provincial Hospitals in Eighteenth-Century England." In *The Hospital in History,* edited by Roy Porter and Lindsay Patricia Granshaw, 149–78. London: Routledge, 1989.

———. *Health for Sale: Quackery in England, 1660–1850*. Manchester: Manchester University Press, 1989.

———, ed. *Patients and Practitioners: Lay Perceptions of Medicine in Pre-Industrial Society*. Cambridge: Cambridge University Press, 1985.

Porter, Roy, and John Brewer, eds. *Consumption and the World of Goods*. London: Routledge, 1993.

Porter, Roy, and Lindsay Patricia Granshaw, eds. *The Hospital in History*. London: Routledge, 1989.

Porter, Theodore M. "Statistics and the Career of Public Reason: Engagement and Detachment in a Quantified World." In *Statistics and the Public Sphere: Numbers and the People in Modern Britain, c. 1800–2000*, edited by Tom Crook and Glen O'Hara, 32–47. New York: Routledge, 2011.

———. *Trust in Numbers: The Pursuit of Objectivity in Science and Public Life*. Princeton, NJ: Princeton University Press, 1995.

Prinzing, Friedrich. *Epidemics Resulting from Wars*. Edited by Harald Westergaard. Oxford: Clarendon Press, 1916.

Prior, D. L. "John Zephaniah Howell (1711–1798)." In *Oxford Dictionary of National Biography*. Oxford University Press, 2004–. Accessed 9 Dec. 2006. doi:10.1093/ref:odnb/13622.

Pritchard, James. "From Shipwright to Naval Constructor: The Professionalization of 18th-Century French Naval Shipbuilders." *Technology and Culture* 28:1 (1987): 1–25.

———. "Le problème de l'Amérique du Nord dans la science nautique française aux XVIIe et XVIIIe siècles." In *Les Marines de guerre européennes, XVII–XVIIIe siècles*, edited by Martine Acerra, José Merino, and Jean Meyer, 331–44. Paris: Presses Paris Sorbonne, 1998.

———. *Louis XV's Navy, 1748–1762: A Study of Organization and Administration*. Kingston: McGill-Queen's University Press, 1987.

Rabier, Christelle. "Introduction: Expertise in Historical Perspectives." In *Fields of Expertise: A Comparative History of Expert Procedures in Paris and London, 1600 to Present*, edited by Christelle Rabier, 1–33. Newcastle: Cambridge Scholars Publishing, 2007.

Rabinow, Paul. *French Modern: Norms and Forms of the Social Environment*. Cambridge, MA: MIT Press, 1989.

Ranlet, Philip. "The British, Their Virginian Prisoners, and Prison Ships of the American Revolution." *American Neptune* 60:3 (2000): 253–62.

Razzell, P. E. *The Conquest of Smallpox: The Impact of Inoculation on Smallpox Mortality in Eighteenth Century Britain*. London: Caliban Books, 1977.

Rees, David C., Thomas N. Williams, and Mark T. Gladwin. "Sickle-Cell Disease." *The Lancet* 376:9757 (2010): 2018–203.

Reid, Stuart. "Simon Fraser, Master of Lovat (1726–1782)." In *Oxford Dictionary of National Biography*. Oxford University Press, 2004–. Accessed 9 Dec. 2006. doi: 10.1093/ref:odnb/10124.

Reynolds, W. M. "Inoculation for the Smallpox in Colonial America." *Bulletin of the History of Medicine* 22 (1948): 273–76.

Richter, Daniel. *Facing East from Indian Country: A Native History of Early America.* Cambridge, MA: Harvard University Press, 2001.

Riley, James C. *The Eighteenth-Century Campaign to Avoid Disease.* New York: St. Martin's Press, 1987.

———. *Population Thought in the Age of the Demographic Revolution.* Durham, NC: Carolina Academic Press, 1985.

Risse, Guenter B. *Hospital Life in Enlightenment Scotland: Care and Teaching at the Royal Infirmary of Edinburgh.* Cambridge: Cambridge University Press, 1986.

Ritchie, M. K., and C. I. A. Ritchie. "The Troubles of a Commissary during the Seven Years War." *Journal of the Society for Army Historical Research* 36:148 (1958): 157–64.

Robson, Eric. "The Armed Forces and the Art of War." In *The New Cambridge Modern History*, vol. 7, *The Old Regime, 1713–1763*, edited by J. O. Lindsay, 163–90. Cambridge: Cambridge University Press, 1957.

Rodger, N. A. M. *The Command of the Ocean: A Naval History of Britain.* London: Penguin, 2005.

———. "La mobilisation navale au XVIIIe siècle." In *État, marine et société*, edited by Martine Acerra et al., 365–74. Paris: Presses de l'Université de Paris-Sorbonne, 1995.

———. "Le scorbut dans la Royal Navy pendant la guerre de Sept Ans, 1756–1763." In *Les hommes et la mer dans l'Europe du Nord-Ouest de l'antiquité à nos jours: Actes du colloque de Boulogne-sur-Mer, 15–17 Juin 1984*, edited by Jean Claude Hocquet, Stéphane Lebecq, and Alain Lottin, 455–62. Villeneuve-d'Ascq, France: Revue du Nord, 1986.

———. "Medicine and Science in the British Navy of the Eighteenth Century." In *L'homme, la santé et la mer: Actes du colloque international tenu à l'Institut catholique de Paris les 5 et 6 décembre 1995*, edited by Christian Buchet, 333–44. Paris: H. Champion, 1997.

———. "The Victualling of the British Navy during the Seven Years' War." *Bulletin du Centre d'Histoire des Espaces Atlantiques* 2 (1985): 37–53.

———. *The Wooden World: An Anatomy of the Georgian Navy.* London: Fontana, 1988.

Rogers, Clifford J., ed. *The Military Revolution Debate: Readings on the Military Transformation of Early Modern Europe.* Boulder, CO: Westview, 1995.

Rogers, Nicholas. *Whigs and Cities: Popular Politics in the Age of Walpole and Pitt.* Oxford: Oxford University Press, 1989.

Rogers, Nicholas, and Gerald Jordan. "Admirals as Heroes: Patriotism and Liberty in Hanoverian England." *Journal of British Studies* 28:3 (1989): 20124.

Rublack, Ulinka. "Fluxes: The Early Modern Body and the Emotions." Translated by Pamela Selwyn. *History Workshop Journal* 53 (2002): 1–16.

Rusnock, Andrea. *Vital Accounts: Quantifying Health and Population in Eighteenth-Century England and France.* Cambridge: Cambridge University Press, 2002.

Ryan, A. N. "The Royal Navy and the Blockade of Brest, 1689–1805: Theory and Practice." In *Les Marines de guerre européennes, XVII–XVIIIe siècles*, edited by Martine Acerra, José Merino, and Jean Meyer, 175–93. Paris: Presses de l'Université de Paris-Sorbonne, 1985.

Sankey, Margaret. *Jacobite Prisoners of the 1715 Rebellion: Preventing and Punishing Insurrection in Early Hanoverian Britain*. Aldershot, UK: Ashgate, 2005.

Sardet, Michel. *L'École de chirurgie du port de Rochefort (1722–1789): Un modèle sous l'Ancien Régime*. Vincennes: Service historique de la Marine, 2000.

Savory, Reginald. "The Convention of Écluse, 1759–1762." *Journal for the Society of Army Historical Research* 42 (1964): 68–77.

———. *His Britannic Majesty's Army in Germany during the Seven Years War*. Oxford: Clarendon Press, 1966.

Schaffer, Simon. "Self-Evidence." In *Questions of Evidence: Proof, Practice, and Persuasion across the Disciplines*, edited by James K. Chandler, Arnold Ira Davidson, and Harry D. Harootunian, 56–91. Chicago: University of Chicago Press, 1994.

Schumann, Matt, and Karl W. Schweizer. *The Seven Years War: A Transatlantic History*. London: Routledge, 2007.

Scott, Hamish M. "The Fiscal-Military State and International Rivalry during the Long Eighteenth Century." In *The Fiscal-Military State in Eighteenth-Century Europe: Essays in Honour of P. G. M. Dickson*, edited by Christopher Storrs, 23–54. Farnham, UK: Ashgate, 2009.

———. "The Seven Years' War and Europe's *Ancien Regime*." *War in History* 18:4 (2011): 419–55.

Scott, H. M., and Brendan Simms, eds. *Cultures of Power in Europe during the Long Eighteenth Century*. Cambridge: Cambridge University Press, 2007.

Scott, Susan, S. R. Duncan, and C. J. Duncan. "The Dynamics of Smallpox Epidemics in Britain, 1550–1800." *Demography* 30:3 (1993): 405–23.

———. "An Hypothesis for the Periodicity of Smallpox Epidemics as Revealed by Time Series Analysis." *Journal of Theoretical Biology* 160 (1993): 231–48.

Scouller, R. E. *The Armies of Queen Anne*. Oxford: Clarendon Press, 1966.

Selesky, Harold E. *War and Society in Colonial Connecticut*. New Haven, CT: Yale University Press, 1990.

Selinger, Evan, and Robert P. Crease, eds. *The Philosophy of Expertise*. New York: Columbia University Press, 2006.

Shapin, Steven. *A Social History of Truth: Civility and Science in Seventeenth-Century England*. Chicago: University of Chicago Press, 1994.

Shapin, Steven, and Simon Schaffer. *Leviathan and the Air-Pump: Hobbes, Boyle, and the Experimental Life*. Princeton, NJ: Princeton University Press, 2011.

Showalter, Dennis E. *The Wars of Frederick the Great*. London: Longman, 1996.

Shukla, R. N., and B. R. Solanki. "Sickle-Cell Trait in Central India." *The Lancet* 1:7015 (1958): 297–98.

Shy, John. *Toward Lexington: The Role of the British Army in the Coming of the American Revolution*. Princeton, NJ: Princeton University Press, 1965.

Simms, Brendan. "'Ministers of Europe': British Strategic Culture, 1714–1760." In *Cultures of Power in Europe during the Long Eighteenth Century*, edited by H. M. Scott and Brendan Simms, 110–57. Cambridge: Cambridge University Press, 2007.

———. *Three Victories and a Defeat: The Rise and Fall of the First British Empire*. London: Penguin, 2008.

Skaggs, David Curtis, and Larry L. Nelson, eds. *The Sixty Years' War for the Great Lakes, 1754–1814*. East Lansing: Michigan State University Press, 2001.

Slack, Paul. *From Reformation to Improvement: Public Welfare in Early Modern England*. Oxford: Clarendon Press, 1998.

Smelser, Marshall. *The Campaign for the Sugar Islands, 1759: A Study of Amphibious Warfare*. Chapel Hill: University of North Carolina Press, 1955.

Snyder, John C. "Typhus Fever Rickettsiae." In *Viral and Rickettsial Infections of Man*, edited by Frank L. Harsfall and Igor Tamm, 1059–94. 4th ed. Philadelphia: Lippincott, 1965.

Solkin, David H. *Painting for Money: The Visual Arts and the Public Sphere in Eighteenth-Century England*. New Haven, CT: Yale University Press, 1993.

———. "Portraiture in Motion: Edward Penny's 'Marquis of Granby' and the Creation of a Public for English Art." *Huntington Library Quarterly* 49 (1986): 1–23.

Speelman, Patrick J. "Conclusion: Father of the Modern Age." In *The Seven Years' War: Global Views*, edited by Mark H. Danley and Patrick J. Speelman, 519–36. Leiden: Brill, 2012.

Springer, Paul J. *America's Captives: Treatment of POWs from the Revolutionary War to the War on Terror*. Lawrence: University Press of Kansas, 2010.

Stacey, C. P. *Quebec, 1759: The Siege and the Battle*. Edited and revised by Donald E Graves. Toronto: Robin Brass Studio, 2002.

Steele, Ian K. *Guerillas and Grenadiers: The Struggle for Canada, 1689–1760*. Toronto: Ryerson Press, 1969.

———. "Surrendering Rites: Prisoners on Colonial North American Frontiers." In *Hanoverian Britain and Empire: Essays in Memory of Philip Lawson*, edited by Stephen Taylor et al., 137–57. Woodbridge, UK: Boydell Press, 1998.

Stein, Stanley J., and Barbara H. Stein. *Apogee of Empire: Spain and New Spain in the Age of Charles III, 1759–1789*. Baltimore: Johns Hopkins University Press.

Stepan, Nancy. "Race, Gender, Science and Citizenship." *Gender and History* 10:1 (1998): 26–52.

———. "Tropical Medicine and Public Health in Latin America." *Medical History* 42 (1998): 104–12.

Stern, Philip J. *The Company-State: Corporate Sovereignty and the Early Modern Foundations of the British Empire in India*. Oxford: Oxford University Press, 2011.

Stevenson, Christine. *Medicine and Magnificence: British Hospital and Asylum Architecture, 1660–1815*. New Haven, CT: Yale University Press, 2000.

Stevenson, L. G. "A Note on the Relation of Military Service to Licensing in the History of British Surgery." *Bulletin of the History of Medicine* 27 (1953): 420–27.

Stewart, Larry. "Experimental Spaces and the Knowledge Economy." *History of Science* 45 (2007): 155–77.

———. *The Rise of Public Science: Rhetoric, Technology, and Natural Philosophy in Newtonian Britain, 1660–1750*. Cambridge: Cambridge University Press, 1992.

Stewart, Larry, and Margaret C. Jacob. *Practical Matter: Newton's Science in the Service of Industry and Empire*. Cambridge, MA: Harvard University Press, 2004.

Stoler, Ann Laura. *Race and the Education of Desire: Foucault's History of Sexuality and the Colonial Order of Things*. Durham, NC: Duke University Press, 1995.

Stone, Lawrence, ed. *An Imperial State at War: Britain from 1689 to 1815*. London: Routledge, 1994.

Storrs, Christopher, ed. *The Fiscal-Military State in Eighteenth-Century Europe: Essays in Honour of P. G. M. Dickson*. Farnham, UK: Ashgate, 2009.

———. "Introduction: The Fiscal-Military State in the 'Long' Eighteenth Century." In Storrs, *The Fiscal-Military State in Eighteenth-Century Europe*, 1–22.

Stott, Anne. *Hannah More: The First Victorian*. Oxford: Oxford University Press, 2003.

Strachan, Hew. *European Armies and the Conduct of War*. London: Allen & Unwin, 1983.

Sutherland, Lucy Stuart. *The East India Company in Eighteenth-Century Politics*. Oxford: Clarendon Press, 1952.

Sutton, Jean. *Lords of the East: The East India Company and Its Ships, 1600–1874*. New ed. London: Conway Maritime Press, 2000.

Syrett, David. "American Provincials and the Havana Campaign of 1762." *New York History* 49 (1968): 375–90.

———. "The Methodology of British Amphibious Operations during the Seven Years and American Wars." *Mariner's Mirror* 58 (1972): 269–80.

———. *Shipping and Military Power in the Seven Years War: The Sails of Victory*. Exeter: University of Exeter Press, 2008.

Szabo, Franz A. J. *The Seven Years War in Europe, 1756–1763*. Harlow, UK: Pearson Longman, 2008.

Taylor, G. "Clinical Manifestations of Vitamin Deficiencies." In *Starving Sailors: The Influence of Nutrition upon Naval and Maritime History*, edited by J. Watt, E. J. Freeman, and W. F. Bynum, 35–50. London: National Maritime Museum, 1981.

Teltscher, Kate. "'The Fearful Name of the Black Hole': The Fashioning of an Imperial Myth." In *Writing India, 1757–1990: The Literature of British India*, edited by B. J. Moore-Gilbert, 30–51. Manchester: Manchester University Press, 1996.

Thick, Malcolm. "Market Gardening in England and Wales." In *The Agrarian History of England and Wales*, vol. 5.2, *1640–1750: Agrarian Change*, edited by Jane Thirsk, 506–30. Cambridge: Cambridge University Press, 1985.

Tilly, Charles. *Coercion, Capital and European States, A.D. 990–1992*. Oxford: Blackwell, 1992.

Tomori, Oyewale. "Yellow Fever: The Recurring Plague." *Critical Reviews in Clinical Laboratory* 41:4 (2004): 391–427.

Topley, W. W. C., G. R. Smith, and C. S. F. Easman, eds. *Topley and Wilson's Principles of Bacteriology, Virology and Immunology*. 8th ed. London: Edward Arnold, 1990.

Travers, Robert. "Death and the Nabob: Imperialism and Commemoration in Eighteenth-Century India." *Past and Present* 196 (2007): 97–107.

———. *Ideology and Empire in Eighteenth-Century India*. Cambridge: Cambridge University Press, 2007.

Tröhler, Ulrich. *"To Improve the Evidence of Medicine": The 18th Century British Ori-*

gins of a Critical Approach. Edinburgh: Royal College of Physicians of Edinburgh, 2000.

Truxes, Thomas. *Defying Empire: Trading with the Enemy in Colonial New York*. New Haven, CT: Yale University Press, 2008.

Tuck, Richard. *The Rights of War and Peace: Political Thought and the International Order from Grotius to Kant*. Oxford: Oxford University Press, 1999.

Tunstall, Brian. *Admiral Byng and the Loss of Minorca*. London: P. Allan, 1928.

Turner, B. S. "The Rationalization of the Body: Reflections on Modernity and Discipline." In *The Body: Critical Concepts in Sociology*, edited by Andrew Blaikie, 320–40. London: Routledge, 2004.

Turner, Michael Edward, J. V Beckett, and B. Afton, eds. *Farm Production in England, 1700–1914*. Oxford: Oxford University Press, 2001.

Van Buskirk, Judith L. *Generous Enemies: Patriots and Loyalists in Revolutionary New York*. Philadelphia: University of Pennsylvania Press, 2002.

Van Orden, Kate. *Music, Discipline, and Arms in Early Modern France*. Chicago: University of Chicago Press, 2005.

Veyssière, Laurent, and Bertrand Fonck, eds. *La guerre de Sept Ans en Nouvelle-France*. Quebec City: Éditions du Septentrion, 2011.

Vigarello, Georges. *Concepts of Cleanliness: Changing Attitudes in France since the Middle Ages*. Translated by Jean Birrell. Cambridge: Cambridge University Press, 1988.

von Arni, Eric Gruber. *Hospital Care and the British Standing Army, 1660–1714*. Aldershot, UK: Ashgate, 2006.

Wahrman, Dror. *The Making of the Modern Self: Identity and Culture in Eighteenth-Century England*. New Haven, CT: Yale University Press, 2004.

Ward, Matthew C. *The Battle for Quebec, 1759*. Stroud, UK: Tempus, 2005.

———. *Breaking the Backcountry: The Seven Years' War in Virginia and Pennsylvania, 1754–1765*. Pittsburgh: University of Pittsburgh Press, 2003.

———. "Understanding Native American Alliances." In *The Seven Years' War: Global Views*, edited by Mark H. Danley and Patrick J. Speelman, 47–72. Leiden: Brill, 2012.

Webb, W. W. "Richard Huck Saunders (1720–1785)." Revised by Jeffrey S. Reznick. In *Oxford Dictionary of National Biography*. Oxford University Press, 2004–. Accessed 9 Aug. 2012. doi:10.1093/ref:odnb/24703.

Weiss, Kimberly. "The Role of Rickettsioses in History." In *Biology of Rickettsial Diseases*, edited by David H. Walker, 1–14. Boca Raton, FL: CRC Press, 1988.

Wheeler, Roxann. *The Complexion of Race: Categories of Difference in Eighteenth-Century British Culture*. Philadelphia: University of Pennsylvania Press, 2000.

Whitworth, Rex. *William Augustus, Duke of Cumberland: A Life*. London: Leo Cooper, 1992.

Wickremesekera, Channa. *"Best Black Troops in the World": British Perception and the Making of the Sepoy, 1746–1805*. New Delhi: Manohar, 2002.

Wilkinson, Clive. *The British Navy and the State in the Eighteenth Century*. Woodbridge, UK: Boydell Press in association with the National Maritime Museum, 2004.

Wilson, Jon E. *The Domination of Strangers: Modern Governance in Eastern India, 1780–1835*. Basingstoke, UK: Palgrave Macmillan, 2008.

Wilson, Kathleen. *The Island Race: Englishness, Empire, and Gender in the Eighteenth Century*. London: Routledge, 2003.

———. *The Sense of the People: Politics, Culture and Imperialism in England, 1715–1785*. Cambridge: Cambridge University Press, 1995.

Wilson, Leonard G. "Fevers." In *Companion Encyclopedia of the History of Medicine*, edited by W. F. Bynum and Roy Porter, 1:382–411. London: Routledge, 1993.

Wilson, Peter H. "Prisoners in Early Modern European Warfare." In *Prisoners in War*, edited by Sibylle Scheipers, 39–56. Oxford: Oxford University Press, 2010.

Woodward, J. H. *"To do the Sick no Harm": A Study of the British Voluntary Hospital System to 1875*. London: Routledge & Kegan Paul, 1974.

Wootton, David. *Bad Medicine: Doctors Doing Harm since Hippocrates*. Oxford: Oxford University Press, 2006.

Worboys, Michael. "The Emergence of Tropical Medicine." In *Perspectives on the Emergence of Scientific Disciplines*, edited by Gérard Lemaine, Roy Macleod, Michael Mulkay, and Peter Weingart, 75–98. The Hague: Mouton, 1976.

———. "Tropical Diseases." In *Companion Encyclopedia of the History of Medicine*, edited by W. F. Bynum and Roy Porter, 1:512–36. London: Routledge, 1993.

Zinsser, Hans. *Rats, Lice, & History: Being a Study in Biography, which, after Twelve Preliminary Chapters Indispensable for the Preparation of the Lay Reader, Deals with the Life History of Typhus Fever*. London: Routledge, 1935.

Unpublished Works

Baugh, Daniel. "A War on Water: The Role of the Geographical Extremities in British Success, 1755–1763." Plenary lecture presented at the conference "A War for Empire: The Seven Years War in Context," London, 13 July 2006.

Berry, Amanda. "Patronage, Funding and the Hospital Patient, c. 1750–1815: Three English Regional Case Studies." D.Phil. thesis, University of Oxford, 1995.

Harding, Richard. "The Royal Navy in the West Indies: Expectations and Outcomes for Control of the Sea in Peace and War, 1713–1748." Paper presented at the annual meeting for the Society for Military History, New Orleans, Louisiana, 14–17 March 2013.

Little, H. M. "The Treasury, the Commissariat and the Supply of the Combined Army in Germany during the Seven Years War (1756–1763)." Ph.D. thesis, University of London, 1981.

Marshall, Tabitha. "The Health of the British Soldier in America, 1775–1781." PhD diss., McMaster University, 2006.

Meier, Henry. "Smallpox in Stuart London: Causes and Effects of an Emerging Disease." D.Phil. thesis, University of Oxford, 2009.

Norris, Sorcha. "The Administration of Prisoners of War based in Exeter during the Seven Years War." Undergraduate thesis, University of Oxford, 2012.

Siena, Kevin. "Investigating Westminster Prison Deaths, 1762–1799." Paper presented at the annual meeting for the American Association for the History of Medicine, Cleveland, Ohio, 23–26 April 2009.

Steppler, Glenn A. "The Common Soldier in the Reign of George III, 1760–1793." D.Phil. thesis, University of Oxford, 1984.

Williams, Mark. "Encountering the French: A New Approach to National Identity in England in the Eighteenth Century." PhD diss., University of Sussex, 2010.

INDEX

Académie de Marine (French), 137
acclimatization, 13, 19–20, 193; seasoned troops, 66–67, 70, 83–84
Account of the Manner of Inoculating for the Small Pox in the East Indies (Holwell), 149–50, 154, 158
administration, military, 100–109
administration, naval, 120–21, 130–31, 134–35. *See also* Admiralty, Royal Navy
Admiralty, Royal Navy, 127, 131, 134–35, 140; Sick and Hurt Board, 126, 130–38, 139, 152, 176; Victualing Board, 126–27
Albemarle, 3rd Earl of (George Keppel), 54, 66–67, 69–77, 80, 105, 107
American identity, 9, 48–52, 68, 80–81
American War of Independence, 47, 50–51, 79, 80, 100; prisoners of war, 189–90; returns, 106, 108
Amherst, Jeffrey: correspondence, 32–33, 107; Pontiac's War, 80, 216n149; provincials, 41, 46–49; scurvy, 25, 27–28; West Indian campaign, 67–70, 74, 76, 79–80
Anson, George, 22, 84, 125–27
auxiliaries: disease, 14, 16–17, 40–51, 74, 169–70, 192–93; Highlanders, 31, 39–40, 208n83; Native Americans, 20, 29, 45; provincial soldiers, 47–51, 67–70 (*see also* provincials); Rangers, 40, 46; recruitment, 12, 17, 66–67, 169–71, 192; sepoys, 162–63, 169–70

Barrington, John, 62–65
Barrington, 2nd Viscount (William Wildman), 62, 100–103, 106, 114–15
Bills of Mortality, 44, 109. *See also* quantitative methods
black vomit. *See* yellow fever
blue-water policy, 112–14. *See also* foreign policy
Boscawen, Edward, 122, 127, 129
Brocklesby, Richard: career, 97–98, 100; experiments, 99–100; fevers and hospitals, 94, 96; smallpox, 43–44, 48
Byng, John, 108, 115, 122, 140–41

Calcutta, Black Hole of, 142, 159–60, 231n85
Calcutta, retaking of and battle of Plassey (1756–57), 159–61
camp fever, 42, 94. *See also* fevers; typhus
camps, army: conditions, 42; diseases, 40–42, 50, 91–95; regulations, 91–93
Cartagena, battle of (1741), 53, 66
censorship, 81, 115–17
charity. *See* philanthropy
Chelsea, 152
civilian-military relations, 12–13, 89. *See also* prisoners of war; public opinion
cleanliness. *See* sanitation
climate, foreign: German, 101, 113, 118–19; tropical, 13, 57–60, 150, 154–59, 167–68. *See also* tropical medicine
Clive, Robert, 151, 152, 161–63, 167, 169–70
colonial newspapers, 77–79
colonial warfare: compared with European warfare, 119; historiography, 9–10
colonists. *See* empire; provincials
Commissariat, 90, 114–15

constitutions, physical and moral, 14, 41–42, 48–50, 70, 150, 192–94. *See also* acclimatization; race
contracting, 90–91
Coote, Eyre, 161, 162–63, 165–67
correspondence, medical. *See under* medicine, imperial networks; Pringle, John
crowd diseases, 42, 87, 94, 159. *See also* diarrheal diseases; fevers; typhus
Cumberland, Duke of (Prince William Augustus), 11–12, 42–43, 45, 89–90, 118

Death of Wolfe, The (West), 1–2, 28
desertion, 29, 48, 53, 77, 89, 91, 137. *See also* discipline
diarrheal diseases, 12, 42, 72, 91, 93–96. *See also* crowd diseases
discipline, military and naval, 12, 14, 91, 139; camp orders, 91–93; European identity, 169–71
disease: constitutions, 14, 41–42, 48–50, 70, 150, 192–94; differential immunity, 60, 82, 170; as disorder, 4–5, 12, 13–14, 119, 158; retro-diagnosis, 6, 94
disease, rates of: army compared with navy, 139–40; British compared with other nations' forces, 83–84, 137–38, 197–98. *See also* returns
dissections, 34, 35, 155. *See also* observations, medical
Durant, Guy, 61, 62
dysentery. *See* diarrheal diseases

East India Company, the: British state, 10, 143–44; medical care, 152–53; medical careers, 141–48; Poplar Fund, 152; recruitment, 151–52; transportation of troops, 153–54; troops, 151–52
effluvium, 96. *See also* miasma; putrefaction
empire, 8–9, 56–57, 65, 150, 168–69; adaptive, 11; colonial contributions, 67–70, 80–81; theory, 56–57. *See also* blue-water policy; foreign policy
enlistment. *See* recruitment
Essay on Diseases Incidental to Europeans in Hot Climates, An (Lind), 57–60, 154–59, 168, 192–93
Essay towards the Improvement of Physick, An (Bellers), 110
Estimate of the Manners and Principles of the Times, An (Brown), 109–10
experiments, 24, 99–100, 123, 131–36; practitioners' status, 136, 140; onboard HMS *Salisbury*, 22, 121
expertise, definition of, 6–7

Ferdinand, Prince of Brunswick, 89, 91, 111, 114–15
fevers, 12, 42, 59, 61, 87, 93–96, 97, 132, 154, 155–56. *See also* crowd diseases; malaria; typhus; yellow fever
fiscal-military state, 3, 4, 10
flux. *See* diarrheal diseases
foraging, 25, 89–90
foreign policy, 56–57, 86–87, 88–89. *See also* blue-water policy
Foucault, Michel, 192
Fraser, Malcolm, 39. *See also* Highlanders
Fullerton, William, 146–47

gardens, 25
Granby, Marquis of (John Manners), 1, 100–102, 111, 114, 198. See also *Marquis of Granby* (Penny)
Greenwich, 152
Grenville, George, 181, 188
Guadeloupe, campaign of (1758), 61–65

Hanover, 86, 88–89, 112–13. *See also* blue-water policy
Hanway, Jonas, 111, 185
Haslar, 22, 34, 132–33
Havana, expedition to (1762), 65–85
Hawke, Edward, 122–23, 126, 127, 128–30
Hayman, Francis, 2, 5, 198
Highlanders: regiments, 31, 39–40, 208n83; sickness, 38–39, 74
Holwell, John Zephaniah, 142, 149–50, 154, 158
Hopson, Peregrine, 61–63, 82, 107
hospital fever, 24, 93–96. *See also* fevers; typhus
hospitals: Chelsea, 152; claims of mismanagement, 100–102, 114; convalescent soldiers, 97, 101; disease, 95–97; experiments, 98–100, 132–33; Greenwich, 152; Haslar, 22, 34, 132–33; malingering, 97; military compared with civilian, 98–100, 108; naval compared with military, 140; nurses, 99; order, 96–100; practitioners' authority and status, 98–100; reform, 117–18; staff, 97

Howard, John, 117, 191
Huck, Richard, 35, 37, 40, 60, 98
Hulton, Henry, 90, 218n18
hygiene. *See* sanitation

immunity, differential, 60, 82, 170. *See also* constitutions, physical and moral
inoculation. *See under* smallpox
international law. *See* laws of war
irregulars. *See* auxiliaries
Ives, Edward, 148–49, 153, 156, 167

Jacobitism, 39, 183
jail fever, 94. *See also* fevers; prisons; typhus

Lally, Thomas, comte de, 164–66
Law of Nations, The (Vattel), 178–79, 187
laws of war, 178–79, 187
Les sauvages de l'Europe (Lesuire), 186–87
Lind, James: career, 19, 22, 133, 136; *Essay on Diseases Incidental to Europeans in Hot Climates*, 57–60, 146, 154–59, 168, 192–93; *Essay on the Most Effectual Means of Preserving the Health of Seamen*, 57; theory of hot climates, 58–60, 70, 154–59, 168; theory of scurvy, 22–24, 25–26, 33–35, 41, 123–24, 135; *Treatise on the Scurvy*, 22, 34, 123–24, 133–34, 154; trial and lemon juice, 22, 121, 123, 126
logistics. *See* mobilization, naval; provisioning; recruitment, returns
Loudoun, 4th Earl of (John Campbell), 37, 42, 45–46
Louisbourg, siege of (1757–58), 25, 27, 46, 61, 175

malaria, 73, 150, 155–59, 159–60, 166–68. *See also* fevers; climate
malingering, 97
Marine Society, 111, 185
Marquis of Granby (Penny), 1, 2, 5, 198
Martinique, campaign of (1758), 61, 67
Mauduit, Israel, 3, 112–13
meat. *See under* provisions
medicine: hospital, 99–100; imperial, 13, 144–45; indigenous, 12, 26, 148–50; moderation as, 158–59; practice, eighteenth-century, 36; scientific and empirical, 35–36, 98–100, 135–38, 194; structure, eighteenth-century, 6, 36, 55, 98, 195–96. *See also* medicine, military and naval; medicine, imperial networks; tropical medicine
medicine, imperial networks, 35–36, 36–37, 40–41, 59–60, 94
medicine, military and naval: hospitals, 96–100; profession, 97–100; regimental medicine, 37–38; structure, 8, 36. *See also* hospitals; observations, medical; practitioners, military medical; tropical medicine
miasma, 11. *See also* effluvium; putrefaction
military revolution, 3
mobilization, naval, 122. *See also* recruitment
Munro, Donald, 91, 97–98, 100, 110
Murray, James, 29–33, 51

Native Americans: definition, 20; combatants, 20, 29, 45; medicine, 26
networks of medical knowledge. *See under* medicine, imperial networks; Pringle, John
Newcastle, Duke of (Thomas Pelham-Holles), 103, 106, 114–15
newspapers: censorship, 81, 115–17; American colonial, 77–79; disease, 76–79. *See also* public opinion

observations, medical, 35–38, 58, 87, 98; dissections, 34, 35, 155; scientific medicine, 35–36, 98–100, 135–38, 194
Observations on the Changes of the Air . . . in the Island of Barbadoes (Hillary), 35, 60
Observations on the Diseases Incidental to Seamen (Blane), 108
Observations on the Diseases in Long Voyages to Hot Countries (Clark), 157–59
Observations on the Diseases of the Army (Pringle), 95–96, 118
officers: conventions of war, 166, 174, 179; medical treatment, 166–68; public opinion, 1–3, 5, 86, 198; reports, 114, 116 (*see also* returns); responsibilities, 1–3, 5, 8, 11–12, 62–63, 81–82, 111, 198

paintings of the Seven Years' War, 1–3, 5, 28, 198. *See also* public opinion
pamphlets, 88, 112–13, 115–16. *See also* public opinion

Parliament (British), 14, 86–87, 104; and quantitative data, 107–8
partisan politics, 112–16
philanthropy: accountability, 182–83; aims, 111; British patriotism, 185–86, 187; British state, 183–85; organization, 182–83
physicians. *See* practitioners, military medical
pillage, 89, 91, 97. *See also* discipline; provisioning
Pitt, William: correspondence, 33, 47, 49, 56, 61–64; foreign policy, 10, 61, 67, 89–90, 112; partisan politics, 89–90, 115
Plains of Abraham, battle of (1759), 19, 28–29
Plassey, battle of (1757), 159–61
political arithmetic, 14, 107, 109–10. *See also* quantitative methods
Pondicherry, siege of (1760–61), 165–66
Poplar Fund, 152
Porter, Roy, 7, 202n16
practitioners, military medical: careers, 36–38, 97–100, 102–3; distinction between surgeons and physicians, 36–37, 145–46; qualifications, 36; role gathering intelligence, 146–48. *See also under* East India Company; hospitals
Prado, Juan de, 70–71
Pringle, John, 19, 24, 93, 98; medical correspondence, 34–35, 36–37, 40–41, 59–60, 94; *Observations on the Diseases of the Army,* 95–96, 118
prisoners of war: agents, 176; cartels and exchanges, 175, 178–81; Committee on French Prisoners, 182; conventions, 166, 175; financial administration, 176–77; guards, 177; mortality, 186; negotiations, 178–81; numbers, 172, 174–75; reimbursement, 188–89; Royal Bounty, 173, 175, 177, 181–82; strategy, 180–81, 187
prisons: disease, 87, 96, 122, 159; nature of eighteenth-century, 179, 189; reform, 87, 117, 191
privateering, 56, 180–81
professions, medical. *See* medicine; medicine, military and naval; practitioners, military medical
provincials: definition, 20, 205n2, 208n87; problems raising, 67–70; public opinion, 77–81; Rangers, 40, 46; sickness, 14, 16–17, 40–51; social background, 50; soldiers, 47–51
provisioning: Commissariat, 90, 114–15; contracting, 90–91; foraging, 25, 89–90; fresh provisions, 25, 27, 31, 64, 123–24, 127–30; gardens, 25; meat, 23, 33–34, 124, 127–28, 133, 226n48; pillaging, 89, 91, 97; portable soup, 131; ships, 127–30, 153–54; vegetables, 25, 123, 127, 133, 226n48; Victualing Board, 126–27
public opinion: colonial compared with British, 77–81; laws of war, 186–87, 190–91; newspapers, 81, 116, 76–79; paintings, 1–3, 198; pamphlets, 88, 112–13, 115–16; prisoners of war, 183–88; war, 5, 14, 16, 81–82, 86–87, 109–17
public sphere, 3–4, 79, 86–87, 109, 111–12. *See also* public opinion
putrefaction, 22–24, 34, 59, 96, 123–24

quantitative methods, 14, 103–10, 197. *See also* returns
Quebec, siege of (1759–60), 28–38
Quiberon Bay, battle of (1759), 129–30

race, 14, 41–42, 171, 193–94. *See also* constitutions, physical and moral
Rangers, 40, 46
recruitment, 4, 66, 101, 192; East India Company troops, 151–52; native and colonial populations, 12, 17, 66–67, 169–71, 192; resistance, 67–70, 81. *See also* mobilization
returns, 14, 30, 51, 62, 66, 71–72, 73–75, 103–9
Royal Academy of Science (French), 137
Royal College of Physicians (British), 36, 98
Royal Society (British), 98, 108

Sainte-Foy, battle of (1760), 19, 32
sanitation, 14, 91–93, 149, 191. *See also* discipline
scurvy: incidence, 12, 19, 61, 153–54, 224n11; remedies, 24–28, 31, 33, 123–24, 133–34; siege of Quebec, 30–31, 33; theories, 19, 21–24, 34, 41, 123–24
seasoning. *See* acclimatization
sepoys, 162–63, 169–70
Shebbeare, John, 88, 112
ship fever, 94, 122. *See also* fevers; typhus
Sick and Hurt Board. *See under* Admiralty

siege warfare, 11, 163–66
Siraj ud-Daula, 142, 159, 161–62
smallpox: immunity, 43–44; incidence, 19, 42–46, 48, 50–51, 61; inoculation, 43–44, 46–47, 51, 109, 209n109; military strategy, 45, 50–51; purposeful spreading, 216n149; theories, 48–49
Society for the Encouragement of the British Troops in Germany and North America, 98
spruce beer, 24, 26–28, 33
state: fiscal-military, 3, 4, 10; formation, 3, 10, 199–200; responsive, 7, 16. *See also* empire
surgeons. *See* practitioners, military medical

Townshend, George, 74, 91, 104–5
Treatise of Military Discipline, A (Bland), 91–92, 97
Treaty of Paris (Franco-British peace treaty of 1763), 76, 188–89
trials. *See* experiments
tropical climates. *See under* climate, foreign
tropical medicine, 7, 57–61, 84, 146, 154–59, 166–68, 192–93
typhus, 87, 93–96, 122

Ursulines (Quebec), 40

vegetables. *See under* provisions
veterans, 144, 152
Victualing Board. *See under* Admiralty

War of Austrian Succession: Cartagena, 53, 66; conditions, 115; medical practice and observation, 38, 96, 98, 118; prisoners of war, 175, 180, 186; Western Squadron, 125
War of Spanish Succession, 175, 178
Watson, Charles, 153, 161–62, 167
Western Squadron: health, 125–26; strategy, 125, 138–39, 140–41; victualing, 127–30
wilderness warfare. *See* colonial warfare

yellow fever, 12, 35, 53, 59–61, 70–72, 74, 80; remedies, 60–61, 83; strategy, 53–54, 66. *See also* climate, foreign; fevers; tropical medicine